CONTENTS AT A GLANCE

T0253127

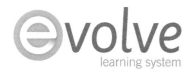 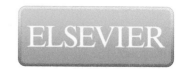

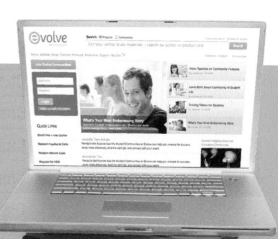

YOU'VE JUST PURCHASED
MORE THAN A TEXTBOOK

ACTIVATE THE COMPLETE LEARNING EXPERIENCE THAT COMES WITH YOUR BOOK BY REGISTERING AT

http://evolve.elsevier.com/Muscolino/knowthebody

Once you register, you will have access to your

STUDENT RESOURCES:

- Video Clips
  - Muscle palpations covered in the book are demonstrated on video on the Evolve site.
- Audio Files
  - Listen to author, Joe Muscolino, read aloud muscle names, attachments, and actions for every muscle covered in the book. Files are downloadable to MP3 devices and CDs for convenient study anywhere you go.
- Interactive Content Review Activities
  - Terminology crossword puzzles and bony landmark identification matching exercises help you review content through fun activities!
- Body Spectrum Electronic Coloring Book
  - Includes over 80 illustrations you can color online or offline!

INSTRUCTOR RESOURCES:

- Image Collection
- TEACH Instructor Resource Manual, with Lesson Plans and PowerPoint presentations for each chapter
- Test Bank in ExamView format
- Answers to end-of-chapter questions and case studies

REGISTER TODAY!

KNOW THE BODY

Muscle, Bone, and Palpation Essentials

JOSEPH E. MUSCOLINO

Instructor, Purchase College
State University of New York
Purchase, New York

Owner, The Art and Science of Kinesiology
Stamford, Connecticut

ELSEVIER

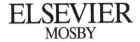

3251 Riverport Lane
Maryland Height, Missouri 63043

KNOW THE BODY: MUSCLE, BONE, AND PALPATION
ESSENTIALS, First Edition

ISBN 978-0-323-08684-4

Notice

ISBN 978-0-323-08684-4

Vice President: Linda Duncan
Executive Content Strategist: Kellie White
Senior Content Development Specialist: Jennifer Watrous
Content Coordinator: Emily Thomson
Publishing Services Manager: Gayle May
Design Direction: Teresa McBryan

Printed in the United States of America

Last digit is the print number: 9 8 7 6 5 4

This book is dedicated to all students of manual and movement therapies who are taking their rightful place in the field of Integrative Healthcare.

Preface

Know the Body: Muscle, Bone, and Palpation Essentials, is meant to be the best single source for all the essential knowledge about the musculoskeletal system that a massage therapist or any manual or movement therapist needs. Attachments (origins and insertions), actions (regular and stabilization functions), and palpation are covered for all the major muscles and muscle groups of the body, as well as applications to treatment. In addition, this book contains five introductory chapters that cover basic kinesiology terminology, bones and bony landmarks, how muscles function, how to palpate, and palpation of bones and bony landmarks. All the essentials that you need to know are contained in this one book, along with online demonstration videos on how to palpate individual muscles and an interactive CD at the back of the book that allows the viewer to place any combination of muscles on the skeleton to learn not just each individual muscle, but also the relative relationship of muscles!

WHO WILL BENEFIT FROM THIS BOOK?

This book is written primarily for students and practicing therapists of manual and movement therapies, including massage therapy, physical therapy, occupational therapy, chiropractic, osteopathy, orthopedics, athletic training, yoga, Pilates, and Feldenkrais. However, anyone who needs to learn the skeletal muscles of the body will find this book invaluable and an essential resource. This book will be your guide as you first learn the muscles of the body, and it will remain an invaluable resource on your bookshelf for as long as you are in practice.

CONCEPTUAL APPROACH

The approach taken by *Know the Body: Muscle, Bone, and Palpation Essentials* is to clearly and concisely present all the essential information that needs to be learned about the musculoskeletal system. The beginning chapters set the framework for how muscles work and how to palpate, as well as offer a five-step approach to learning muscles. The later chapters then provide the application of this knowledge to the bones

and muscles of the body. The goal of this book is to enable the student, therapist, trainer, or physician to be able to critically think through muscle functioning when working clinically with clients and patients.

ORGANIZATION

Know the Body is organized into two major parts.

Part One

Chapter 1 covers all the essential kinesiology terminology that a therapist needs to be able understand and communicate about the musculoskeletal system.

Chapter 2 is an atlas of the skeletal system, covering all the bones, bony landmarks, muscle attachment sites, and joints of the body.

Chapter 3 is a critically important chapter because it explains clearly and concisely how the muscular system functions. This chapter not only provides a strong foundation to be able to learn the muscles of the body, but it also teaches the reader to critically think through muscle function and apply it in clinical settings.

Chapter 4 is another critically important chapter because it teaches the art and science of palpation. With the knowledge presented in this chapter, the therapist will learn how to reason through muscle palpation protocols instead of simply memorizing them.

Chapter 5 is an atlas of palpation of the bones and major bony landmarks of the body—all with clear and simple illustrations.

Part Two

Chapters 6 through 11 are the meat of this book. They divide the body into regions and cover all the essentials for every major muscle and muscle group within the region. Each chapter contains beautiful cutting-edge illustrations of the muscles of the region drawn onto a skeleton and placed over a photograph of a real person. Functional guidelines present how to reason through the actions of the groups of muscles presented. Each muscle or muscle group are then presented individually, with attachments (origins and insertions), actions, stabilization functions, innervation, palpation, and treatment considerations given. Review questions and case studies are also provided at the end of each chapter.

Chapter 6 covers the muscles of the shoulder girdle and arm.

Chapter 7 covers the muscles of the forearm and hand.

Chapter 8 covers the muscles of the spine and rib cage.

Chapter 9 covers the muscles of the head.

Chapter 10 covers the muscles of the pelvis and thigh.

Chapter 11 covers the muscles of the leg and foot.

An illustrated stretching atlas concludes the book, featuring drawings of stretches for all major muscles.

DISTINCTIVE FEATURES

Know the Body has many distinctive features:

- The most thorough yet concise muscle atlas for attachments, actions, and palpation
- Palpation of the bones and bony landmarks
- Explanations and guidelines that promote critical thinking to understand muscle actions
- Beautiful illustrations in which the bones and muscles are placed on a photograph of a real person
- Large group illustrations for every functional muscle group
- Online video coverage of the palpation protocols for individual muscles of the body
- Treatment considerations for application to clinical settings
- An interactive CD that allows for any combination of muscles to be placed on the skeleton and body

LEARNING AIDS

- *Know the Body* is meant to be used not only as a textbook but also as an in-class manual.
- Arrows are placed over the muscle for each individual muscle illustration so that the line of pull of the muscle can be seen and visually understood. This feature allows for the actions of the muscle to be understood instead of memorized.
- A "Treatment Considerations" section is provided that offers interesting insights to each muscle. Many of these are clinical applications that flesh out and make learning the muscle more interesting.
- Review questions and case studies are placed at the end of each chapter to help the reader grasp how well he or she understands the content.
- A companion student workbook is available that provides multiple learning exercises and follows *Know the Body: Muscle, Bone, and Palpation Essentials,* chapter for chapter.

COMPANION CD

Know the Body includes a unique, interactive CD. A base photograph of the region of the body is presented with the skeleton drawn in. A list of every muscle of that region is given; and you can choose any combination of muscles and place them onto the illustration, allowing you to not only see that muscle's attachments, but, more importantly, to be able to see the relationship between all the muscles of the region. Any combination of muscles can be chosen!

EVOLVE ONLINE RESOURCES

Know the Body is supported by an Evolve website that includes the following student resources:

- Downloadable audio pronunciations of muscle names, attachments, and actions
- Palpation video clips covering skeletal muscles of the human body
- Crossword puzzles
- Bony palpation matching activities
- Electronic coloring book

Access these resources at http://evolve.elsevier.com/ Muscolino/knowthebody.

RELATED PUBLICATIONS

Know the Body: Muscle, Bone, and Palpation Essentials is supported by an excellent student workbook, *Workbook for Know the Body,* that provides multiple learning exercises for learning the content. Not only does the student workbook follow *Know the Body* chapter by chapter, providing cross reference page numbers for all of the content covered by the exercises, each chapter of the workbook is divided into sections that amount to roughly 1 week's amount of content. This workbook allows for periodic and regular review of the material being learned!

For more information on the musculoskeletal system, see Dr. Joe Muscolino's other publications:

- *The Muscular System Manual: The Skeletal Muscles of the Human Body,* third edition: the most thorough muscle atlas on the market.
- *Kinesiology: The Skeletal System and Muscle Function,* second edition: the most straightforward and thorough book on how the musculoskeletal system functions written for manual and movement therapists.
- *The Muscle and Bone Palpation Manual: With Trigger Points, Referral Patterns, and Stretching:* the authoritative guide to muscle palpation, trigger points, and stretching.

- *Musculoskeletal Anatomy Flashcards*, second edition: supports *The Muscular System Manual: The Skeletal Muscles of the Human Body*, third edition.
- *Flashcards for Bones, Joints, and Actions of the Human Body*, second edition: supports *Kinesiology: The Skeletal System and Muscle Function*, second edition.
- *Flashcards for Palpation, Trigger Points, and Referral Patterns*: supports *The Muscle and Bone Palpation Manual: With Trigger Points, Referral Patterns, and Stretching*.
- *Mosby's Trigger Point Flip Chart, with Referral Patterns and Stretching*.

NOTE TO THE STUDENT

Learning the musculoskeletal system can often feel overwhelming at first. This book presents the content in an approachable manner that will make learning this material fun! It also presents the content in a clear and straightforward manner that encourages you to think through the content so that you better understand it and can apply it to your clients when you are in practice. This makes learning not just fun and easy but better! Whether as an in-class manual or a reference text for your bookshelf, you will find this book to be an ideal and essential book now and into the future!

Acknowledgments

One name sits on the front cover of this book; but this is very misleading because the contribution of so many people have made this book possible. Acknowledgments are the author's opportunity to thank all these wonderful people.

Know the Body: Muscle, Bone, and Palpation Essentials is a melding of the "essential" components of a number of my other books, all wrapped into one guide for students. As such, I need to start by thanking every individual who contributed to every one of those books. Thank you again!

In addition, I must single out the wonderful art team that created the artwork in this book—Jean Luciano of Connecticut, Jeanne Robertson of Missouri, Frank Forney and David Carlson of Colorado, Peter Bull of England, and Jodie Bernard and Giovanni Rimasti of Lightbox Visuals from our wonderful neighbor to the north, Canada. Superb photography was done by Yanik Chauvin, also out of Canada.

My team at Mosby of Elsevier was, as usual, amazing and wonderful to work with. At this point in time, they feel like family and include Kellie White, my acquisitions editor, Emily Thomson, editorial assistant, Gayle May and Dana Peick, production managers, and Jennifer Watrous, my developmental editor. Jennifer shares so much of my book projects with me; at some point, I will simply need to add her name to the front cover. Thank you also to Kenneth Hewes, Jeffrey Simancek, and Wanda Reyes for reviewing the initial outline of this book and helping mold its format, and again to Kenneth Hewes for contributing to the case studies. A special thank you goes to Chris Jones and Selena Anduze for stepping in at the last moment and helping me organize much of the workbook content.

A continual thank you to William Courtland, a previous student and now fellow instructor, who one day, many years ago said, "You should write a book." Those words launched my writing career.

As always, my tremendous love and appreciation to everyone in my family, especially Simona Cipriani, my angel, my love, and my partner in life.

About the Author

Dr. Joe Muscolino has been a massage and manual and movement therapy educator for 25 years. He teaches anatomy, physiology, kinesiology, pathology, assessment, and treatment courses both in core curriculum and in continuing education. Currently, he is an adjunct professor at Purchase College, State University of New York, where he teaches anatomy, physiology, and nutrition. Dr. Muscolino has also published the following texts:

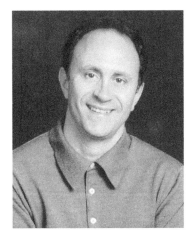

- *The Muscular System Manual: The Skeletal Muscles of the Human Body*, third edition
- *Kinesiology: The Skeletal System and Muscle Function*, second edition
- *The Muscle and Bone Palpation Manual, with Trigger Points, Referral Patterns, and Stretching*
- *Musculoskeletal Anatomy Coloring Book*, second edition
- *Musculoskeletal Anatomy Flashcards*, second edition
- *Flashcards for Bones, Joints, and Actions of the Human Body*, second edition
- *Flashcards for Palpation, Trigger Points, and Referral Patterns*
- *Mosby's Trigger Point Flip Chart with Referral Patterns and Stretching*

His texts have been translated into seven foreign languages.

Dr. Muscolino writes the column article, "Body Mechanics," in *The Massage Therapy Journal (MTJ)*. He has also written for the *Journal of Bodywork and Movement Therapies (JBMT)*, *Massage Magazine*, *Massage Today*, and several massage journals in Australia and New Zealand.

Dr. Muscolino teaches continuing education workshops on such topics as body mechanics, deep tissue massage, stretching and advanced stretching, joint mobilization, palpation, orthopedic assessment, musculoskeletal pathologic conditions, anatomy and physiology, kinesiology, and cadaver workshops. He offers a Certificate Program in Clinical Orthopedic Massage Therapy (COMT), and he also runs instructor in-services for kinesiology instructors. He is an approved provider of continuing education (CE); and CE credit is available through the NCBTMB for Massage Therapists and Bodyworkers toward certification renewal.

Dr. Joe Muscolino holds a Bachelor of Arts degree in Biology from the State University of New York at Binghamton, Harpur College. He attained his Doctor of Chiropractic Degree from Western States Chiropractic College in Portland, Oregon, and is licensed in Connecticut, New York, and California. Dr. Muscolino has been in private practice in Connecticut for more than 26 years and incorporates soft tissue work into his chiropractic practice for all of his patients.

If you would like further information regarding *Know the Body: Muscle, Bone, and Palpation Essentials*, or any of Dr. Muscolino's other publications, or if you are an instructor and would like information regarding the many supportive materials such as PowerPoint slides, test banks of questions, or TEACH instructor's manuals, please visit http://www.elsevieradvantage.com. If you would like information regarding Dr. Muscolino's workshops or if you would like to contact Dr. Muscolino directly, please visit his website: www.learnmuscles.com. You can also follow him on his Facebook page, The Art and Science of Kinesiology.

Contents

Basic Kinesiology Terminology

1

Discussing muscle function without fluency in the language of kinesiology is not possible (Box 1-1). Specific kinesiology terms exist to help us avoid the ambiguities of lay language. Therefore embracing and using these terms is extremely important in the field of health care, where a person's health depends on clear communication. The purpose of this chapter is to provide an overview of the basic terms of kinesiology. (For an in-depth and thorough discussion of the terminology of kinesiology, see *Kinesiology: The Skeletal System and Muscle Function*, 2nd edition [Elsevier, 2011].)

BOX 1-1

The term *kinesiology* literally means the study of motion. Given that motion of our body occurs when bones move at joints, and that muscles are the primary creator of the forces that move the bones, kinesiology is the study of the musculoskeletal system. Because the muscles are controlled and directed by the nervous system, it might be more accurate to expand kinesiology to be the study of the neuromusculoskeletal system.

■ MAJOR BODY PARTS

Motions of the body involve the movement of body parts. To be able to describe the motion of body parts, each part must be accurately named. Figure 1-1 illustrates the major divisions and body parts of the human body. The axial body and the appendicular body are the two major divisions. The appendicular body can be divided into the upper and the lower extremities.

The names of most body parts are identical to the lay English names. However, a few cases exist where kinesiology terms are very specific and need to be observed. For example, the term *arm* is used to refer to the region of the upper extremity that is located between the shoulder and elbow joints. The term *forearm* refers to the body part that is located between the elbow and wrist joints; the forearm is a separate body part and is not considered to be part of the arm. Similarly, the term *leg* describes the region of the lower extremity that is located between the knee and ankle joints, whereas the term *thigh* is used to describe an entirely separate body part that is located between the hip and knee joints; the thigh is not part of the leg. The precise use of these terms is essential so that movements of the leg and thigh are not confused with one another, and movements of the arm and forearm are not confused with one another. *Pelvis* is another term that should be noted. The pelvis is a separate body part from the trunk and is located between the trunk and thighs.

■ ANATOMIC POSITION

Anatomic position is a standard reference position that is used to define terms that describe the physical location of structures of the body and points on the body. In anatomic position, the person is standing erect, facing forward, with the arms at the sides, the palms facing forward, and the fingers and toes extended (Figure 1-2).

Note: Given that movement terminology is based on location terminology, anatomic position is ultimately the foundation for movement terminology as well.

■ LOCATION TERMINOLOGY

Now that anatomic position has been defined, it can be used as the reference position for location terms that describe the relative locations of body parts, structures, and points on the body to each other. Location terminology is made up of directional terms that come in pairs, each member of the pair being the opposite of the other.

Pairs of Terms

Anterior/Posterior

Anterior means farther to the front; *posterior* means farther to the back. These terms can be used for the entire body, axial and appendicular.

Note: The term *ventral* is sometimes used for anterior, and the term dorsal is sometimes used for posterior. The true definition of ventral is the soft belly surface of a body part; dorsal refers to the harder surface on the other side of the body part. In the lower extremity, anterior/ventral and posterior/dorsal are not synonymous. The ventral surface of the thigh is the medial surface; of the leg is the posterior surface; of the foot is the plantar surface.

Medial/Lateral

Medial means closer to an imaginary midline that divides the body into the left and right halves. *Lateral* means farther from this imaginary midline. These terms can be used for the entire body, axial and appendicular.

Superior/Inferior

Superior means above (toward the head). *Inferior* means below (away from the head). These terms are usually used for the axial body only.

Proximal/Distal

Proximal means closer (i.e., more proximity) to the axial body; *distal* means farther (i.e., more distant) from the axial body. These terms are only used for the appendicular body.

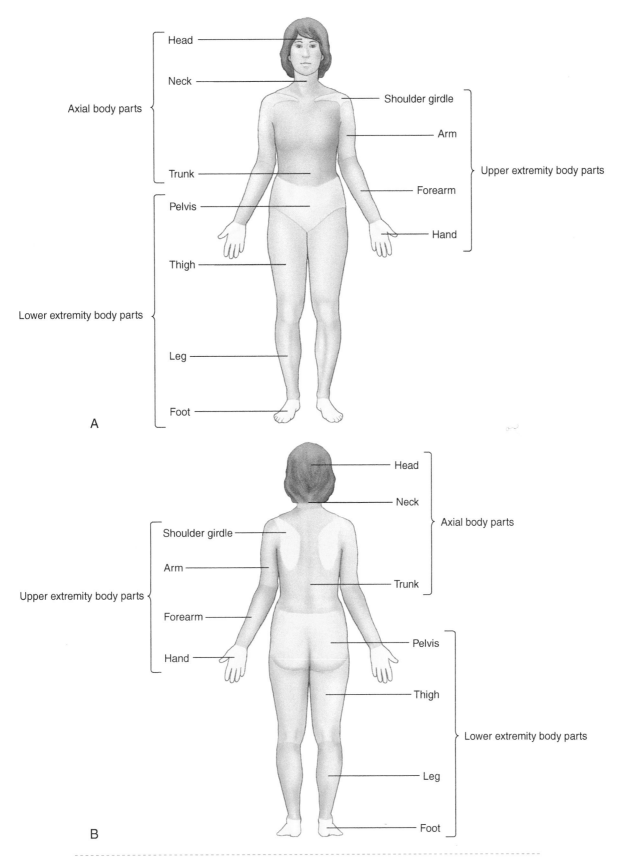

FIGURE 1-1 The three major divisions of the body are the axial body and the two divisions of the appendicular body. The appendicular body is composed of the upper extremities and lower extremities. The body parts within these major divisions are shown. **A,** Anterior view. **B,** Posterior view.

Continued

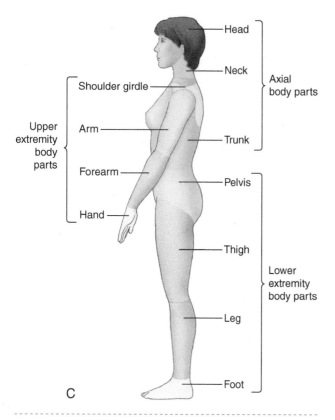

FIGURE 1-1, cont'd **C,** Lateral view.

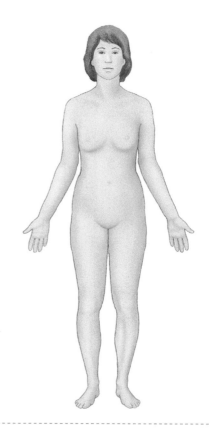

FIGURE 1-2 Anatomic position is a reference position of the body in which the person is standing erect, facing forward, with the arms at the sides, the palms facing forward, and the fingers and toes extended.

Superficial/Deep

Superficial means closer to the surface of the body. *Deep* means farther from the surface of the body (i.e., more internal). These terms can be used for the entire body, axial and appendicular.

> Note: When using the terms *superficial* and *deep*, stating the perspective from which you are viewing the body is always recommended.

Radial/Ulnar

The terms *radial* and *ulnar* can be used for the forearm and hand in place of the terms *lateral* and *medial*, respectively. The radius is the lateral bone of the forearm; the ulna is the medial bone.

Tibial/Fibular

The terms *tibial* and *fibular* can be used for the leg and sometimes the foot in place of the terms *medial* and *lateral*, respectively. The tibia is the medial bone of the leg; the fibula is the lateral bone.

Palmar/Dorsal

The terms *palmar* and *dorsal* can be used for the hand in place of the terms anterior and posterior, respectively.

Plantar/Dorsal

The terms *plantar* and *dorsal* can be used for the foot. The plantar surface of the foot is the undersurface that is planted on the ground. The dorsal surface is the top or dorsum of the foot.

Cranial/Caudal

Cranial means toward the head; *caudal* means toward the "tail" of the body. These terms are only used for the axial body.

Combining Terms of Location

Similar to combining terms such as *north* and *west* to create *northwest*, location terms can be combined. When doing this, the end of the first word is usually dropped, and the letter *o* is placed to connect the two words. For example, anterior and lateral combine to become *anterolateral*. Although no hard and fast rule exists, anterior and posterior are usually placed first when combined with other terms. Figure 1-3 is an anterior view of a person, illustrating the terms of relative location as they pertain to the body.

ANATOMIC POSITION

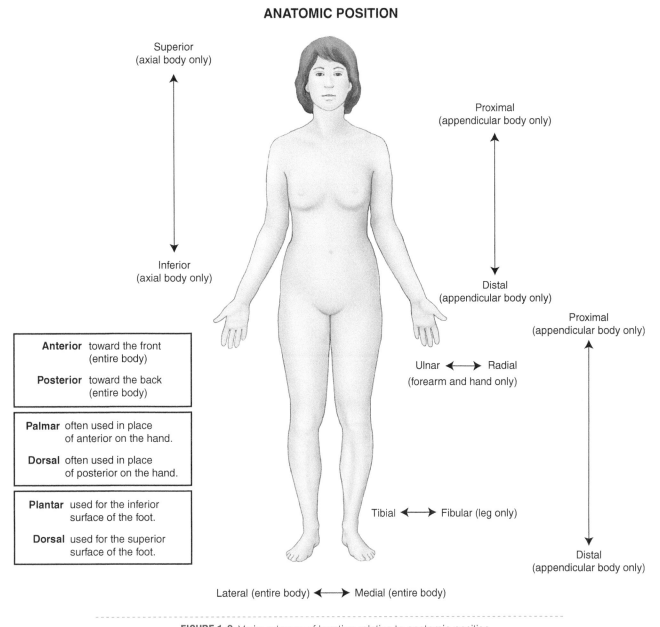

Anterior toward the front (entire body)

Posterior toward the back (entire body)

Palmar often used in place of anterior on the hand.

Dorsal often used in place of posterior on the hand.

Plantar used for the inferior surface of the foot.

Dorsal used for the superior surface of the foot.

Superior (axial body only)

Inferior (axial body only)

Proximal (appendicular body only)

Distal (appendicular body only)

Proximal (appendicular body only)

Ulnar ←→ Radial (forearm and hand only)

Tibial ←→ Fibular (leg only)

Distal (appendicular body only)

Lateral (entire body) ←→ Medial (entire body)

FIGURE 1-3 Various terms of location relative to anatomic position.

PLANES

Planes are flat surfaces that cut through and can be used to map three-dimensional space. Because space is three-dimensional, three major planes, known as cardinal planes, exist. The three cardinal planes are (1) sagittal, (2) frontal, and (3) transverse planes (Box 1-2). The sagittal plane divides the body into left and right portions. The frontal plane divides the body into front and back (anterior and posterior) portions. The transverse plane divides the body into upper and lower (superior and inferior or proximal and distal) portions. Each of these three cardinal planes

is perpendicular to the other two planes. Any plane that is not perfectly sagittal, frontal, or transverse is described as an oblique plane. Therefore an oblique plane has components of two or three cardinal planes. Figure 1-4 illustrates two examples each of the three cardinal planes and an oblique plane.

BOX 1-2

The frontal plane is also known as the coronal plane. The transverse plane is also known as the horizontal plane.

1

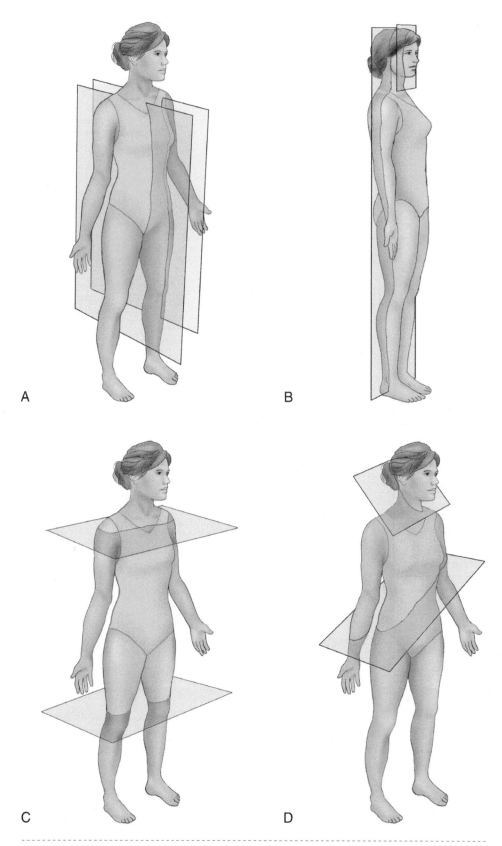

A

B

C

D

FIGURE 1-4 Anterolateral views of the body illustrate the three cardinal planes (sagittal, frontal, and transverse) and oblique planes. **A,** Two examples of sagittal planes. **B,** Two examples of frontal planes. **C,** Two examples of transverse planes. **D,** Two examples of oblique planes. The upper oblique plane has frontal and transverse components; the lower oblique plane has sagittal and transverse components.

Motion of the Body within Planes

Planes become extremely important when we describe the motion of a body part through space, because the body part moves within a plane. Hence, by defining the planes of space, we can describe the path of motion of a body part when it moves. Note that the sagittal and frontal planes are vertical and the transverse plane is horizontal. Therefore motions within the sagittal and frontal planes move vertically up and down and motions within the transverse plane move horizontally. Figure 1-5 illustrates examples of motion within the three cardinal planes and an oblique plane.

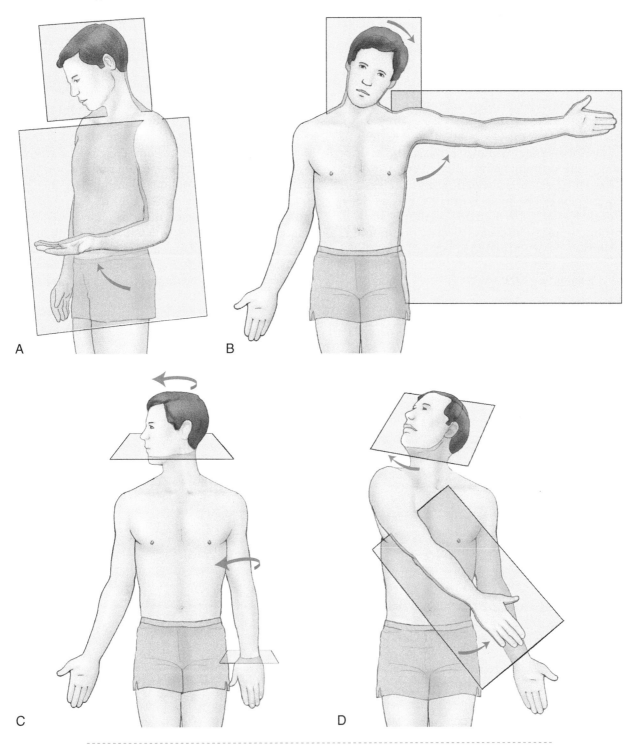

FIGURE 1-5 Examples of motion of body parts within planes. **A,** Motions of the head and neck and forearm within sagittal planes. **B,** Motions of the head and neck and arm within frontal planes. **C,** Motions of the head and neck and arm within transverse planes. **D,** Motions of the head and neck and arm within oblique planes.

AXES

An *axis* (plural: *axes*) is an imaginary line around which a body part moves. If a body part moves in a circular path around an axis, it is described as an axial motion. If the body part moves in a straight line, it is described as a nonaxial motion. Both axial and nonaxial motions of a body part move within a plane. However, an axial motion moves within a plane and moves around an axis. The orientation of an axis for movement is always perpendicular to the plane within which the movement is occurring.

Each plane has its own corresponding axis; therefore there are three cardinal axes. The axis for sagittal plane movements is oriented side to side and described as the mediolateral axis, the axis for frontal plane movements is oriented front to back and described as anteroposterior, and the axis for transverse plane movements is oriented up and down and described as superoinferior or simply vertical. Each oblique plane also has its own corresponding axis, which is perpendicular to it. Figure 1-6 illustrates axial motions that occur within planes and around their corresponding axes.

MOVEMENT TERMINOLOGY

Using anatomic position, we are able to define terms that describe static locations on the body. We now need to define terms that describe dynamic movements of the body. These movement terms are called *joint actions*. Similar to location terms, they come in pairs in which each member of the pair is the opposite of the other (Box 1-3). However, different from location terms, movement terms do not describe a static location; rather, they describe a direction of motion. The major pairs of joint action terms are defined here.

It should be noted that joint actions usually describe cardinal plane motions of a body part. For example, the brachialis muscle brings the forearm anteriorly in the sagittal plane at the elbow joint; therefore its action is described as flexion of the forearm at the elbow joint. If a muscle creates an oblique plane motion, then this motion is described by breaking it into its component cardinal plane joint action motions. An example is the coracobrachialis muscle, which moves the arm anteriorly (in the sagittal plane) and medially (in the frontal plane). When describing this motion, it is said that the coracobrachialis flexes and adducts the arm at the

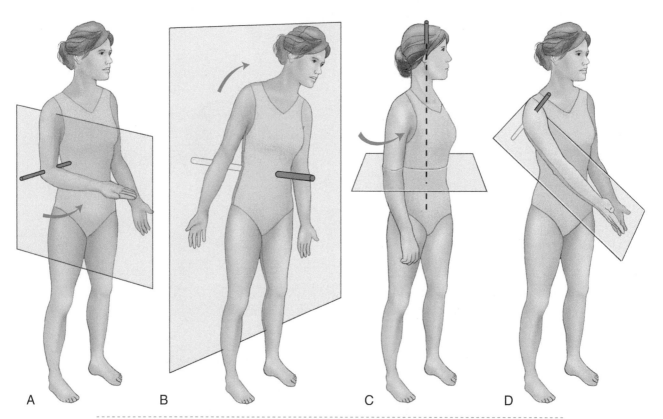

A   B   C   D

FIGURE 1-6 Anterolateral views illustrate the corresponding axes for the three cardinal planes and an oblique plane; the axes are shown as red tubes. Note that an axis always runs perpendicular to the plane in which the motion is occurring. **A,** Motion occurring in the sagittal plane around the mediolateral axis. **B,** Motion occurring in the frontal plane around the anteroposterior axis. **C,** Motion occurring in the transverse plane around the superoinferior axis or, more simply, the vertical axis. **D,** Motion occurring in an oblique plane around an axis that is running perpendicular to that plane (i.e., it is the oblique axis for this oblique plane).

BOX 1-3

Pointing out that joint action terms describe cardinal plane motions is extremely important. For example, flexion and extension of the arm at the shoulder (glenohumeral) joint occur within the sagittal plane, abduction and adduction of the arm at the glenohumeral joint occur within the frontal plane, and right rotation and left rotation of the arm at the glenohumeral joint occur within the transverse plane. If the arm were to move in an oblique plane, then to describe its motion, its cardinal plane motion components must be stated. For example, if the arm moves in a straight line that is forward and toward the midline, it would be described as flexing and adducting, even though it moves in only one direction.

shoulder (glenohumeral) joint. It actually causes one motion, but this one motion is described as having two cardinal (sagittal and frontal) plane components. (For more information on this, see *Kinesiology: The Skeletal System and Muscle Function*, 2nd edition [Elsevier, 2011].)

Following the definitions of joint action terms is a joint action atlas that contains illustrations that demonstrate all the joint actions of the body.

Pairs of Terms

Flexion/Extension

Flexion is generally an anterior movement of a body part within the sagittal plane; *extension* is generally a posterior movement within the sagittal plane.

Exceptions include movements of the legs, feet, toes, and thumbs. From the knee joint and farther distally, flexion of a body part moves posteriorly (extension is therefore an anterior movement). The thumb moves medially within the frontal plane when it flexes and laterally within the frontal plane when it extends. The terms *flexion* and *extension* can be used for the entire body, axial and appendicular.

Abduction/Adduction

Abduction is generally a lateral movement within the frontal plane that is away from the imaginary midline of the body; *adduction* is a medial movement toward the midline.

Exceptions include the toes and fingers, including the thumbs.

The toes adduct toward an imaginary line through the center of the second toe when the second toe is in anatomic position; they abduct away from this imaginary line. Toe number two can only abduct; it can perform tibial abduction and fibular abduction.

Fingers two through five adduct toward an imaginary line that goes through the center of the middle finger when the middle finger is in anatomic position; they abduct away from this imaginary line. The middle finger can only abduct; it can perform radial abduction and ulnar abduction.

The thumb abducts within the sagittal plane by moving away from the palm of the hand; it adducts within the frontal plane by moving back toward the palm. The terms *abduction* and *adduction* are used only for the appendicular body.

Right Lateral Flexion/Left Lateral Flexion

Right lateral flexion is a side-bending movement of the head, neck, and/or trunk toward the right within the frontal plane. *Left lateral flexion* is the opposite. These terms are used only for the axial body.

Lateral Rotation/Medial Rotation

Lateral rotation is a movement within the transverse plane in which the anterior surface of the body part moves to face more laterally (away from the midline); *medial rotation* moves the anterior surface to face more medially (toward the midline).

Lateral rotation is also known as external rotation; medial rotation is also known as internal rotation. These terms are used only for the appendicular body.

Right Rotation/Left Rotation

Right rotation is a movement within the transverse plane in which the anterior surface of the body part moves to face more to the right; *left rotation* moves the anterior surface to face more to the left. These terms are used for the axial body only.

> Note: The terms *ipsilateral rotator* and *contralateral rotator* are often used to describe muscles that produce right or left rotation. Ipsilateral and contralateral rotations are not joint action terms. Rather, they are ways to describe that a muscle on one side of the body either produces rotation to that same (ipsilateral) side or to the opposite (contralateral) side.

Elevation/Depression

Elevation is a movement wherein the body part moves superiorly; *depression* occurs when the body part moves inferiorly.

Protraction/Retraction

Protraction is a movement wherein the body part moves anteriorly; *retraction* is a posterior movement of the body part.

Right Lateral Deviation/Left Lateral Deviation

Lateral deviation is a linear movement that occurs in the lateral direction.

Pronation/Supination

The terms *pronation* and *supination* can be applied to motion of the forearm at the radioulnar joints and motion of the foot at the subtalar (tarsal) joint.

Pronation of the forearm results in the posterior surface of the radius facing anteriorly (when in anatomic position); supination is the opposite.

> Note: Forearm pronation is easily confused with medial rotation of the arm at the glenohumeral joint and forearm supination with lateral rotation of the arm.

Pronation of the foot at the subtalar joint is a triaxial motion that is made up primarily of eversion; it also includes dorsiflexion and lateral rotation (also known as abduction) of the foot at the subtalar joint. Supination of the foot is primarily made up of inversion; it also includes foot plantarflexion and medial rotation (also known as adduction) at the subtalar joint.

Inversion/Eversion

The foot inverts at the subtalar joint when it turns its plantar surface toward the midline of the body; it everts when its plantar surface is turned outward away from the midline. Inversion is the principal component of supination of the foot; eversion is the principal component of pronation of the foot.

Dorsiflexion/Plantarflexion

The foot dorsiflexes when it moves superiorly (in the direction of its dorsal surface); it plantarflexes when it moves inferiorly (in the direction of its plantar surface). Technically, dorsiflexion is extension and plantarflexion is flexion.

Opposition/Reposition

The thumb opposes at the saddle (carpometacarpal) joint when its pad meets the pad of another finger; it repositions when it returns back toward anatomic position. Opposition is actually a composite of abduction, flexion, and medial rotation of the thumb; reposition is a composite of adduction, extension, and lateral rotation of the thumb.

> Note: Medial rotation and lateral rotation in the transverse plane cannot occur in isolation; they must occur in conjunction with flexion and extension, respectively,

The little finger can also oppose and reposition at its carpometacarpal joint. Little finger opposition is composed of flexion, adduction, and lateral rotation of the little finger; little finger reposition is composed of extension, abduction, and medial rotation.

Upward Rotation/Downward Rotation

The scapula upwardly rotates when its glenoid fossa is moved to face more superiorly; downward rotation is the opposite motion. The clavicle upwardly rotates when its inferior surface moves to face anteriorly; downward rotation is the opposite motion.

> Note: These actions of the scapula and clavicle cannot be isolated. Rather, they must couple with motions of the arm at the glenohumeral joint.

Lateral Tilt/Medial Tilt and Upward Tilt/Downward Tilt

The scapula laterally tilts when its medial border lifts away from the body wall; medial tilt is the opposite motion during which the medial border moves back toward the body wall.

The scapula upwardly tilts when its inferior angle lifts away from the body wall; downward tilt is the opposite motion during which the inferior angle moves back toward the body wall.

Horizontal Flexion/Horizontal Extension

Horizontal flexion is a movement of the arm or thigh in which it begins in a horizontal position (i.e., abducted to 90 degrees) and then moves anteriorly toward the midline of the body. Horizontal extension is the movement in the opposite direction.

> Note: Horizontal flexion is also known as horizontal adduction; horizontal extension is also known as horizontal abduction.

Hyperextension and Circumduction

Hyperextension

The term *hyperextension* is often used to describe extension beyond anatomic position. This text does not use hyperextension in this manner. Extension beyond anatomic position is called *extension*, just as flexion and abduction beyond anatomic position are called *flexion* and *abduction*. The prefix *hyper* denotes excessive, therefore the term *hyperextension* would be better and more consistently defined as a range of extension motion that occurs beyond what is normal or beyond what is healthy.

Circumduction

Circumduction is not a joint action. Rather, circumduction is a sequence of four joint actions performed one after the other. For example, if a person moves his or her arm at the glenohumeral joint into flexion, then abduction, then extension, and then adduction, and does this by rounding the corners of the four motions, it creates a circular motion pattern that is called *circumduction*. It should also be noted that circumduction does not contain any rotation motion. Any joint that allows motion within two or more planes (biaxial or triaxial joints) can allow circumduction to occur.

JOINT ACTION ATLAS

Upper Extremity

Scapula at the Scapulocostal Joint

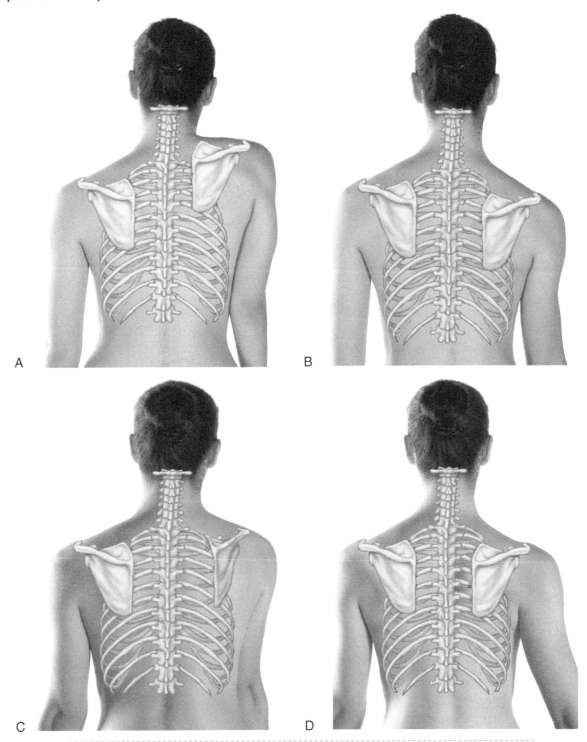

A

B

C

D

FIGURE 1-7 Nonaxial actions of elevation/depression and protraction/retraction of the scapula at the scapulocostal joint. *A,* Elevation. *B,* Depression. *C,* Protraction. *D,* Retraction. The left scapula is in anatomic position in all figures. (Note: All views are posterior.)

1

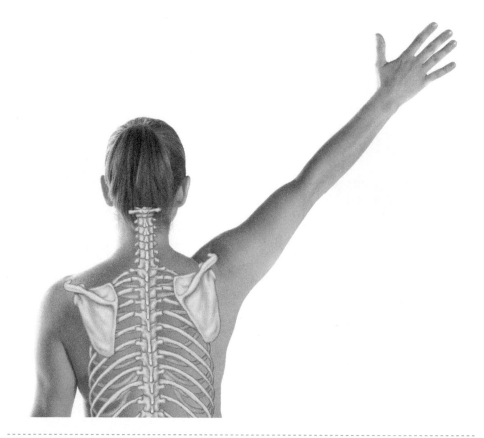

FIGURE 1-8 Upward rotation of the right scapula at the scapulocostal joint. The left scapula is in anatomic position, which is full downward rotation. (Note: Scapular actions of upward and downward rotation cannot be isolated. They must accompany humeral motion. In this case, the humerus is abducted at the glenohumeral joint.) (Note: This is a posterior view.)

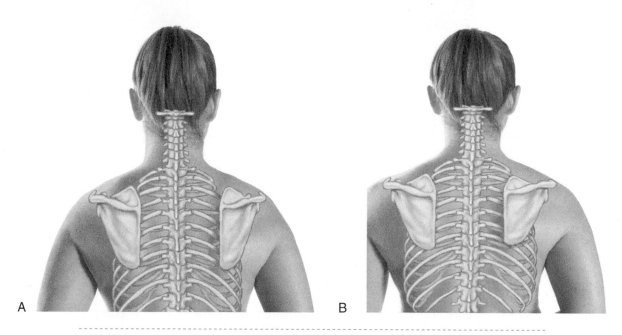

A

B

FIGURE 1-9 Tilt actions of the right scapula at the scapulocostal joint. ***A,*** Lateral tilt: the left scapula is in anatomic position of medial tilt. ***B,*** Upward tilt: the left scapula is in anatomic position of downward tilt. (Note: Both views are posterior.)

Clavicle at the Sternoclavicular Joint

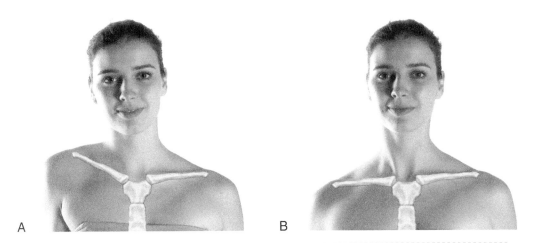

FIGURE 1-10 *A,* Elevation of the right clavicle at the sternoclavicular joint. ***B,*** Depression of the right clavicle. (Note: The left clavicle is in anatomic position. Both views are anterior.)

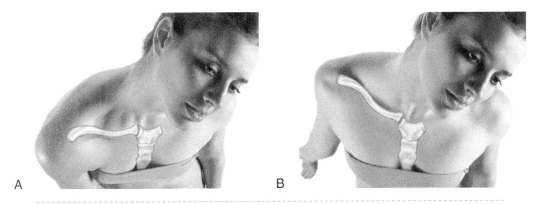

FIGURE 1-11 *A,* Protraction of the right clavicle at the sternoclavicular joint. ***B,*** Retraction of the right clavicle. (Note: Both views are anteroinferior.)

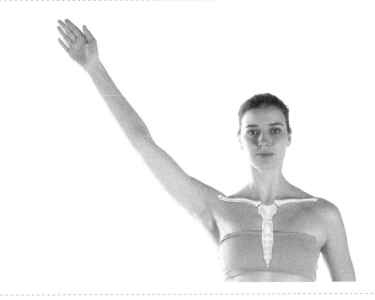

FIGURE 1-12 Anterior view illustrates upward rotation of the right clavicle at the sternoclavicular joint; the left clavicle is in anatomic position, which is full downward rotation. (Note: Upward rotation of the clavicle cannot be isolated. In this figure the arm is abducted at the glenohumeral joint, resulting in the scapula upwardly rotating, which results in upward rotation of the clavicle.)

Arm at the Glenohumeral Joint

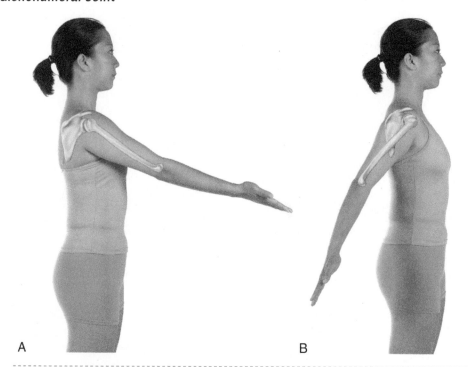

FIGURE 1-13 Sagittal plane actions of the arm at the glenohumeral joint. *A,* Flexion. *B,* Extension. (Note: Both views are lateral.)

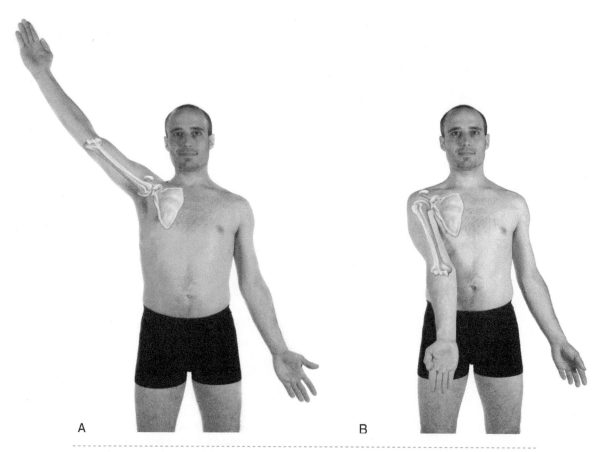

FIGURE 1-14 Frontal plane actions of the arm at the glenohumeral joint. *A,* Abduction. *B,* Adduction. (Note: Both views are anterior.)

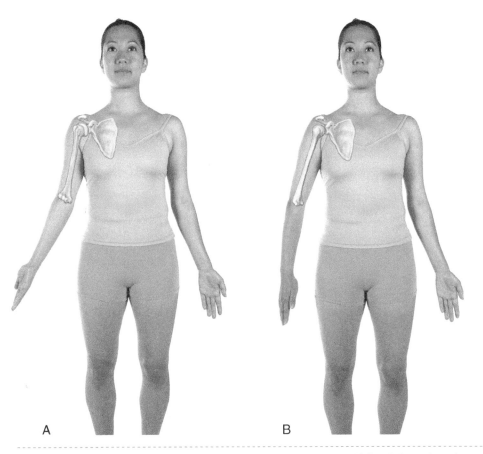

FIGURE 1-15 Transverse plane actions of the arm at the glenohumeral joint. **A,** Lateral rotation. **B,** Medial rotation. (Note: Both views are anterior.)

Reverse Action of the Scapula and Trunk at the Glenohumeral Joint

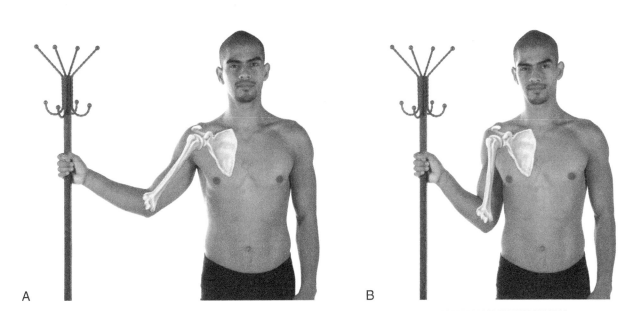

FIGURE 1-16 Reverse actions in which the trunk moves relative to the arm at the glenohumeral (GH) joint are also possible. In these illustrations, the trunk is seen to move relative to the arm at the GH joint. **A** and **B** illustrate neutral position and right lateral deviation of the trunk at the right GH joint, respectively.

Continued

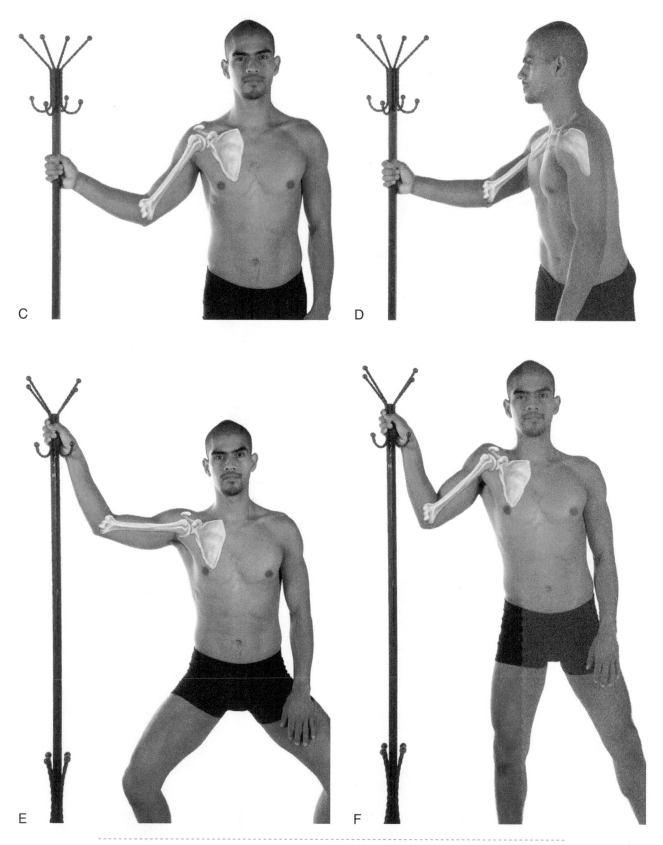

FIGURE 1-16, cont'd *C* and *D* illustrate neutral position and right rotation of the trunk at the right GH joint, respectively; and *E* and *F* illustrate neutral position and elevation of the trunk at the right GH joint, respectively. In all three cases, note the change in angulation between the arm and trunk at the GH joint (for lateral deviation *B* and elevation *F,* the elbow joint has also flexed). (Note: All views are anterior.)

Forearm at the Elbow and Radioulnar Joints

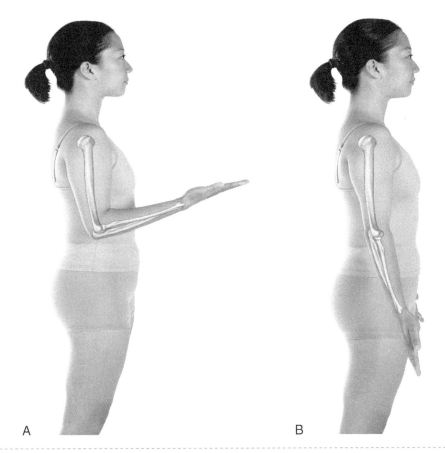

FIGURE 1-17 Motions of the right forearm at the elbow joint. *A,* Flexion. *B,* Extension. (Note: Both views are lateral.)

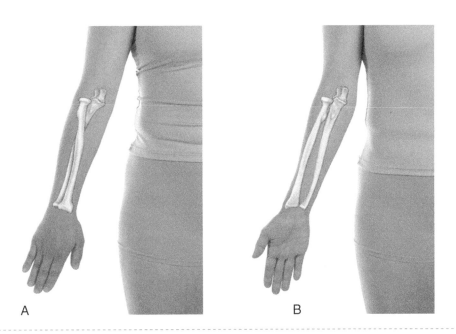

FIGURE 1-18 Pronation and supination of the right forearm at the radioulnar joints. *A,* Pronation. *B,* Supination, which is anatomic position for the forearm. (Note: Both views are anterior.)

Hand at the Wrist Joint

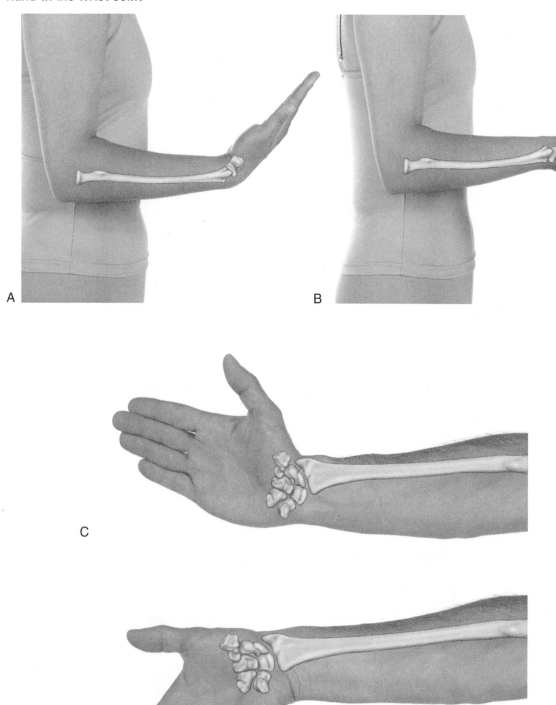

FIGURE 1-19 Motions of the right hand at the wrist joint (radiocarpal and midcarpal joints). **A** and **B,** Lateral views illustrate flexion and extension of the hand, respectively. **C** and **D,** Anterior views illustrate radial deviation and ulnar deviation, respectively. Radial deviation of the hand is also known as *abduction*; ulnar deviation is also known as *adduction*.

Fingers Two through Five at the Metacarpophalangeal and Interphalangeal Joints

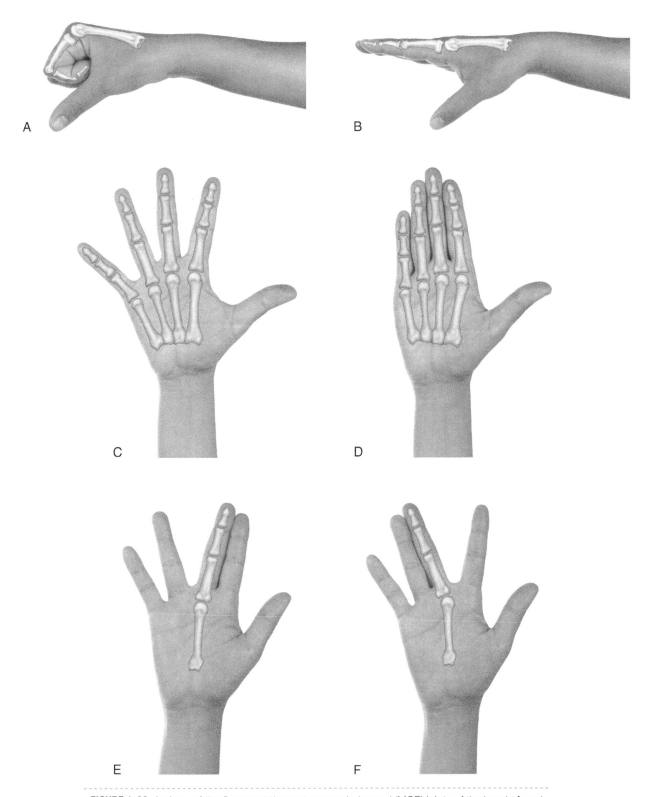

FIGURE 1-20 Actions of the fingers at the metacarpophalangeal (MCP) joints of the hand. *A* and *B,* Radial (i.e., lateral) views illustrate flexion and extension, respectively, of fingers two through five at the MCP joints. Flexion of the fingers at the interphalangeal joints is also seen. *C* and *D,* Anterior views illustrate abduction and adduction of fingers two through four at the MCP joints, respectively. *E* and *F,* Anterior views illustrate radial abduction and ulnar abduction of the middle finger at the third MCP joint, respectively.

1

Thumb at the Carpometacarpal Joint

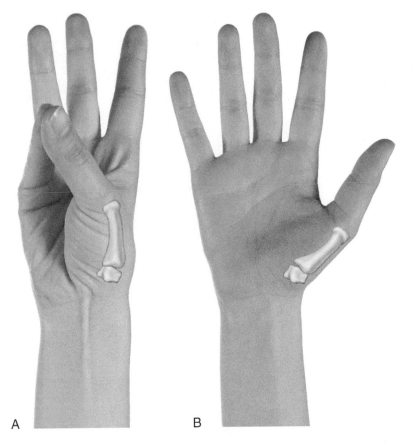

FIGURE 1-21 Actions of the thumb at the first carpometacarpal (CMC) joint (also known as the *saddle joint of the thumb*). ***A*** and ***B,*** Anterior views illustrate opposition and reposition of the thumb, respectively. ***C*** and ***D,*** Anterior views illustrate flexion and extension, respectively; these actions occur within the frontal plane. ***E*** and ***F,*** Lateral views illustrate abduction and adduction, respectively; these actions occur within the sagittal plane. (Note: Flexion of the phalanges of the thumb and/or little finger at metacarpophalangeal joint is also seen in ***A*** and ***C;*** flexion of the thumb at the interphalangeal joint is also seen in ***C.***)

A   B

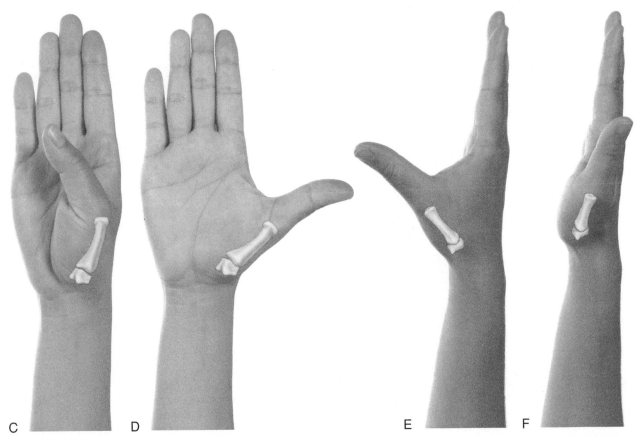

C   D   E   F

Axial Body

Head at the Atlanto-Occipital Joint

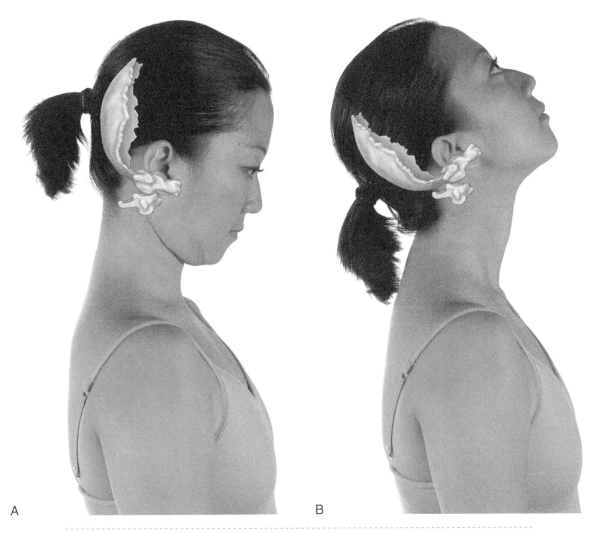

A B

FIGURE 1-22 Lateral views illustrate sagittal plane motions of the head at the atlanto-occipital joint. *A,* Flexion. *B,* Extension.

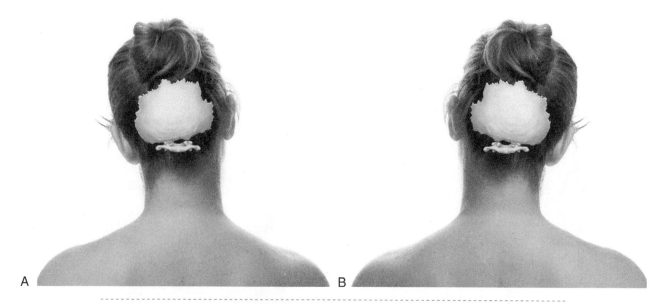

A   B

FIGURE 1-23 Posterior views illustrate frontal plane lateral flexion motions of the head at the atlanto-occipital joint. **A,** Left lateral flexion. **B,** Right lateral flexion.

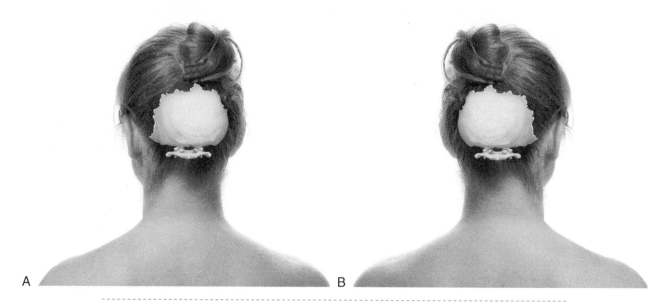

A   B

FIGURE 1-24 Posterior views illustrate transverse plane rotation motions of the head at the atlanto-occipital joint. **A,** Left rotation; **B,** Right rotation.

Neck at the Cervical Spinal Joints

FIGURE 1-25 Motions of the neck at the spinal joints. **A** and **B** are lateral views that depict flexion and extension in the sagittal plane, respectively. **C** and **D** are posterior views that depict left lateral flexion and right lateral flexion in the frontal plane, respectively. **E** and **F** are anterior views that depict right rotation and left rotation in the transverse plane, respectively. Note: **A** to **F** depict motions of the entire craniocervical region (i.e., the head at the atlanto-occipital joint and the neck at the spinal joints).

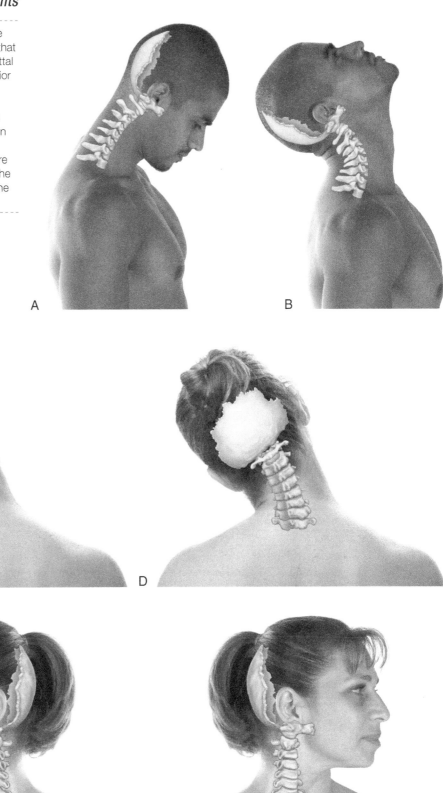

A

B

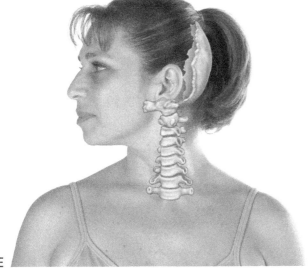

C

D

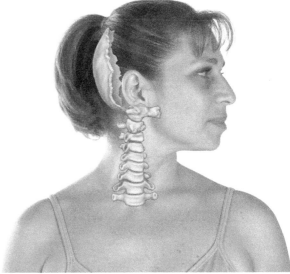

E

F

Trunk at the Thoracolumbar Spinal Joints

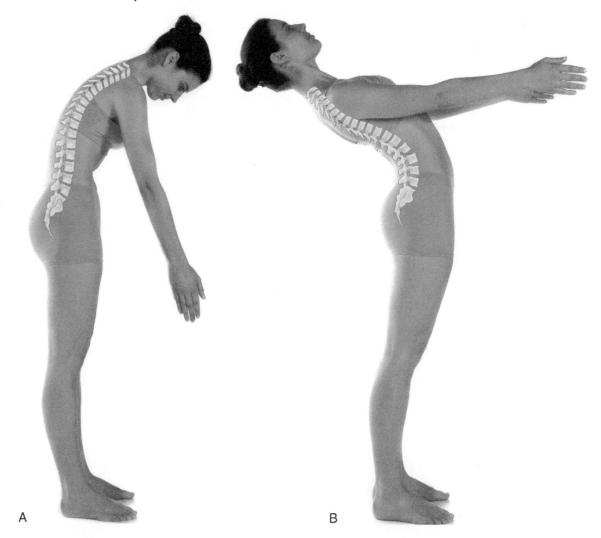

A   B

FIGURE 1-26 Motions of the thoracolumbar spine (trunk) at the spinal joints. *A* and *B,* Lateral views illustrate flexion and extension of the trunk, respectively, in the sagittal plane.

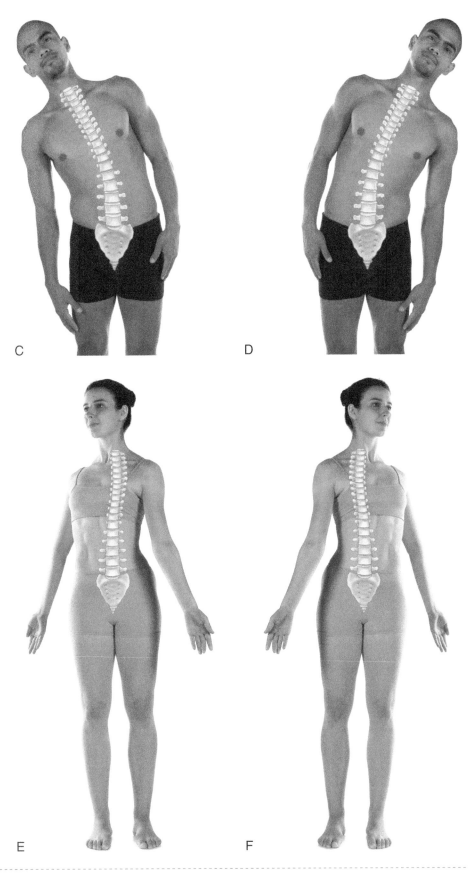

FIGURE 1-26, cont'd *C* and *D,* Anterior views illustrate right lateral flexion and left lateral flexion of the trunk, respectively, in the frontal plane. *E* and *F,* Anterior views illustrate right rotation and left rotation of the trunk, respectively, in the transverse plane.

Pelvis at the Lumbosacral Joint

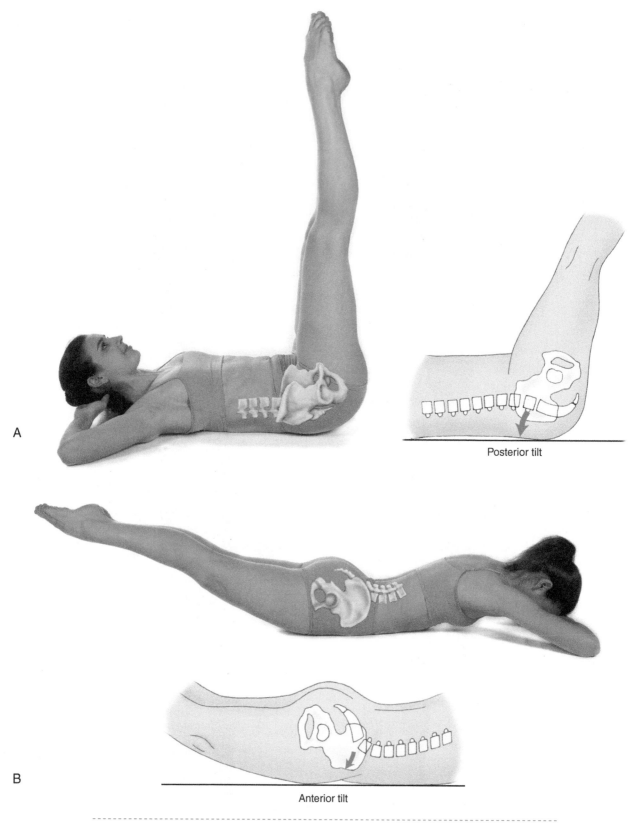

A

Posterior tilt

B

Anterior tilt

FIGURE 1-27 Motion of the pelvis at the lumbosacral joint. *A* and *B,* Lateral views illustrate posterior tilt and anterior tilt, respectively. (Note: In *A* and *B,* no motion is occurring at the hip joints; therefore the thighs are seen to "go along for the ride," resulting in the lower extremities changing their orientation.)

1

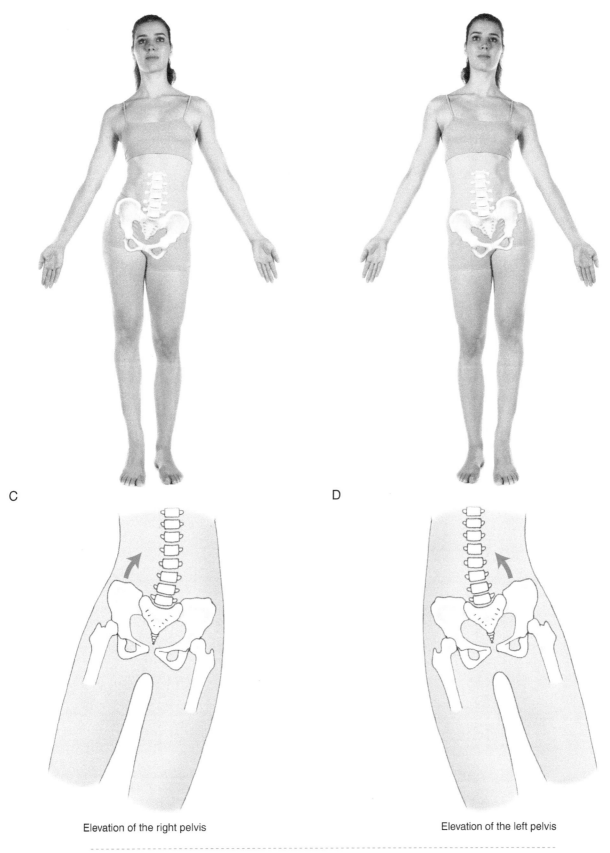

Elevation of the right pelvis

Elevation of the left pelvis

FIGURE 1-27, cont'd *C* and *D,* Anterior views illustrate elevation of the right pelvis and elevation of the left pelvis, respectively, at the lumbosacral joint. (Note: In illustrations of *C* and *D,* no motion is occurring at the hip joints; therefore the thighs are seen to "go along for the ride," resulting in the lower extremities changing their orientation.)

Continued

1

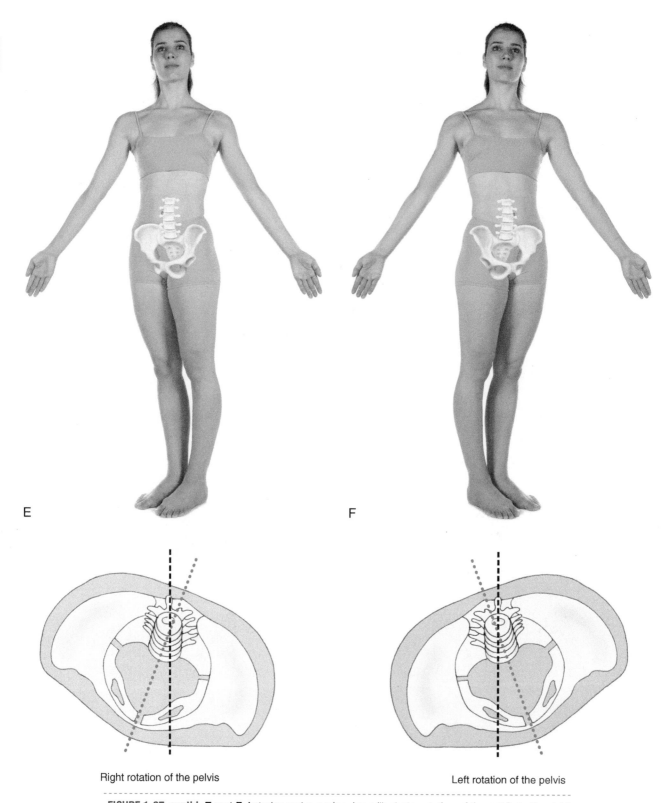

E

F

Right rotation of the pelvis

Left rotation of the pelvis

FIGURE 1-27, cont'd *E* and *F,* Anterior and superior views illustrate rotation of the pelvis to the right and rotation to the left, respectively, at the lumbosacral joint. (Note: In *E* and *F* the dashed black line represents the orientation of the spine and the red dotted line represents the orientation of the pelvis. Given the different directions of these two lines, the pelvis has clearly rotated relative to the spine; this motion has occurred at the LS joint.)

Mandible at the Temporomandibular Joints (TMJs)

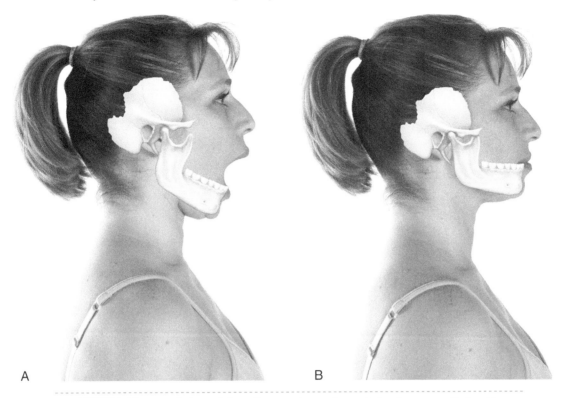

A   B

FIGURE 1-28 **A** and **B**, Lateral views illustrate depression and elevation, respectively, of the mandible at the temporomandibular joints (TMJs). These are axial motions.

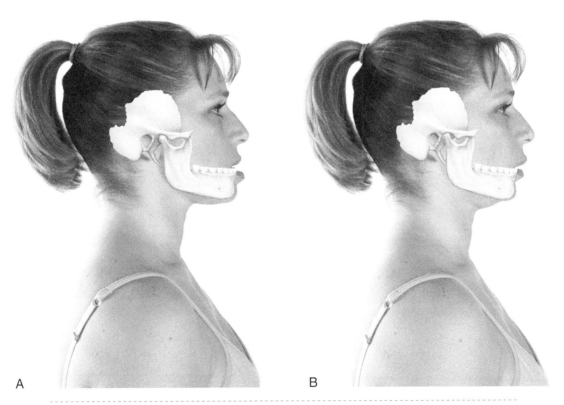

A   B

FIGURE 1-29 **A** and **B**, Lateral views illustrate protraction and retraction, respectively, of the mandible at the temporomandibular joints (TMJs). These are nonaxial glide motions.

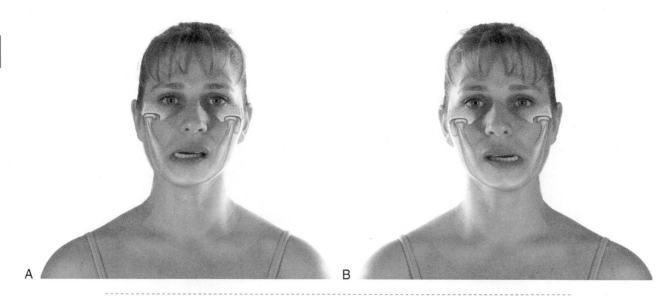

A   B

FIGURE 1-30 *A* and ***B,*** Anterior views illustrate right lateral deviation and left lateral deviation, respectively, of the mandible at the temporomandibular joints (TMJs). These are nonaxial glide motions.

Lower Extremity

Thigh at the Hip Joint

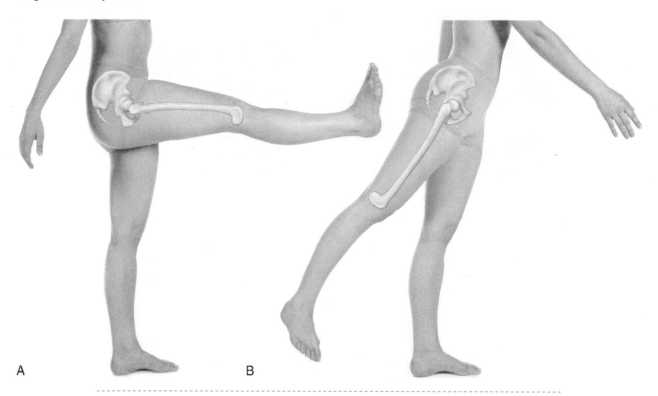

A   B

FIGURE 1-31 Motions of the right thigh at the hip joint. ***A*** and ***B,*** Lateral views illustrate flexion and extension, respectively.

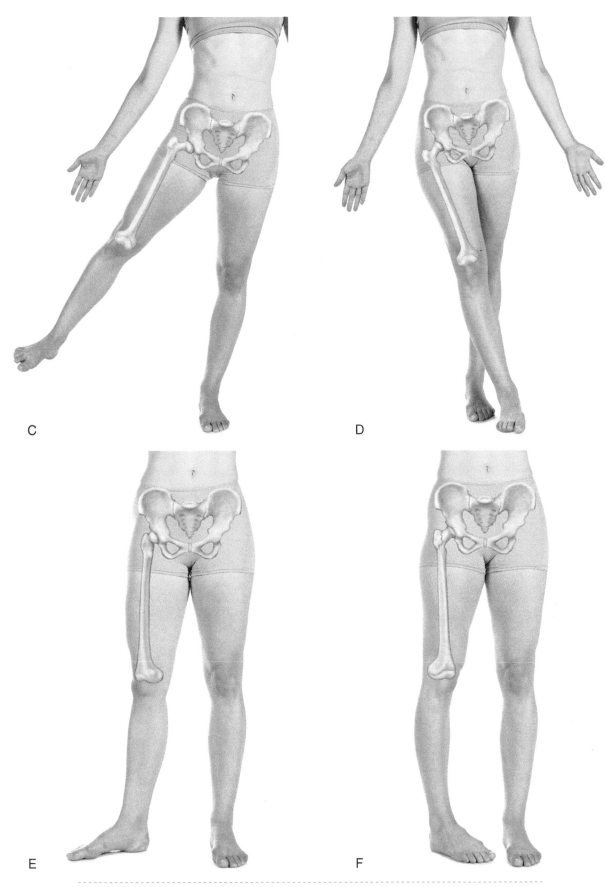

C

D

E

F

FIGURE 1-31, cont'd *C* and *D,* Anterior views illustrate abduction and adduction, respectively. *E* and *F,* Anterior views illustrate lateral rotation and medial rotation, respectively.

1

Pelvis at the Hip Joint

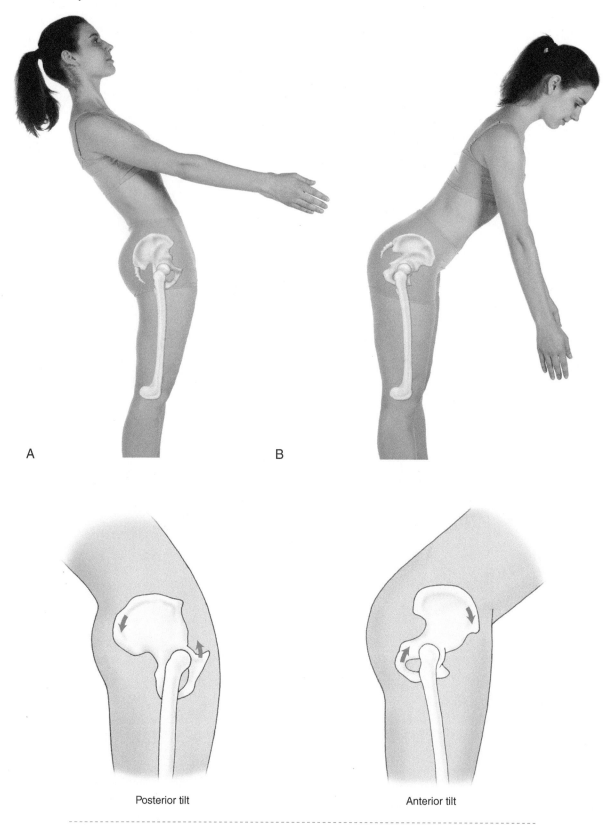

A

B

Posterior tilt

Anterior tilt

FIGURE 1-32 Motion of the pelvis at the hip joints. (Note: No motion is occurring in **A** to **D** at the lumbosacral joint; therefore the trunk is seen to "go along for the ride," resulting in the upper body changing its orientation.) **A** and **B,** Lateral views illustrate posterior tilt and anterior tilt, respectively.

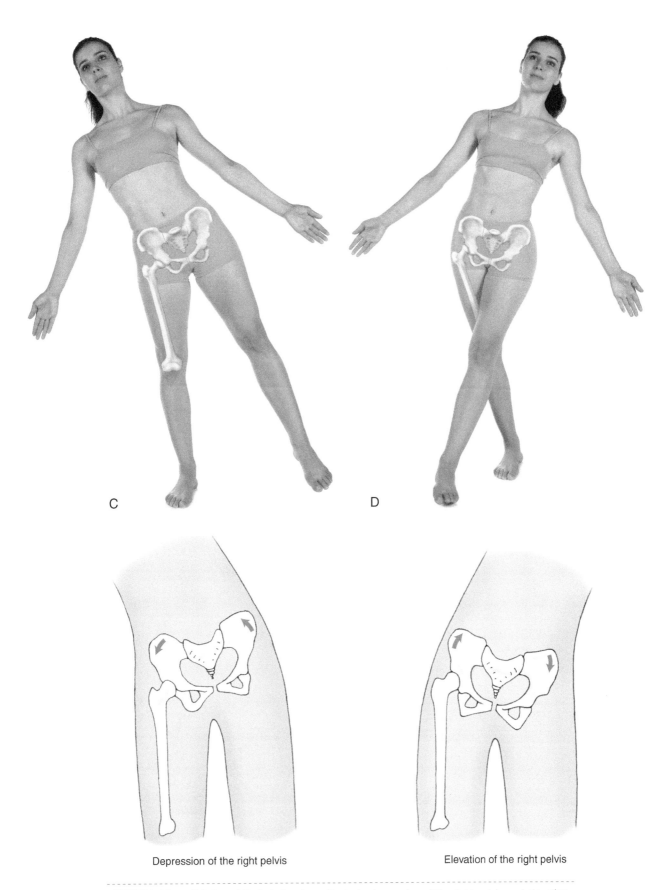

Depression of the right pelvis

Elevation of the right pelvis

FIGURE 1-32, cont'd *C* and *D,* Anterior views illustrate depression of the right pelvis and elevation of the right pelvis, respectively. (Note: When the pelvis elevates on one side, it depresses on the other, and vice versa.)

Continued

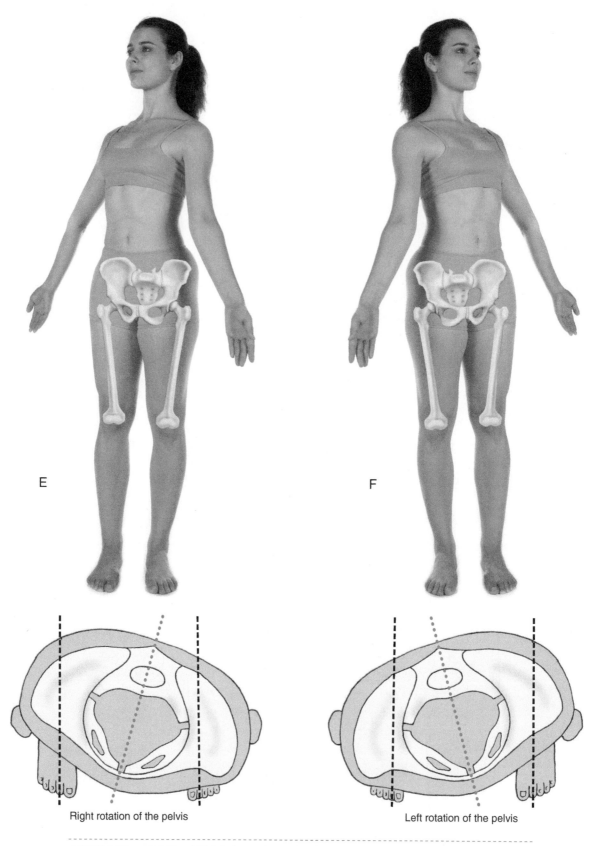

E

F

Right rotation of the pelvis

Left rotation of the pelvis

FIGURE 1-32, cont'd *E* and *F*, Anterior and superior views illustrate rotation of the pelvis to the right and rotation to the left, respectively. (Note: In *E* and *F* the black dashed line represents the orientation of the thighs and the red dotted line represents the orientation of the pelvis. Given the different directions of these lines, the pelvis has clearly rotated relative to the thighs; this motion has occurred at the hip joints.)

Leg at the Knee Joint

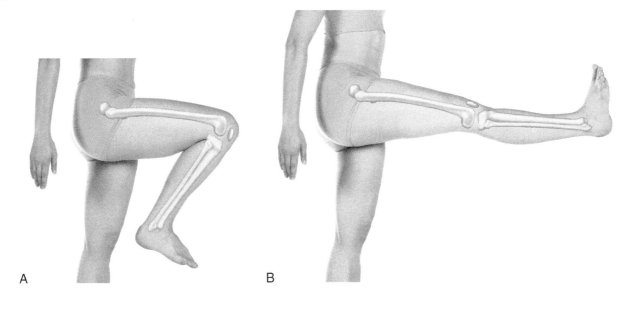

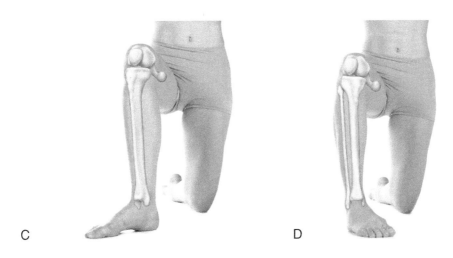

FIGURE 1-33 Motions possible at the right tibiofemoral (i.e., knee) joint. **A** and **B,** Lateral views illustrate flexion and extension of the right leg at the knee joint, respectively. **C** and **D,** Anterior views illustrate lateral and medial rotation of the right leg at the knee joint, respectively. (Note: The knee joint can only rotate if it is first flexed.)

Foot at the Ankle Joint

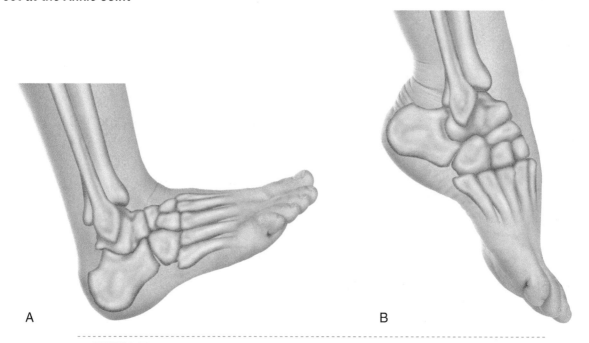

A   B

FIGURE 1-34 *A* and *B,* Lateral views illustrate dorsiflexion and plantarflexion of the right foot at the talocrural (i.e., ankle) joint, respectively.

Foot at the Subtalar (Tarsal) Joint

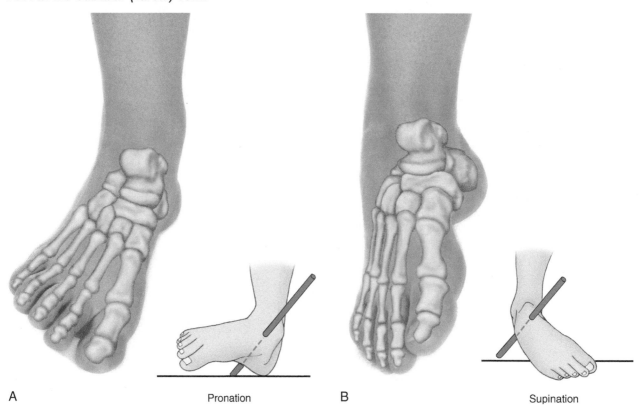

A   Pronation   B   Supination

FIGURE 1-35 *A* and *B,* Motions of the right foot at the subtalar (tarsal) joint. *A,* Pronation. The principal component of pronation is eversion. *B,* Supination. The principal component of supination is inversion.

Foot at the Subtalar and Ankle Joints

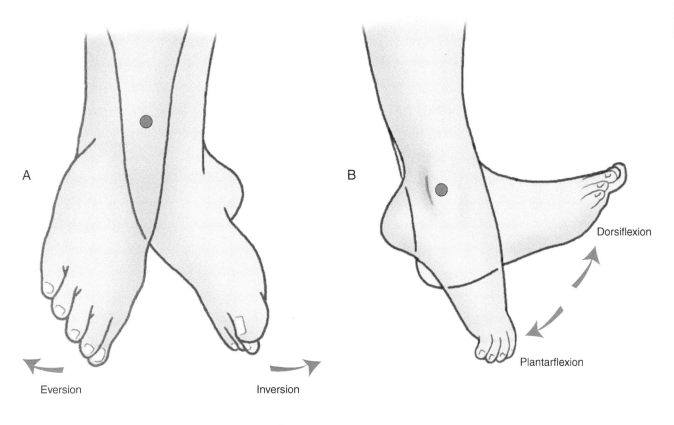

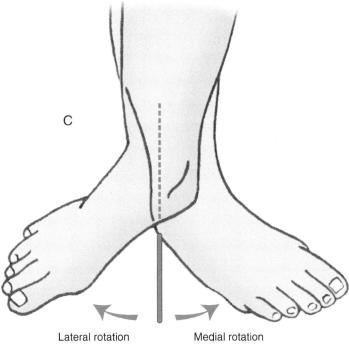

FIGURE 1-36 Cardinal plane components of right foot motion at the subtalar and ankle joints. *A,* Frontal plane components of eversion/inversion. *B,* Sagittal plane components of dorsiflexion/plantarflexion. *C,* Transverse plane components of lateral rotation/medial rotation (abduction/adduction). (Note: In *A* and *B,* the axis is represented by the red dot.)

1

Toes at the Metatarsophalangeal and Interphalangeal Joints

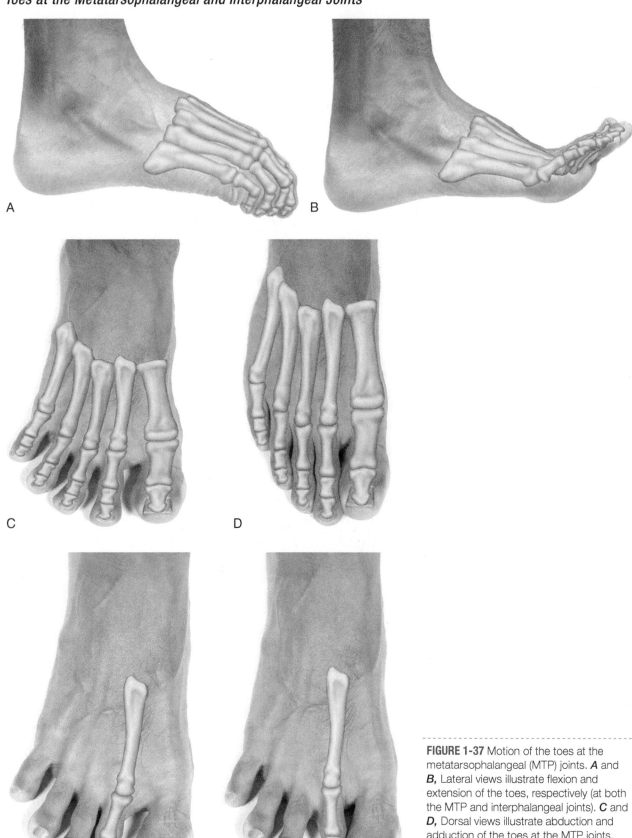

FIGURE 1-37 Motion of the toes at the metatarsophalangeal (MTP) joints. *A* and *B,* Lateral views illustrate flexion and extension of the toes, respectively (at both the MTP and interphalangeal joints). *C* and *D,* Dorsal views illustrate abduction and adduction of the toes at the MTP joints. *E,* Fibular abduction of the second toe at the MTP joint. *F,* Tibial abduction of the second toe at the MTP joint.

REVIEW QUESTIONS

Circle or fill in the correct answer for each of the following questions or statements. More study resources are provided on the Evolve website at http://evolve.elsevier.com/Muscolino/knowthebody.

1. **The arm begins at the _____ joint, and ends at the _____ joint.**

2. **What are the three cardinal planes?**

   _____

   _____

   _____

3. **What are the three cardinal axes?**

   _____

   _____

   _____

4. **The leg begins at the _____ joint, and ends at the _____ joint(s).**
   a. Hip; ankle
   b. Hip; toe
   c. Hip; knee
   d. Knee; ankle

5. **What term means closer to the midline of the body?**
   a. Anterior
   b. Superior
   c. Medial
   d. Proximal

6. **Which of the following terms describes the location of the wrist joint relative to the elbow joint?**
   a. Inferior
   b. Medial
   c. Proximal
   d. Distal

7. **Which of the following terms best describes the location of the sternum relative to the hip joint?**
   a. Superomedial
   b. Anterolateral
   c. Deep
   d. Posteromedial

8. **As a general rule, in what direction does a body part move when it flexes?**
   a. Posterior
   b. Anterior
   c. Medial
   d. Lateral

9. **Which of the following joint actions does not occur at the shoulder (glenohumeral) joint?**
   a. Right rotation
   b. Flexion
   c. Abduction
   d. Medial rotation

10. **Which of the following is true regarding circumduction?**
    a. It is always unhealthy.
    b. It is the same as rotation.
    c. It involves rotation.
    d. It is not an action.

The Skeletal System

THE SKELETON

The skeletal system is composed of approximately 206 bones and can be divided into bones of the axial body and bones of the appendicular body. Figure 2-1 is an anterior view of the full skeleton. Figure 2-2 is a posterior view.

JOINTS

Wherever two or more bones come together, in other words, join, a joint is formed.

Structural Classification of Joints

Structurally, the definition of a joint is having the two (or more) bones united by a soft tissue. There are three structural classifications of joints: (1) fibrous, (2) cartilaginous, and (3) synovial (Figure 2-3 on page 44). Fibrous joints are united by dense fibrous fascial tissue, cartilaginous joints are united by fibrocartilage, and synovial joints are united by a thin fibrous capsule that is lined internally by a synovial membrane, enclosing a joint cavity that contains synovial fluid. Only synovial joints possess a joint cavity and have articular cartilage that covers the joint surfaces of the bones.

Functional Classification of Joints

Functionally, a joint is defined by its ability to allow motion between two (or more) bones. There are three functional classifications of joints: (1) synarthrotic, (2) amphiarthrotic, and (3) diarthrotic. Synarthrotic joints permit very little motion; amphiarthrotic joints allow limited-to-moderate motion; and diarthrotic joints allow a great deal of motion.

Generally, a correlation exists between the structural and functional classifications of joints. Fibrous joints are usually classified as synarthrotic because they allow very little motion; cartilaginous joints are usually classified as amphiarthrotic because they allow a limited-to-moderate amount of motion; and synovial joints are usually classified as diarthrotic because they allow a great deal of motion.

Types of Synovial Joints

Diarthrotic synovial joints can be subdivided based on the number of axes around which they permit motion to occur. The four categories are (1) uniaxial, (2) biaxial, (3) triaxial, and (4) nonaxial. These categories can be further subdivided based on the shapes of the bones of the joint.

Uniaxial Joints

There are two types of synovial uniaxial joints: (1) hinge and (2) pivot. Hinge joints act similar to the hinge of a door. One surface is concave and the other is shaped similar to a spool. Flexion and extension are allowed in the sagittal plane around a mediolateral axis. The humeroulnar (elbow) joint is a classic example of a hinge joint (Figure 2-4 on page 44).

The pivot joint is another type of synovial uniaxial joint. A pivot joint allows only rotation (pivot) motions in the transverse plane around a vertical axis. The atlantoaxial joint of the spine is a classic example of a uniaxial pivot joint (Figure 2-5 on page 45).

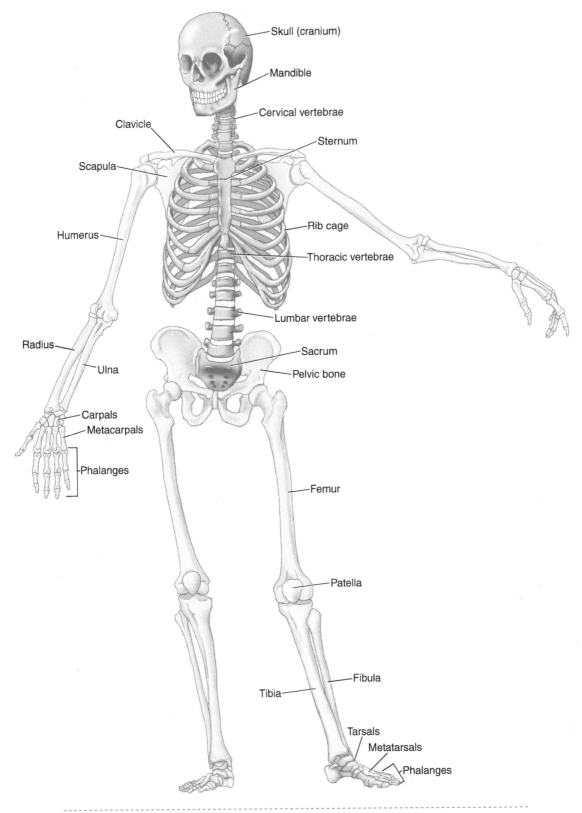

FIGURE 2-1 Full skeleton—anterior view. *Green,* Axial skeleton; *cream,* appendicular skeleton.

2

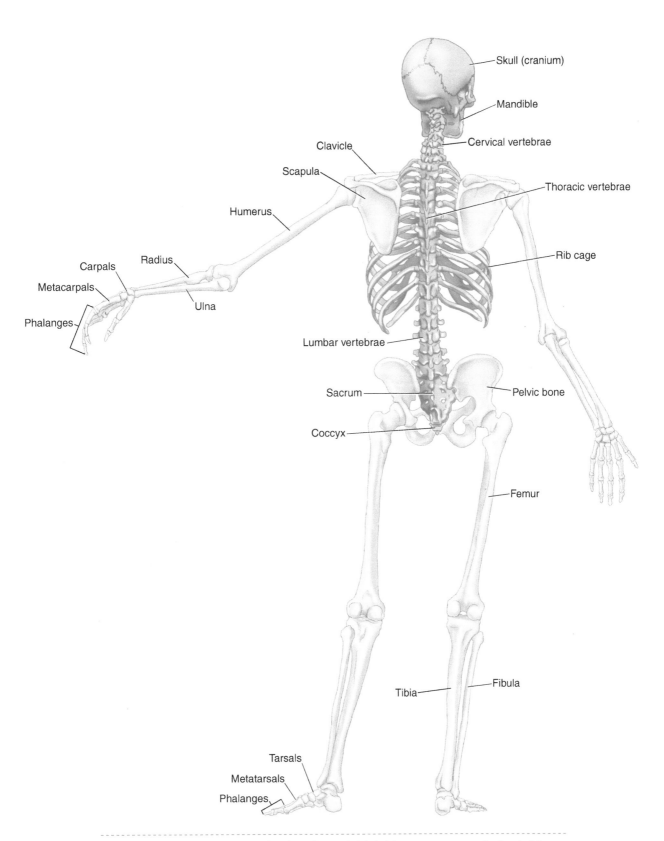

FIGURE 2-2 Full skeleton—posterior view. *Green,* Axial skeleton; *cream,* appendicular skeleton.

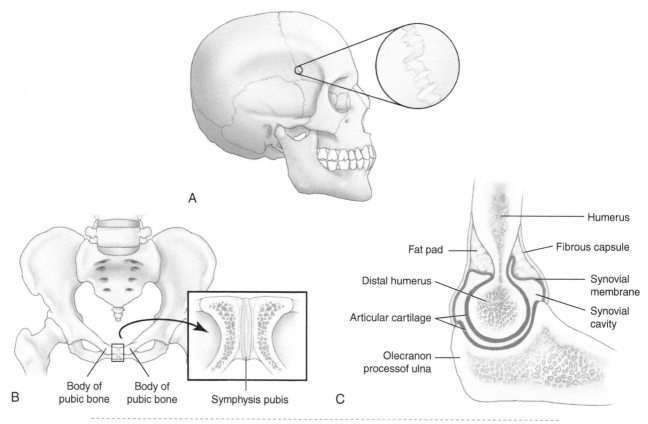

A

B

Body of
pubic bone

Body of
pubic bone

Symphysis pubis

C

Humerus

Fat pad

Fibrous capsule

Distal humerus

Synovial
membrane

Articular cartilage

Synovial
cavity

Olecranon
processof ulna

FIGURE 2-3 Structurally, there are three types of joints: *A,* Fibrous. *B,* Cartilaginous. *C,* Synovial.

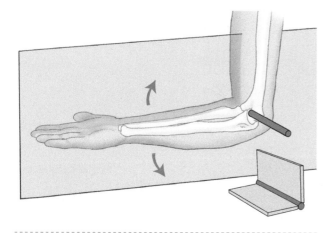

FIGURE 2-4 The humeroulnar joint of the elbow is an example of a synovial, uniaxial hinge joint. It allows flexion and extension within the sagittal plane around a mediolateral axis.

Biaxial Joints

There are two types of synovial biaxial joints: (1) condyloid and (2) saddle. A condyloid joint has one bone whose surface is concave, and the other bone's surface is convex. The convex surface of one bone fits into the concave surface of the other. Flexion and extension are allowed within the sagittal plane around a mediolateral axis, and abduction and adduction are allowed within the frontal plane around an anteroposterior axis. The metacarpophalangeal joint of the hand is an example of a condyloid joint (Figure 2-6).

The other type of synovial biaxial joint is the saddle joint. Both bones of a saddle joint have a convex and concave shape. The convexity of one bone fits into the concavity of the other and vice versa. Flexion and extension are allowed in one plane, and abduction and adduction are allowed in a second plane. Interestingly, a saddle joint also allows medial rotation and lateral rotation to occur in the third plane; therefore some might consider a saddle joint to be triaxial. However, because these rotation actions cannot be actively isolated, a saddle joint is still considered to be biaxial. The carpometacarpal joint of the thumb is a classic example of a saddle joint (Figure 2-7).

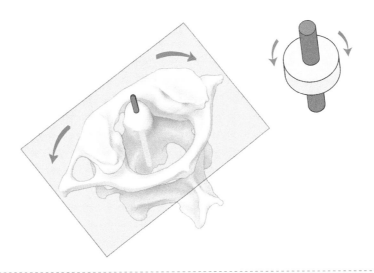

FIGURE 2-5 The atlantoaxial (C1-C2) joint of the spine between the atlas and axis is an example of a synovial, uniaxial pivot joint. It allows right and left rotations within the transverse plane around a vertical axis.

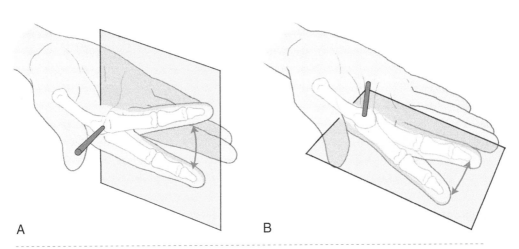

A   B

FIGURE 2-6 The metacarpophalangeal joint of the hand is an example of a synovial, biaxial condyloid joint. It allows flexion and extension in the sagittal joint around a mediolateral axis **(A)** and abduction and adduction in the frontal plane around an anteroposterior axis **(B)**.

Triaxial Joints

There is only one major type of synovial triaxial joint: ball-and-socket. As its name implies, one bone is shaped like a ball and fits into the socket shape of the other bone. A ball-and-socket joint allows the following motions: flexion and extension in the sagittal plane around a mediolateral axis; abduction and adduction in the frontal plane around an anteroposterior axis; and medial rotation and lateral rotation in the transverse plane around a vertical axis. The hip joint is a classic example of a ball-and-socket joint (Figure 2-8).

Nonaxial Joints

Synovial nonaxial joints permit motion within a plane, but the motion is a linear gliding motion and not a circular (axial) motion around an axis. The surfaces of nonaxial joints are usually flat or curved. Intercarpal joints between individual carpal bones of the wrist are examples of nonaxial joints (Figure 2-9).

2

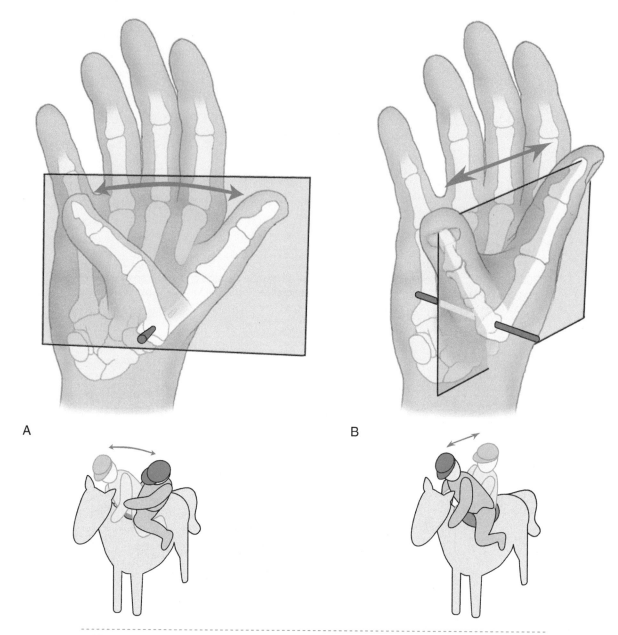

FIGURE 2-7 The carpometacarpal joint of the thumb is an example of a synovial, biaxial saddle joint. It allows flexion and extension *(A);* and abduction and adduction *(B).* It also allows medial and lateral rotation around a third axis; however, these motions cannot be actively isolated. They must be coupled with flexion and extension, respectively. (Adapted from Neumann DA: *Kinesiology of the musculoskeletal system: foundations for physical rehabilitation,* ed 2, St Louis, 2010, Mosby.)

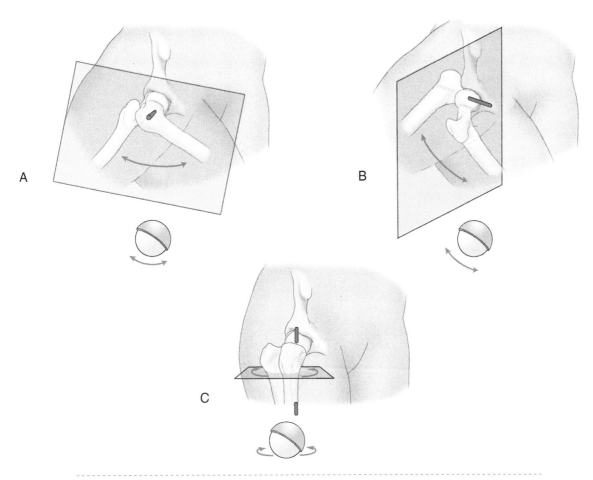

FIGURE 2-8 The hip joint between the head of the femur and the acetabulum of the pelvic bone is an example of a synovial, triaxial ball-and-socket joint. It allows flexion and extension in the sagittal plane around a mediolateral axis **(A),** abduction and adduction in the frontal plane around an anteroposterior axis **(B),** and medial rotation and lateral rotation in the transverse plane around a vertical axis **(C).**

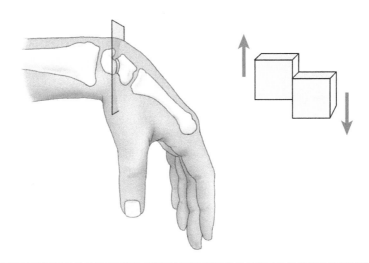

FIGURE 2-9 An intercarpal joint of the wrist is an example of a synovial, nonaxial joint. Linear gliding motion is allowed within a plane, but this motion does not occur around an axis; consequently, it is nonaxial.

ATLAS OF BONY LANDMARKS AND MUSCLE ATTACHMENT SITES ON BONES

Upper Extremity

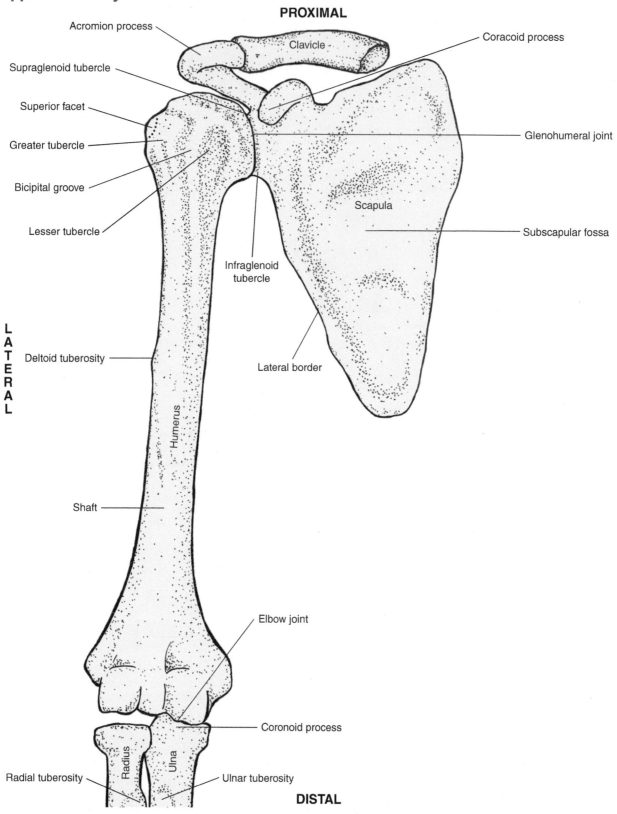

PROXIMAL

Acromion process

Clavicle

Coracoid process

Supraglenoid tubercle

Superior facet

Glenohumeral joint

Greater tubercle

Bicipital groove

Scapula

Lesser tubercle

Subscapular fossa

Infraglenoid tubercle

LATERAL

MEDIAL

Deltoid tuberosity

Lateral border

Humerus

Shaft

Elbow joint

Coronoid process

Radius

Ulna

Radial tuberosity

Ulnar tuberosity

DISTAL

FIGURE 2-10 Anterior view of the bones and bony landmarks of the right scapula/arm.

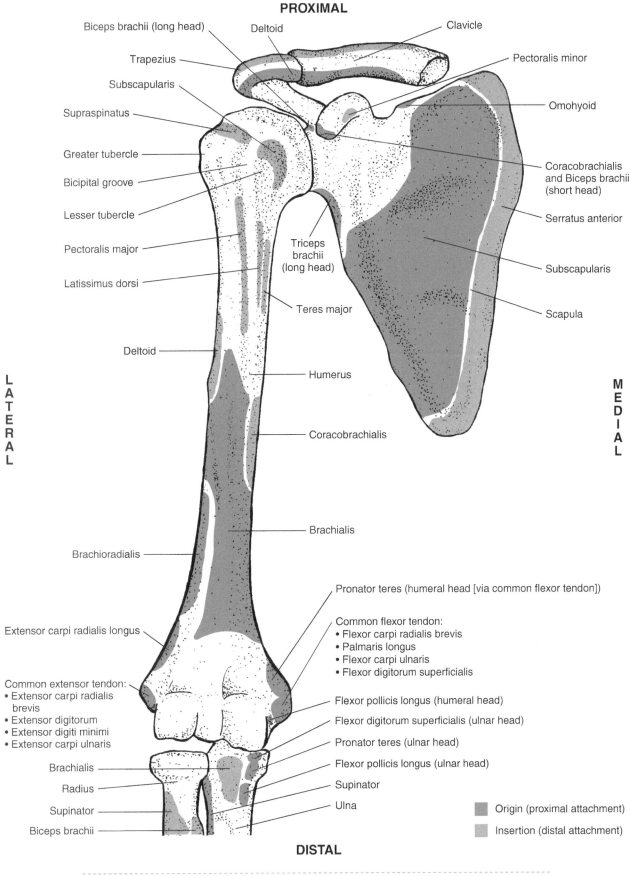

PROXIMAL

Biceps brachii (long head)

Deltoid

Clavicle

Trapezius

Pectoralis minor

Subscapularis

Omohyoid

Supraspinatus

Greater tubercle

Bicipital groove

Coracobrachialis and Biceps brachii (short head)

Lesser tubercle

Serratus anterior

Pectoralis major

Triceps brachii (long head)

Latissimus dorsi

Subscapularis

Teres major

Scapula

Deltoid

Humerus

Coracobrachialis

Brachialis

Brachioradialis

LATERAL

MEDIAL

Pronator teres (humeral head [via common flexor tendon])

Extensor carpi radialis longus

Common flexor tendon:
• Flexor carpi radialis brevis
• Palmaris longus
• Flexor carpi ulnaris
• Flexor digitorum superficialis

Common extensor tendon:
• Extensor carpi radialis brevis
• Extensor digitorum
• Extensor digiti minimi
• Extensor carpi ulnaris

Flexor pollicis longus (humeral head)

Flexor digitorum superficialis (ulnar head)

Pronator teres (ulnar head)

Brachialis

Flexor pollicis longus (ulnar head)

Radius

Supinator

Supinator

Ulna

Biceps brachii

Origin (proximal attachment)

Insertion (distal attachment)

DISTAL

FIGURE 2-11 Anterior view of muscle attachment sites on the right scapula/arm.

2

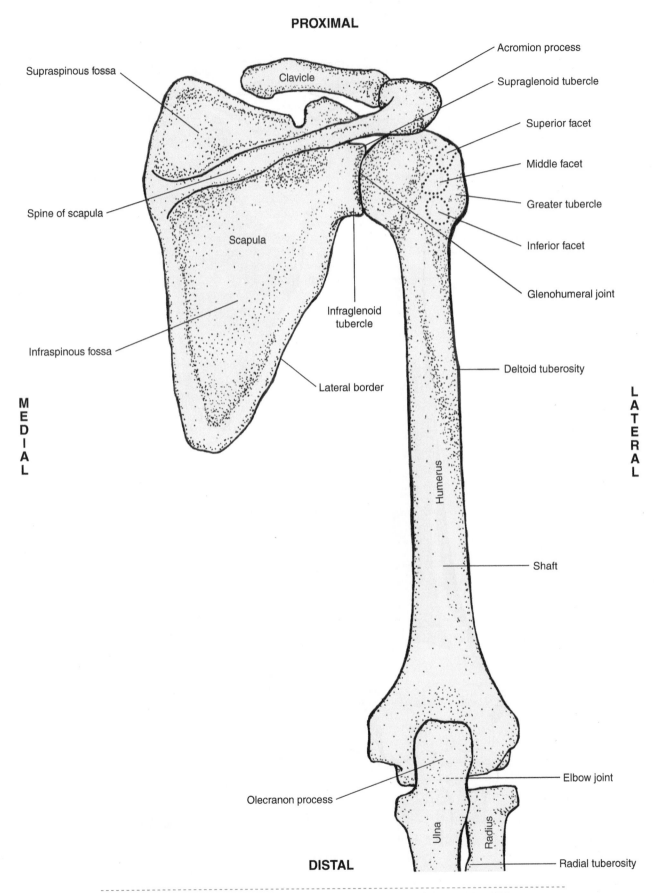

PROXIMAL

Supraspinous fossa

Clavicle

Acromion process

Supraglenoid tubercle

Superior facet

Middle facet

Greater tubercle

Inferior facet

Glenohumeral joint

Spine of scapula

Scapula

Infraglenoid
tubercle

Infraspinous fossa

Lateral border

Deltoid tuberosity

MEDIAL

LATERAL

Humerus

Shaft

Olecranon process

Elbow joint

Ulna

Radius

DISTAL

Radial tuberosity

FIGURE 2-12 Posterior view of bones and bony landmarks of the right scapula/arm.

2

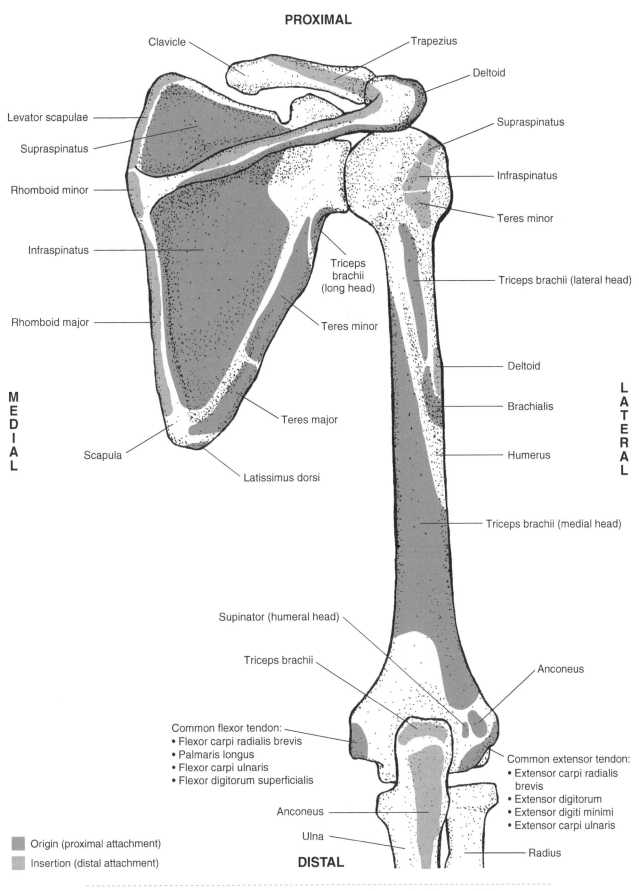

FIGURE 2-13 Posterior view of muscle attachment sites on the right scapula/arm.

2

PROXIMAL

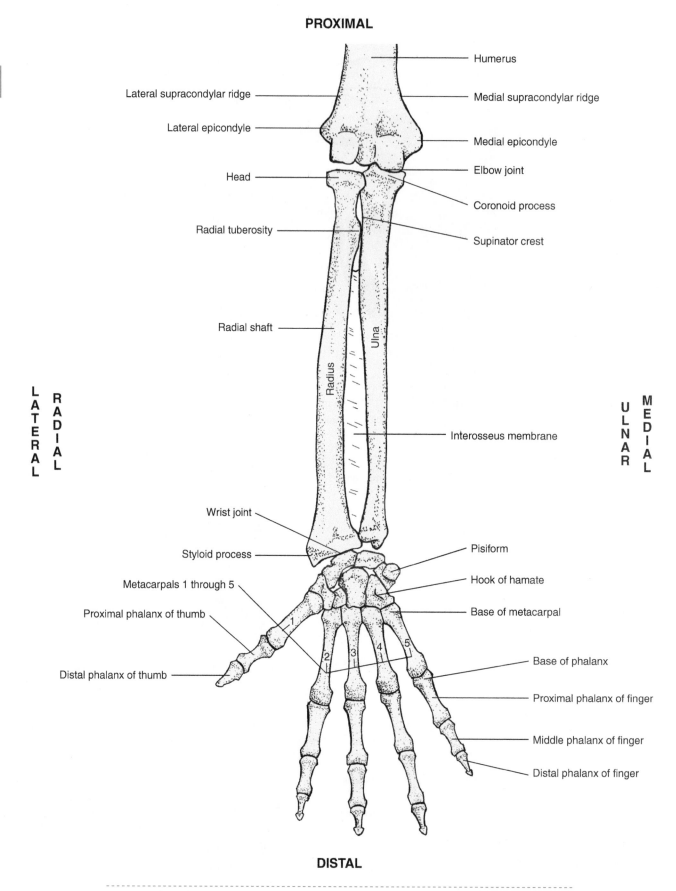

Humerus

Lateral supracondylar ridge

Medial supracondylar ridge

Lateral epicondyle

Medial epicondyle

Head

Elbow joint

Coronoid process

Radial tuberosity

Supinator crest

Radial shaft

Radius

Ulna

Interosseus membrane

L A T E R A L

R A D I A L

U L N A R

M E D I A L

Wrist joint

Styloid process

Pisiform

Hook of hamate

Metacarpals 1 through 5

Base of metacarpal

Proximal phalanx of thumb

Distal phalanx of thumb

Base of phalanx

Proximal phalanx of finger

Middle phalanx of finger

Distal phalanx of finger

DISTAL

FIGURE 2-14 Anterior view of bones and bony landmarks of the right forearm.

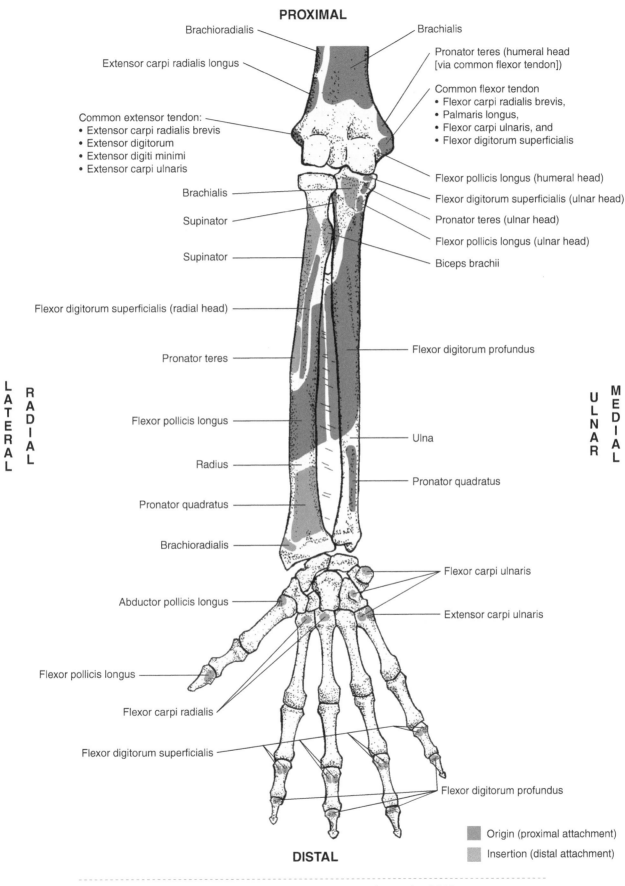

PROXIMAL

Brachioradialis

Brachialis

Extensor carpi radialis longus

Pronator teres (humeral head [via common flexor tendon])

Common flexor tendon
• Flexor carpi radialis brevis,
• Palmaris longus,
• Flexor carpi ulnaris, and
• Flexor digitorum superficialis

Common extensor tendon:
• Extensor carpi radialis brevis
• Extensor digitorum
• Extensor digiti minimi
• Extensor carpi ulnaris

Flexor pollicis longus (humeral head)

Flexor digitorum superficialis (ulnar head)

Brachialis

Pronator teres (ulnar head)

Supinator

Flexor pollicis longus (ulnar head)

Supinator

Biceps brachii

Flexor digitorum superficialis (radial head)

Flexor digitorum profundus

Pronator teres

Flexor pollicis longus

Ulna

Radius

Pronator quadratus

Pronator quadratus

Brachioradialis

Flexor carpi ulnaris

Abductor pollicis longus

Extensor carpi ulnaris

Flexor pollicis longus

Flexor carpi radialis

Flexor digitorum superficialis

Flexor digitorum profundus

LATERAL RADIAL

ULNAR MEDIAL

Origin (proximal attachment)

Insertion (distal attachment)

DISTAL

FIGURE 2-15 Anterior view of muscle attachment sites on the right forearm.

PROXIMAL

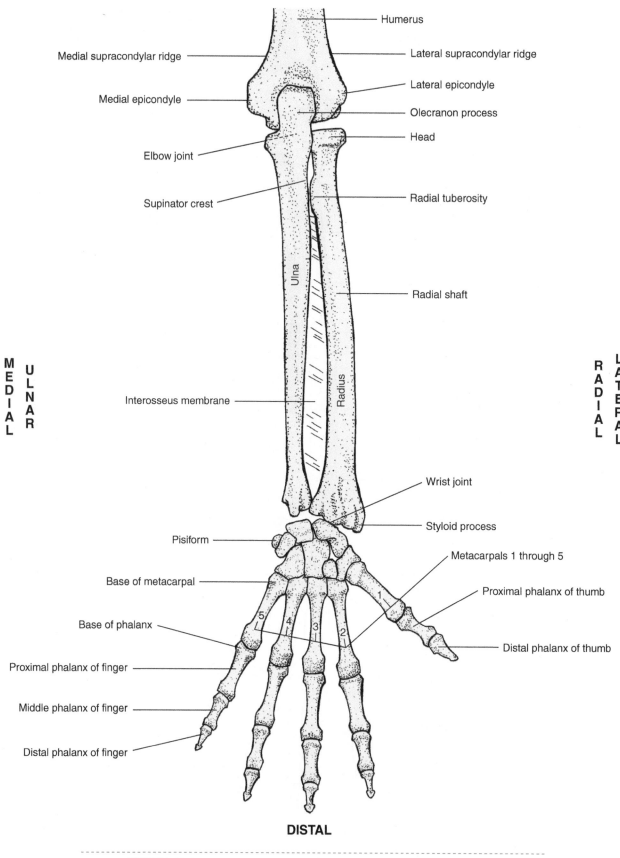

Humerus

Medial supracondylar ridge

Lateral supracondylar ridge

Lateral epicondyle

Medial epicondyle

Olecranon process

Head

Elbow joint

Supinator crest

Radial tuberosity

Ulna

Radius

Radial shaft

M E D I A L   U L N A R

R A D I A L   L A T E R A L

Interosseus membrane

Wrist joint

Styloid process

Pisiform

Metacarpals 1 through 5

Base of metacarpal

Proximal phalanx of thumb

Base of phalanx

Distal phalanx of thumb

Proximal phalanx of finger

Middle phalanx of finger

Distal phalanx of finger

DISTAL

FIGURE 2-16 Posterior view of bones and bony landmarks of the right forearm.

PROXIMAL

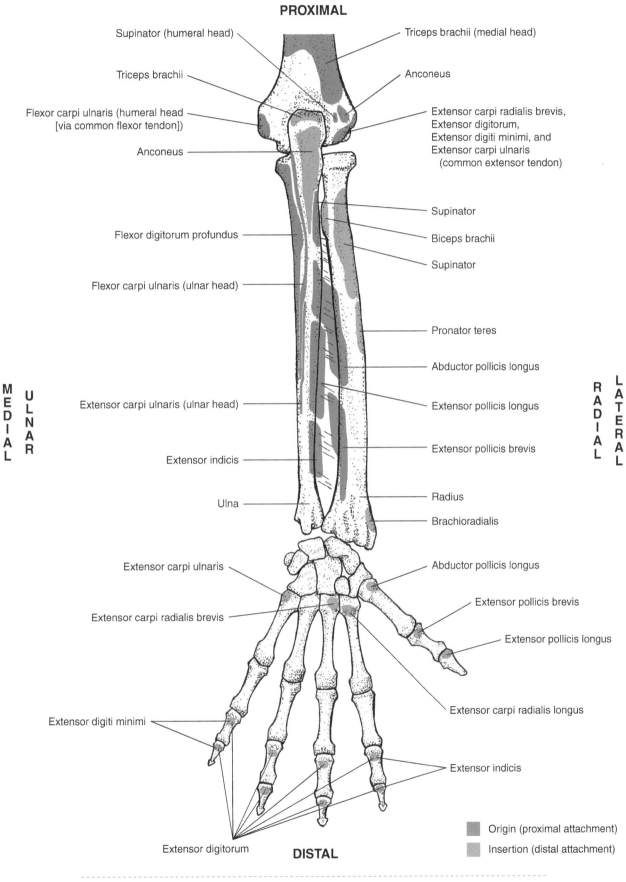

Supinator (humeral head)

Triceps brachii (medial head)

Triceps brachii

Anconeus

Flexor carpi ulnaris (humeral head [via common flexor tendon])

Extensor carpi radialis brevis, Extensor digitorum, Extensor digiti minimi, and Extensor carpi ulnaris (common extensor tendon)

Anconeus

Supinator

Flexor digitorum profundus

Biceps brachii

Supinator

Flexor carpi ulnaris (ulnar head)

Pronator teres

Abductor pollicis longus

M E D I A L

U L N A R

R A D I A L

L A T E R A L

Extensor carpi ulnaris (ulnar head)

Extensor pollicis longus

Extensor indicis

Extensor pollicis brevis

Ulna

Radius

Brachioradialis

Extensor carpi ulnaris

Abductor pollicis longus

Extensor pollicis brevis

Extensor carpi radialis brevis

Extensor pollicis longus

Extensor carpi radialis longus

Extensor digiti minimi

Extensor indicis

Extensor digitorum

DISTAL

Origin (proximal attachment)

Insertion (distal attachment)

FIGURE 2-17 Posterior view of muscle attachment sites on the right forearm.

2

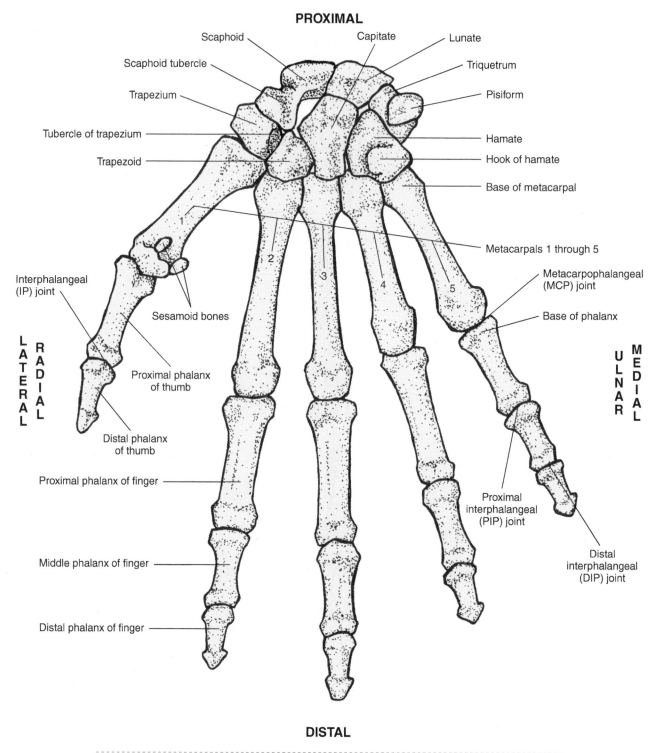

PROXIMAL

Scaphoid

Capitate

Lunate

Scaphoid tubercle

Triquetrum

Trapezium

Pisiform

Tubercle of trapezium

Hamate

Trapezoid

Hook of hamate

Base of metacarpal

1

2

3

4

5

Metacarpals 1 through 5

Interphalangeal
(IP) joint

Metacarpophalangeal
(MCP) joint

Base of phalanx

Sesamoid bones

L
A
T
E
R
A
L

R
A
D
I
A
L

U
L
N
A
R

M
E
D
I
A
L

Proximal phalanx
of thumb

Distal phalanx
of thumb

Proximal phalanx of finger

Proximal
interphalangeal
(PIP) joint

Middle phalanx of finger

Distal
interphalangeal
(DIP) joint

Distal phalanx of finger

DISTAL

FIGURE 2-18 Palmar view of bones and bony landmarks of the right hand.

2

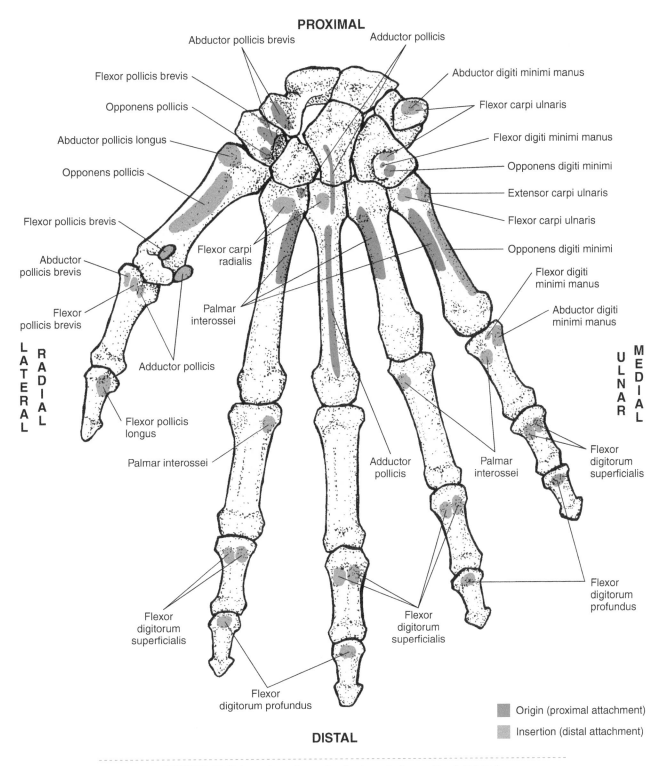

PROXIMAL

Abductor pollicis brevis

Flexor pollicis brevis

Opponens pollicis

Abductor pollicis longus

Opponens pollicis

Flexor pollicis brevis

Abductor pollicis brevis

Flexor pollicis brevis

Flexor carpi radialis

Palmar interossei

Adductor pollicis

Flexor pollicis longus

Palmar interossei

Flexor digitorum superficialis

Flexor digitorum profundus

Adductor pollicis

Abductor digiti minimi manus

Flexor carpi ulnaris

Flexor digiti minimi manus

Opponens digiti minimi

Extensor carpi ulnaris

Flexor carpi ulnaris

Opponens digiti minimi

Flexor digiti minimi manus

Abductor digiti minimi manus

Flexor digitorum superficialis

Adductor pollicis

Palmar interossei

Flexor digitorum superficialis

Flexor digitorum profundus

L A T E R A L

R A D I A L

U L N A R

M E D I A L

Origin (proximal attachment)

Insertion (distal attachment)

DISTAL

FIGURE 2-19 Palmar view of muscle attachment sites on the right hand.

2

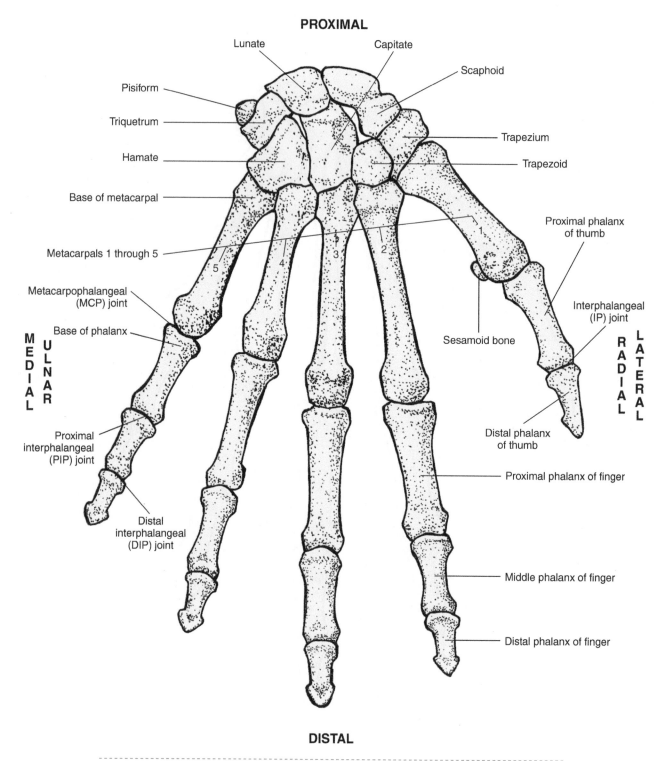

PROXIMAL

Lunate

Capitate

Scaphoid

Pisiform

Triquetrum

Trapezium

Hamate

Trapezoid

Base of metacarpal

Proximal phalanx
of thumb

Metacarpals 1 through 5

Metacarpophalangeal
(MCP) joint

Interphalangeal
(IP) joint

Base of phalanx

Sesamoid bone

M E D I A L **U L N A R**

R A D I A L **L A T E R A L**

Proximal
interphalangeal
(PIP) joint

Distal phalanx
of thumb

Proximal phalanx of finger

Distal
interphalangeal
(DIP) joint

Middle phalanx of finger

Distal phalanx of finger

DISTAL

FIGURE 2-20 Dorsal view of bones and bony landmarks of the right hand.

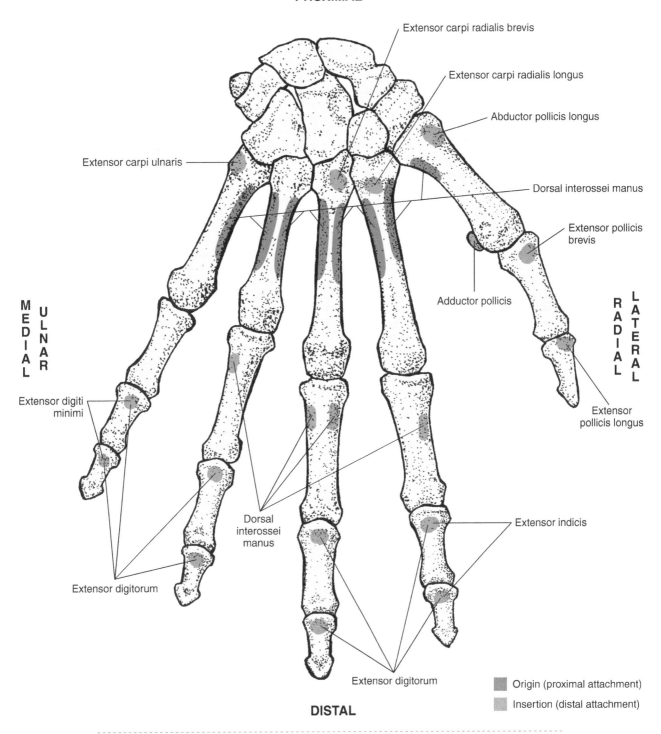

FIGURE 2-21 Dorsal view of muscle attachment sites on the right hand.

Axial Body

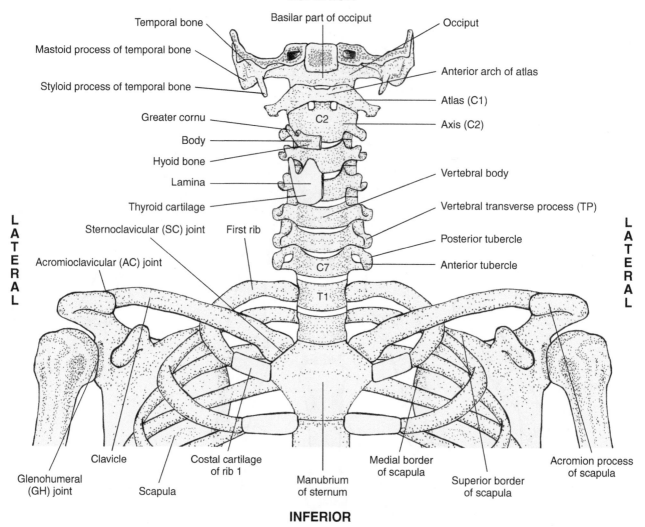

FIGURE 2-22 Anterior view of bones and bony landmarks of the neck.

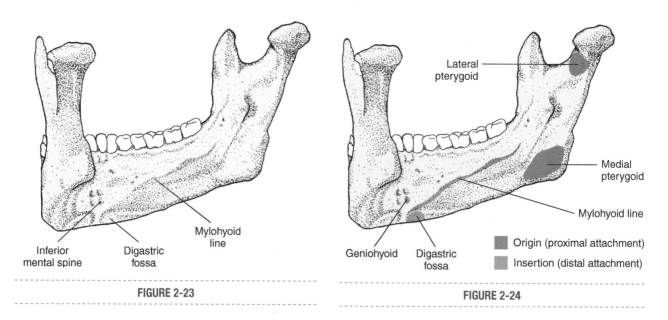

FIGURE 2-23

FIGURE 2-24

2

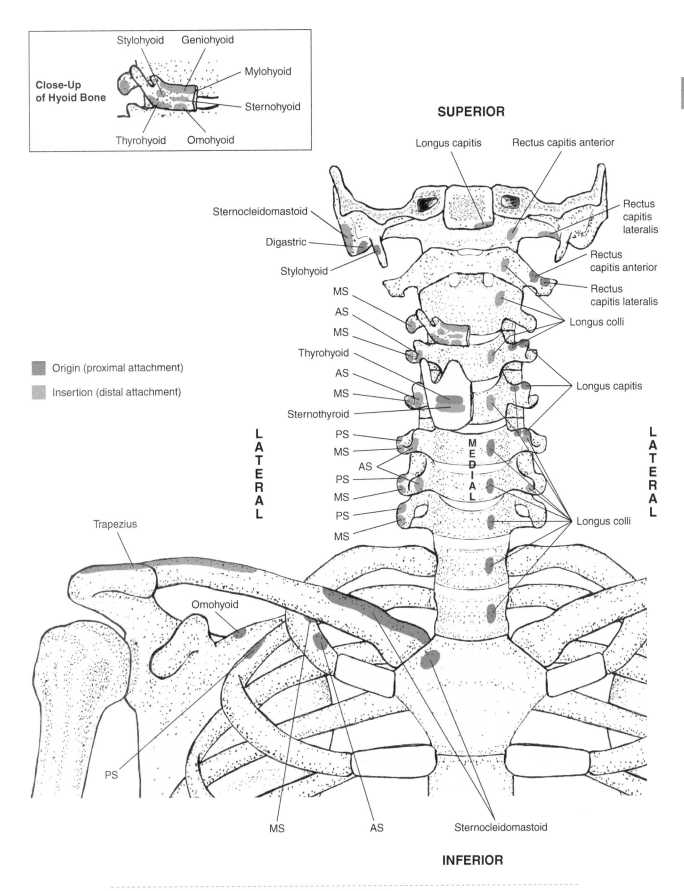

Close-Up of Hyoid Bone

Stylohyoid Geniohyoid
Mylohyoid
Sternohyoid
Thyrohyoid Omohyoid

SUPERIOR

Longus capitis   Rectus capitis anterior

Sternocleidomastoid

Digastric

Stylohyoid

Rectus capitis lateralis

Rectus capitis anterior

Rectus capitis lateralis

Longus colli

MS
AS
MS
Thyrohyoid
AS
MS
Sternothyroid
PS
MS
AS
PS
MS
PS
MS

Longus capitis

MEDIAL

■ Origin (proximal attachment)

▨ Insertion (distal attachment)

LATERAL

LATERAL

Longus colli

Trapezius

Omohyoid

PS

MS   AS   Sternocleidomastoid

INFERIOR

FIGURE 2-25 Anterior view of muscle attachment sites on the neck. *AS,* Anterior scalene; *MS,* middle scalene; *PS,* posterior scalene.

SUPERIOR

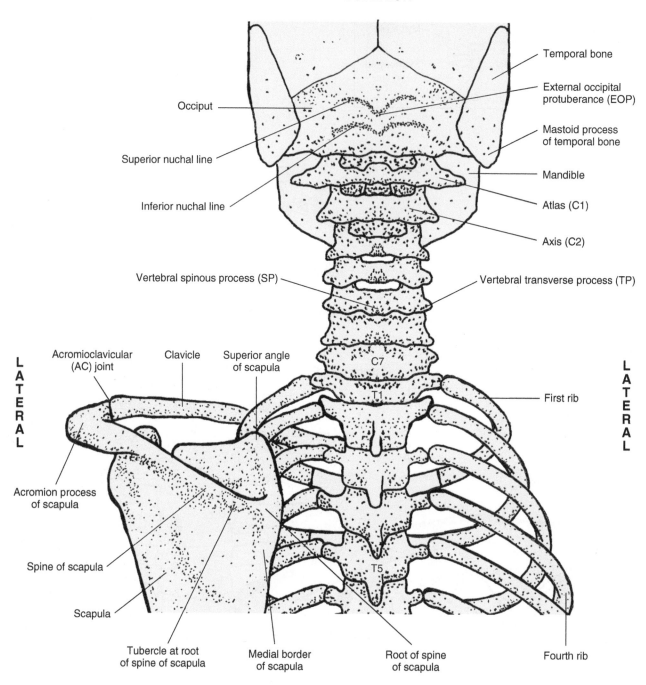

Occiput

Superior nuchal line

Inferior nuchal line

Vertebral spinous process (SP)

Temporal bone

External occipital protuberance (EOP)

Mastoid process of temporal bone

Mandible

Atlas (C1)

Axis (C2)

Vertebral transverse process (TP)

Acromioclavicular (AC) joint

Clavicle

Superior angle of scapula

C7

T1

First rib

T5

Acromion process of scapula

Spine of scapula

Scapula

Tubercle at root of spine of scapula

Medial border of scapula

Root of spine of scapula

Fourth rib

LATERAL

LATERAL

INFERIOR

FIGURE 2-26 Posterior view of bones and bony landmarks of the neck.

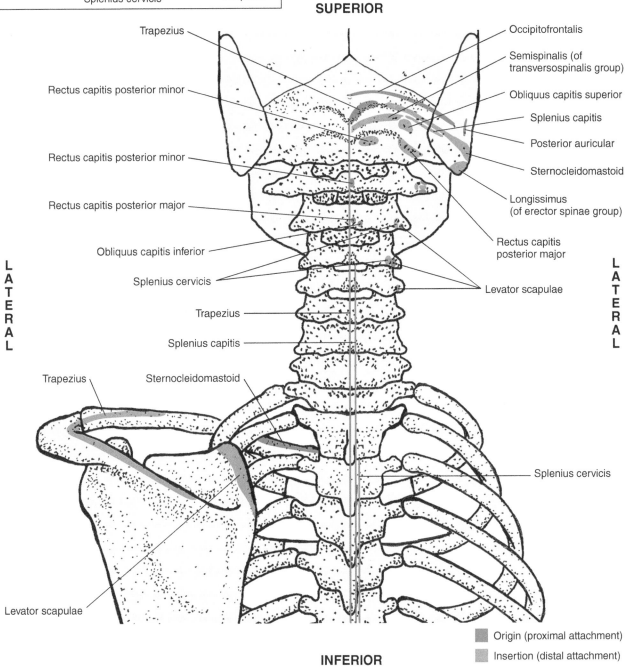

Close-up of Transverse Process of Atlas (C1)

Obliquus capitis superior

Obliquus capitis inferior

Levator scapulae

Splenius cervicis

SUPERIOR

Trapezius

Rectus capitis posterior minor

Rectus capitis posterior minor

Rectus capitis posterior major

Obliquus capitis inferior

Splenius cervicis

Trapezius

Splenius capitis

Trapezius

Sternocleidomastoid

Levator scapulae

Occipitofrontalis

Semispinalis (of transversospinalis group)

Obliquus capitis superior

Splenius capitis

Posterior auricular

Sternocleidomastoid

Longissimus (of erector spinae group)

Rectus capitis posterior major

Levator scapulae

Splenius cervicis

LATERAL

LATERAL

Origin (proximal attachment)

Insertion (distal attachment)

INFERIOR

FIGURE 2-27 Posterior view of muscle attachment sites on the neck.

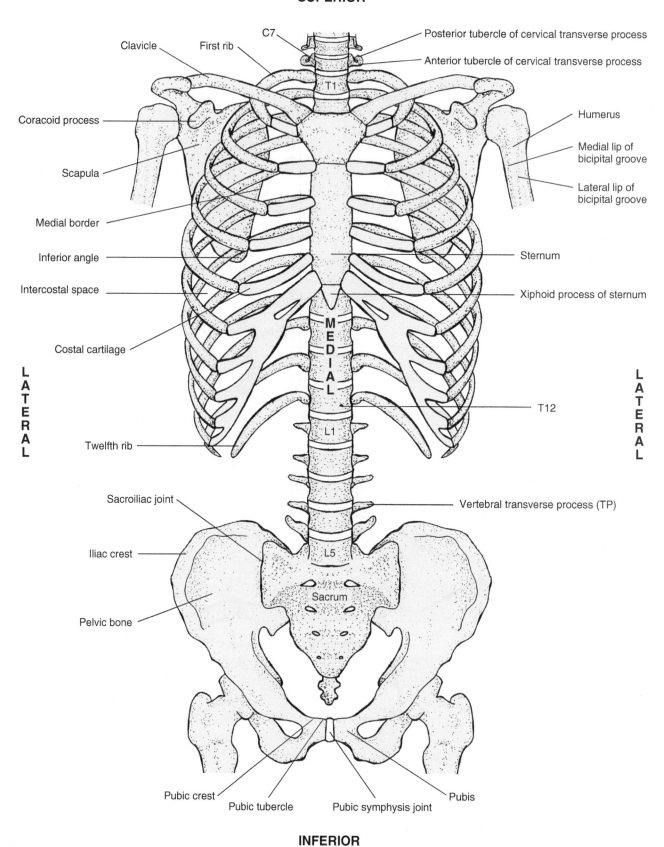

FIGURE 2-28 Anterior view of bones and bony landmarks of the trunk.

SUPERIOR

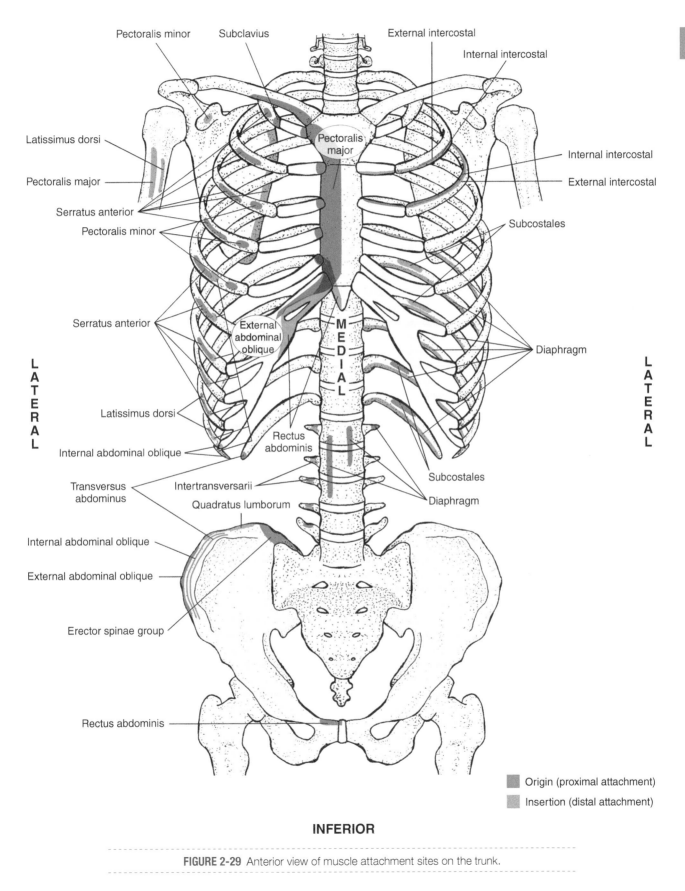

Pectoralis minor

Subclavius

External intercostal

Internal intercostal

Latissimus dorsi

Pectoralis major

Serratus anterior

Pectoralis minor

Pectoralis major

Internal intercostal

External intercostal

Subcostales

Serratus anterior

External abdominal oblique

MEDIAL

Diaphragm

Latissimus dorsi

Internal abdominal oblique

Rectus abdominis

Subcostales

Diaphragm

LATERAL

LATERAL

Transversus abdominus

Intertransversarii

Quadratus lumborum

Internal abdominal oblique

External abdominal oblique

Erector spinae group

Rectus abdominis

Origin (proximal attachment)

Insertion (distal attachment)

INFERIOR

FIGURE 2-29 Anterior view of muscle attachment sites on the trunk.

SUPERIOR

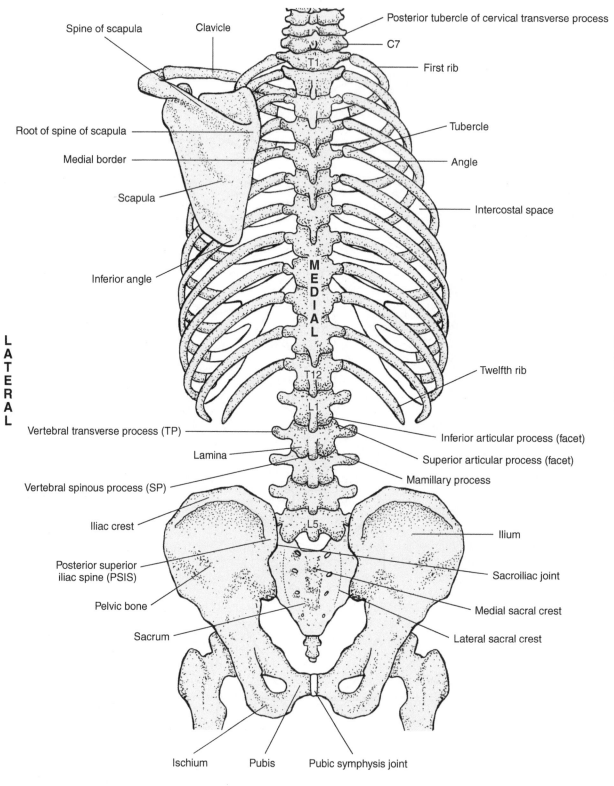

LATERAL

LATERAL

Spine of scapula

Clavicle

Posterior tubercle of cervical transverse process

C7

First rib

Root of spine of scapula

Tubercle

Medial border

Angle

Scapula

Intercostal space

Inferior angle

Twelfth rib

Vertebral transverse process (TP)

Inferior articular process (facet)

Lamina

Superior articular process (facet)

Vertebral spinous process (SP)

Mamillary process

Iliac crest

Ilium

Posterior superior
iliac spine (PSIS)

Sacroiliac joint

Pelvic bone

Medial sacral crest

Sacrum

Lateral sacral crest

Ischium   Pubis   Pubic symphysis joint

MEDIAL

INFERIOR

FIGURE 2-30 Posterior view of bones and bony landmarks of the trunk.

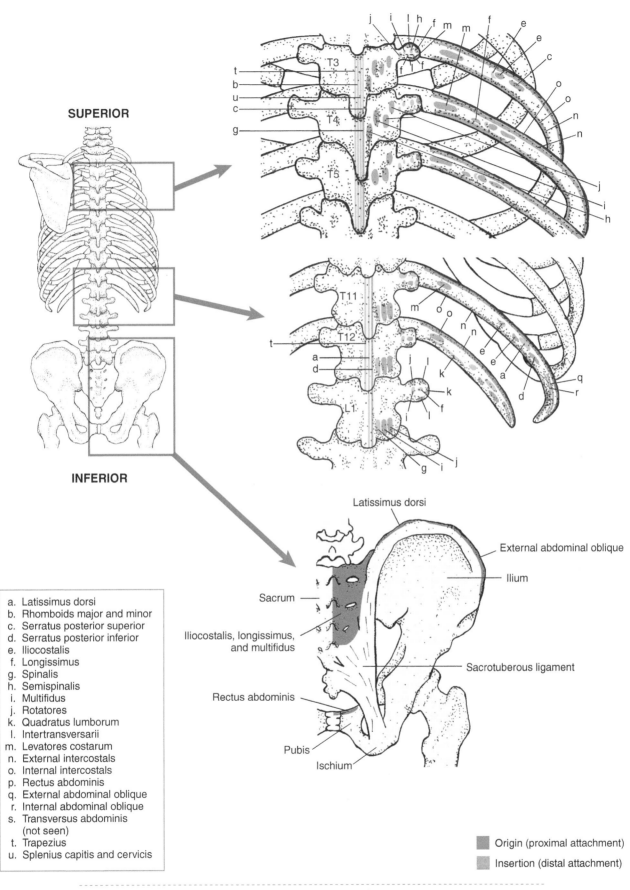

a. Latissimus dorsi
b. Rhomboids major and minor
c. Serratus posterior superior
d. Serratus posterior inferior
e. Iliocostalis
f. Longissimus
g. Spinalis
h. Semispinalis
i. Multifidus
j. Rotatores
k. Quadratus lumborum
l. Intertransversarii
m. Levatores costarum
n. External intercostals
o. Internal intercostals
p. Rectus abdominis
q. External abdominal oblique
r. Internal abdominal oblique
s. Transversus abdominis
   (not seen)
t. Trapezius
u. Splenius capitis and cervicis

Origin (proximal attachment)

Insertion (distal attachment)

FIGURE 2-31 Posterior view of muscle attachment sites on the trunk.

SUPERIOR

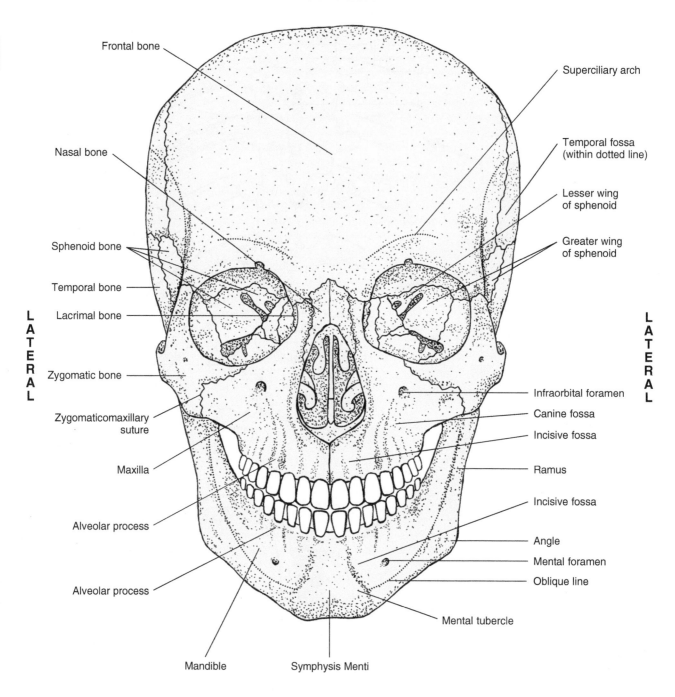

Frontal bone

Superciliary arch

Temporal fossa
(within dotted line)

Nasal bone

Lesser wing
of sphenoid

Greater wing
of sphenoid

Sphenoid bone

Temporal bone

Lacrimal bone

L
A
T
E
R
A
L

L
A
T
E
R
A
L

Zygomatic bone

Infraorbital foramen

Canine fossa

Zygomaticomaxillary
suture

Incisive fossa

Ramus

Maxilla

Incisive fossa

Angle

Alveolar process

Mental foramen

Oblique line

Alveolar process

Mental tubercle

Mandible

Symphysis Menti

INFERIOR

FIGURE 2-32 Anterior view of bones and bony landmarks of the head.

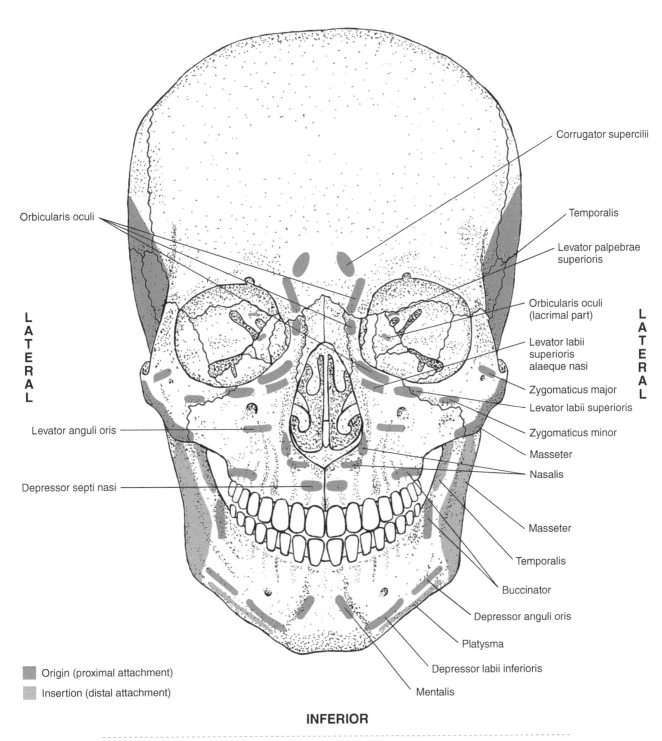

SUPERIOR

Corrugator supercilii

Orbicularis oculi

Temporalis

Levator palpebrae superioris

LATERAL

LATERAL

Orbicularis oculi (lacrimal part)

Levator labii superioris alaeque nasi

Levator anguli oris

Zygomaticus major

Levator labii superioris

Zygomaticus minor

Masseter

Depressor septi nasi

Nasalis

Masseter

Temporalis

Buccinator

Depressor anguli oris

Platysma

Depressor labii inferioris

Mentalis

■ Origin (proximal attachment)
■ Insertion (distal attachment)

INFERIOR

FIGURE 2-33 Anterior view of muscle attachment sites on the head.

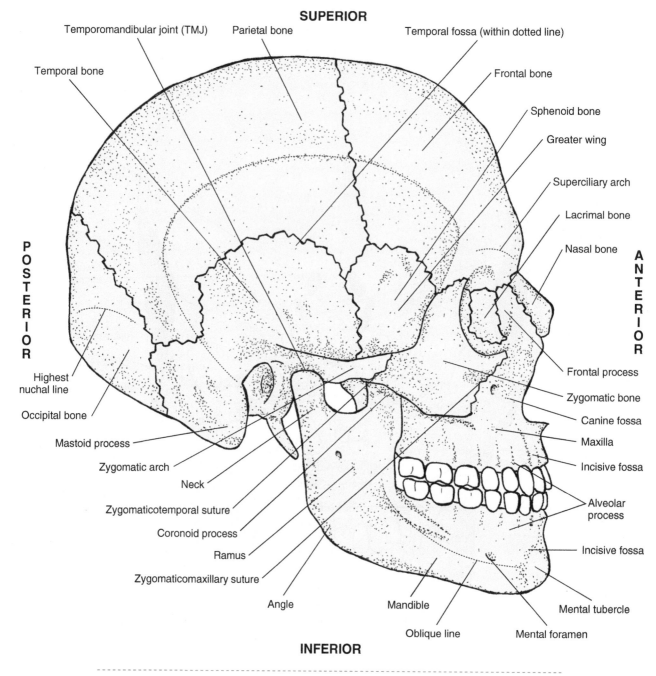

SUPERIOR

Temporomandibular joint (TMJ)

Temporal bone

Parietal bone

Temporal fossa (within dotted line)

Frontal bone

Sphenoid bone

Greater wing

Superciliary arch

Lacrimal bone

Nasal bone

Frontal process

Zygomatic bone

Canine fossa

Maxilla

Incisive fossa

Alveolar process

Incisive fossa

Mental tubercle

Mental foramen

Highest nuchal line

Occipital bone

Mastoid process

Zygomatic arch

Neck

Zygomaticotemporal suture

Coronoid process

Ramus

Zygomaticomaxillary suture

Angle

Mandible

Oblique line

POSTERIOR

ANTERIOR

INFERIOR

FIGURE 2-34 Lateral view of bones and bony landmarks of the head.

2

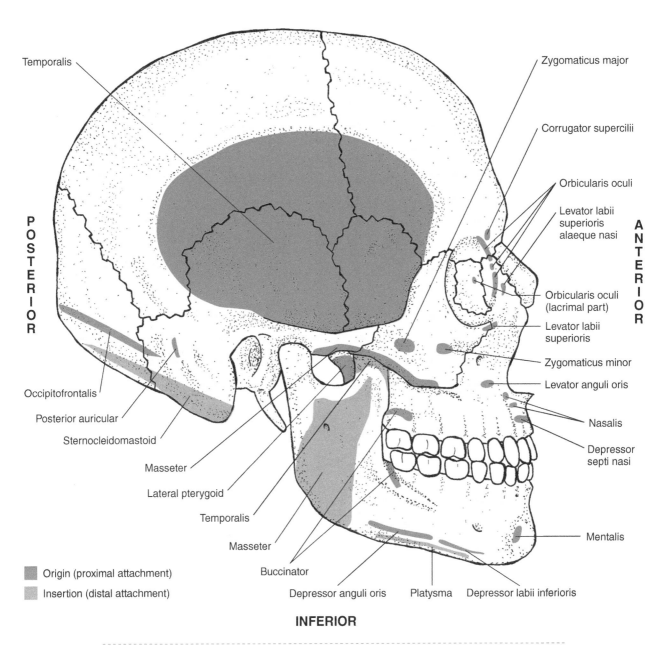

SUPERIOR

Temporalis

Zygomaticus major

Corrugator supercilii

Orbicularis oculi

Levator labii superioris alaeque nasi

Orbicularis oculi (lacrimal part)

Levator labii superioris

Zygomaticus minor

Levator anguli oris

Nasalis

Depressor septi nasi

Mentalis

Occipitofrontalis

Posterior auricular

Sternocleidomastoid

Masseter

Lateral pterygoid

Temporalis

Masseter

Buccinator

Depressor anguli oris   Platysma   Depressor labii inferioris

POSTERIOR

ANTERIOR

■ Origin (proximal attachment)

■ Insertion (distal attachment)

INFERIOR

FIGURE 2-35 Lateral view of muscle attachment sites on the head.

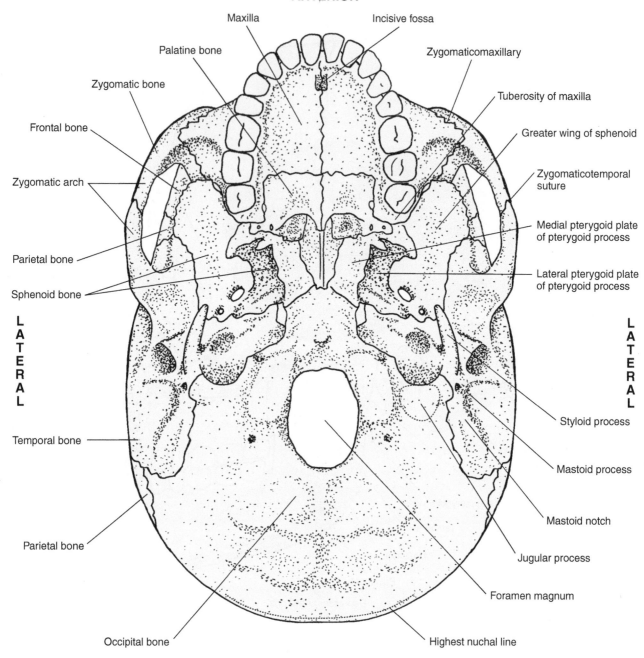

FIGURE 2-36 Inferior view of bones and bony landmarks of the head.

ANTERIOR

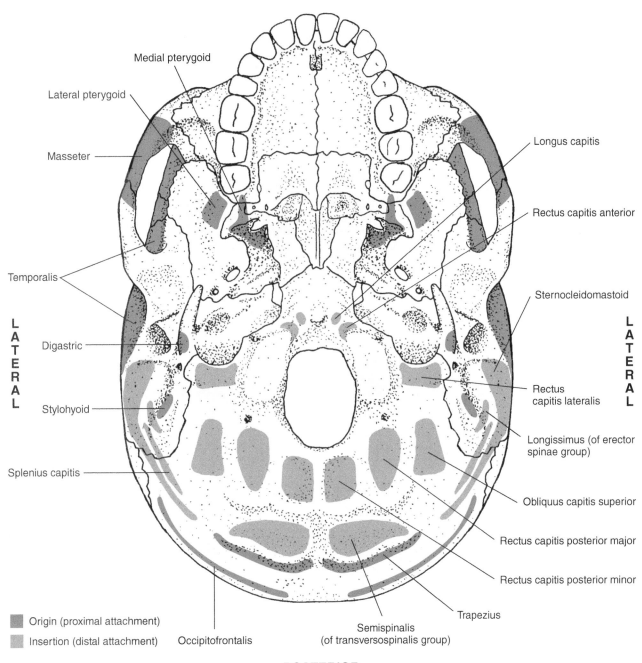

Medial pterygoid

Lateral pterygoid

Masseter

Temporalis

Digastric

Stylohyoid

Splenius capitis

L A T E R A L

Longus capitis

Rectus capitis anterior

Sternocleidomastoid

Rectus capitis lateralis

Longissimus (of erector spinae group)

Obliquus capitis superior

Rectus capitis posterior major

Rectus capitis posterior minor

Trapezius

L A T E R A L

■ Origin (proximal attachment)

■ Insertion (distal attachment)

Occipitofrontalis

Semispinalis (of transversospinalis group)

POSTERIOR

FIGURE 2-37 Inferior view of muscle attachment sites on the head.

Lower Extremity

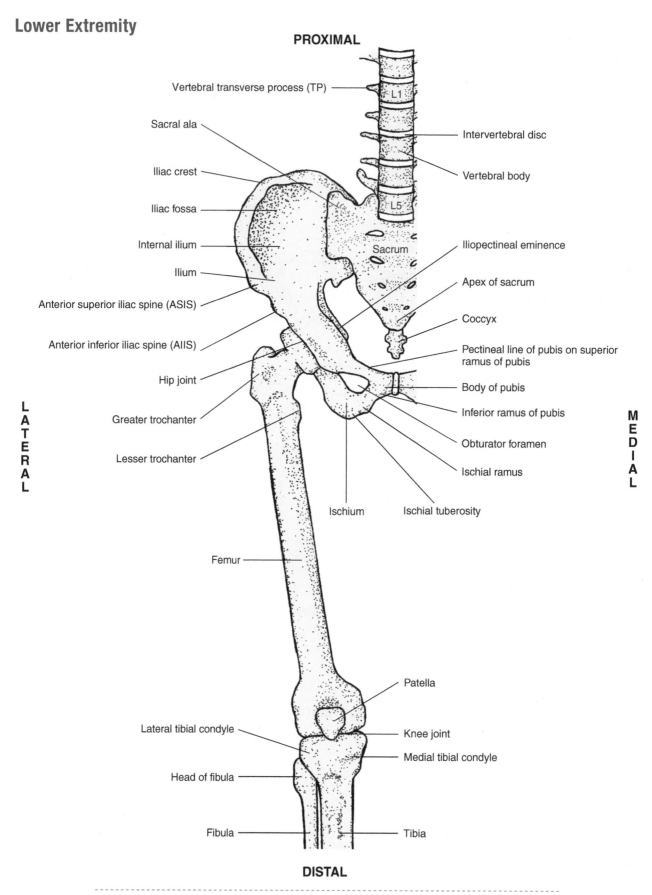

PROXIMAL

Vertebral transverse process (TP)

Sacral ala

Iliac crest

Iliac fossa

Internal ilium

Ilium

Anterior superior iliac spine (ASIS)

Anterior inferior iliac spine (AIIS)

Hip joint

Greater trochanter

Lesser trochanter

Femur

Lateral tibial condyle

Head of fibula

Fibula

L1

Intervertebral disc

Vertebral body

L5

Sacrum

Iliopectineal eminence

Apex of sacrum

Coccyx

Pectineal line of pubis on superior ramus of pubis

Body of pubis

Inferior ramus of pubis

Obturator foramen

Ischial ramus

Ischium

Ischial tuberosity

Patella

Knee joint

Medial tibial condyle

Tibia

LATERAL

MEDIAL

DISTAL

FIGURE 2-38 Anterior view of bones and bony landmarks of the right pelvis and thigh.

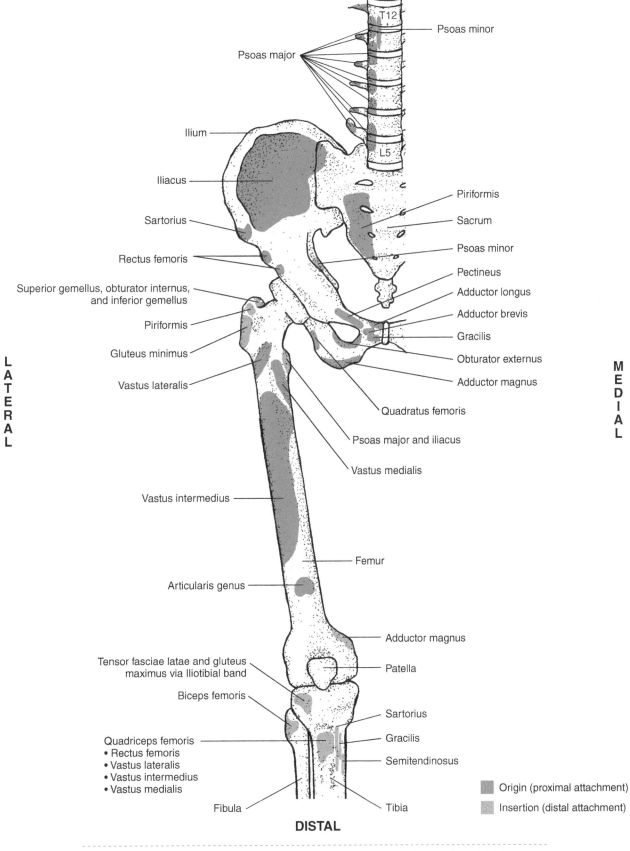

FIGURE 2-39 Anterior view of muscle attachment sites on the right pelvis and thigh.

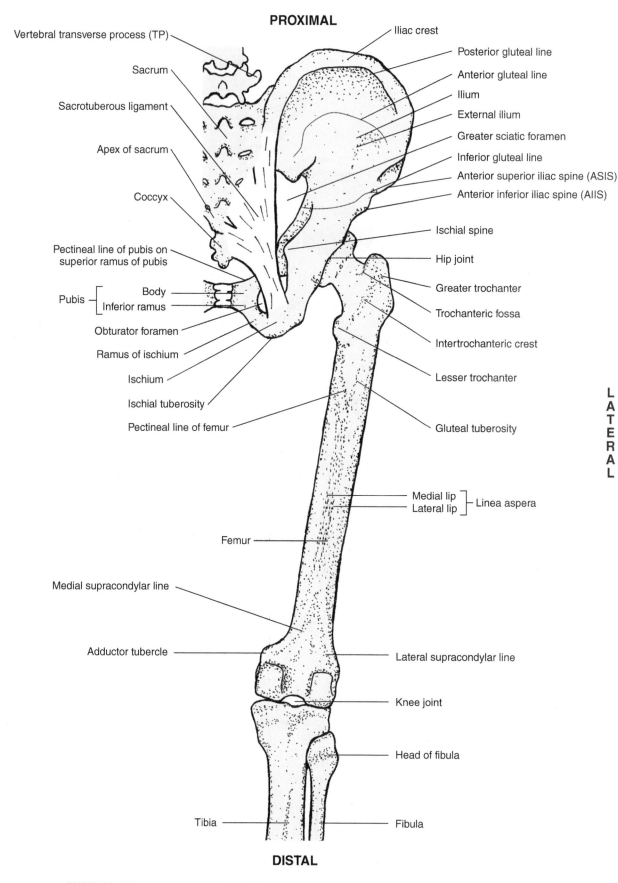

PROXIMAL

Vertebral transverse process (TP)

Sacrum

Sacrotuberous ligament

Apex of sacrum

Coccyx

Pectineal line of pubis on superior ramus of pubis

Pubis — Body / Inferior ramus

Obturator foramen

Ramus of ischium

Ischium

Ischial tuberosity

Pectineal line of femur

Iliac crest

Posterior gluteal line

Anterior gluteal line

Ilium

External ilium

Greater sciatic foramen

Inferior gluteal line

Anterior superior iliac spine (ASIS)

Anterior inferior iliac spine (AIIS)

Ischial spine

Hip joint

Greater trochanter

Trochanteric fossa

Intertrochanteric crest

Lesser trochanter

Gluteal tuberosity

Medial lip / Lateral lip — Linea aspera

Femur

Medial supracondylar line

Adductor tubercle

Lateral supracondylar line

Knee joint

Head of fibula

Tibia

Fibula

MEDIAL

LATERAL

DISTAL

FIGURE 2-40 Posterior view of bones and bony landmarks of the right pelvis and thigh.

PROXIMAL

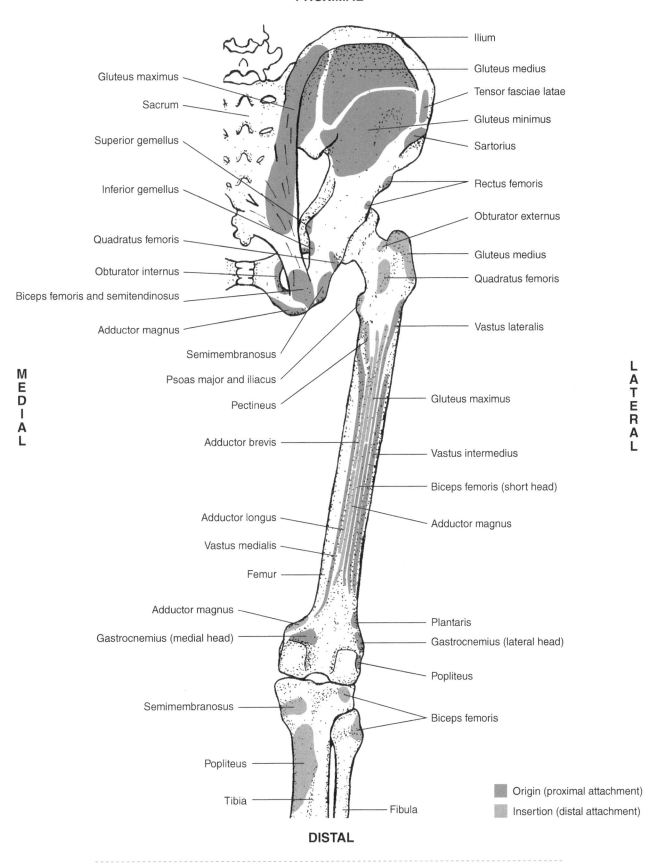

Gluteus maximus
Sacrum
Superior gemellus
Inferior gemellus
Quadratus femoris
Obturator internus
Biceps femoris and semitendinosus
Adductor magnus
Semimembranosus
Psoas major and iliacus
Pectineus
Adductor brevis
Adductor longus
Vastus medialis
Femur
Adductor magnus
Gastrocnemius (medial head)
Semimembranosus
Popliteus
Tibia

Ilium
Gluteus medius
Tensor fasciae latae
Gluteus minimus
Sartorius
Rectus femoris
Obturator externus
Gluteus medius
Quadratus femoris
Vastus lateralis
Gluteus maximus
Vastus intermedius
Biceps femoris (short head)
Adductor magnus
Plantaris
Gastrocnemius (lateral head)
Popliteus
Biceps femoris
Fibula

MEDIAL

LATERAL

Origin (proximal attachment)
Insertion (distal attachment)

DISTAL

FIGURE 2-41 Posterior view of muscle attachment sites on the right pelvis and thigh.

PROXIMAL

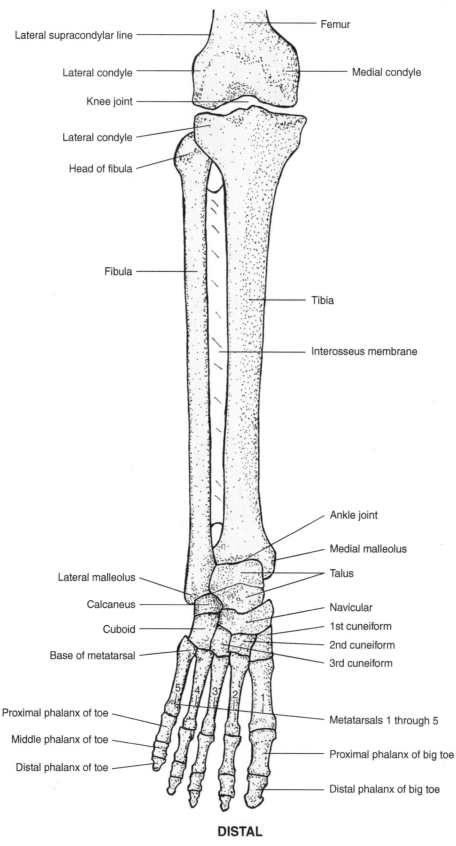

Lateral supracondylar line — Femur

Lateral condyle — Medial condyle

Knee joint —

Lateral condyle —

Head of fibula —

Fibula —

Tibia —

Interosseus membrane —

Ankle joint —

Medial malleolus —

Lateral malleolus — Talus —

Calcaneus — Navicular —

Cuboid — 1st cuneiform —

Base of metatarsal — 2nd cuneiform —

3rd cuneiform —

Proximal phalanx of toe — Metatarsals 1 through 5 —

Middle phalanx of toe —

Proximal phalanx of big toe —

Distal phalanx of toe —

Distal phalanx of big toe —

LATERAL

MEDIAL

DISTAL

FIGURE 2-42 Anterior view of bones and bony landmarks of the right leg.

2

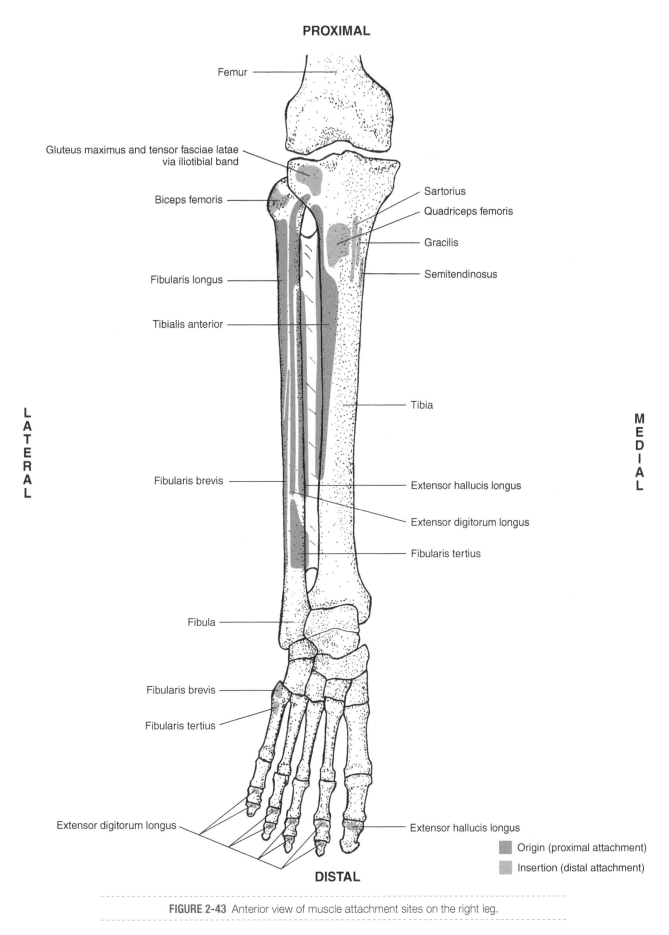

PROXIMAL

Femur

Gluteus maximus and tensor fasciae latae via iliotibial band

Biceps femoris

Sartorius

Quadriceps femoris

Gracilis

Semitendinosus

Fibularis longus

Tibialis anterior

Tibia

LATERAL

MEDIAL

Fibularis brevis

Extensor hallucis longus

Extensor digitorum longus

Fibularis tertius

Fibula

Fibularis brevis

Fibularis tertius

Extensor digitorum longus

Extensor hallucis longus

Origin (proximal attachment)

Insertion (distal attachment)

DISTAL

FIGURE 2-43 Anterior view of muscle attachment sites on the right leg.

2

PROXIMAL

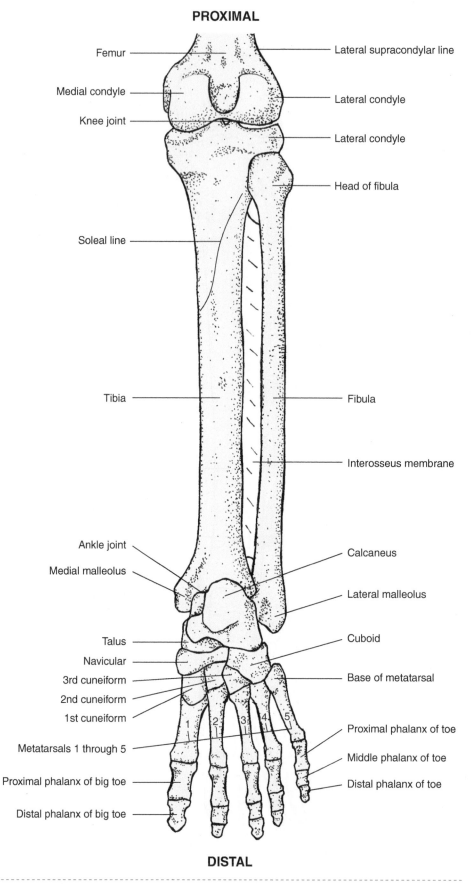

Femur —————————————————— Lateral supracondylar line

Medial condyle ——————————————— Lateral condyle

Knee joint ———————————————— Lateral condyle

—————————————— Head of fibula

Soleal line ——————————

Tibia ———————————————— Fibula

—————————— Interosseus membrane

Ankle joint ————————————— Calcaneus

Medial malleolus ————————— Lateral malleolus

Talus ——————————————— Cuboid

Navicular ——————————

3rd cuneiform ——————— Base of metatarsal

2nd cuneiform ————————

1st cuneiform ————————

Metatarsals 1 through 5 ———— Proximal phalanx of toe

Middle phalanx of toe

Proximal phalanx of big toe —— Distal phalanx of toe

Distal phalanx of big toe ———

MEDIAL

LATERAL

DISTAL

FIGURE 2-44 Posterior view of bones and bony landmarks of the right leg.

PROXIMAL

Femur

Plantaris

Gastrocnemius (lateral head)

Gastrocnemius (medial head)

Popliteus

Semimembranosus

Biceps femoris

Popliteus

Soleus

Tibialis posterior

Flexor digitorum longus

Flexor hallucis longus

MEDIAL

LATERAL

Tibia

Plantaris

Fibularis brevis

Gastrocnemius and soleus
(via calcaneal tendon [Achilles tendon])

Fibula

Tibialis posterior

Tibialis anterior

Fibularis longus

Origin (proximal attachment)

Insertion (distal attachment)

Flexor hallucis longus

Flexor digitorum longus

DISTAL

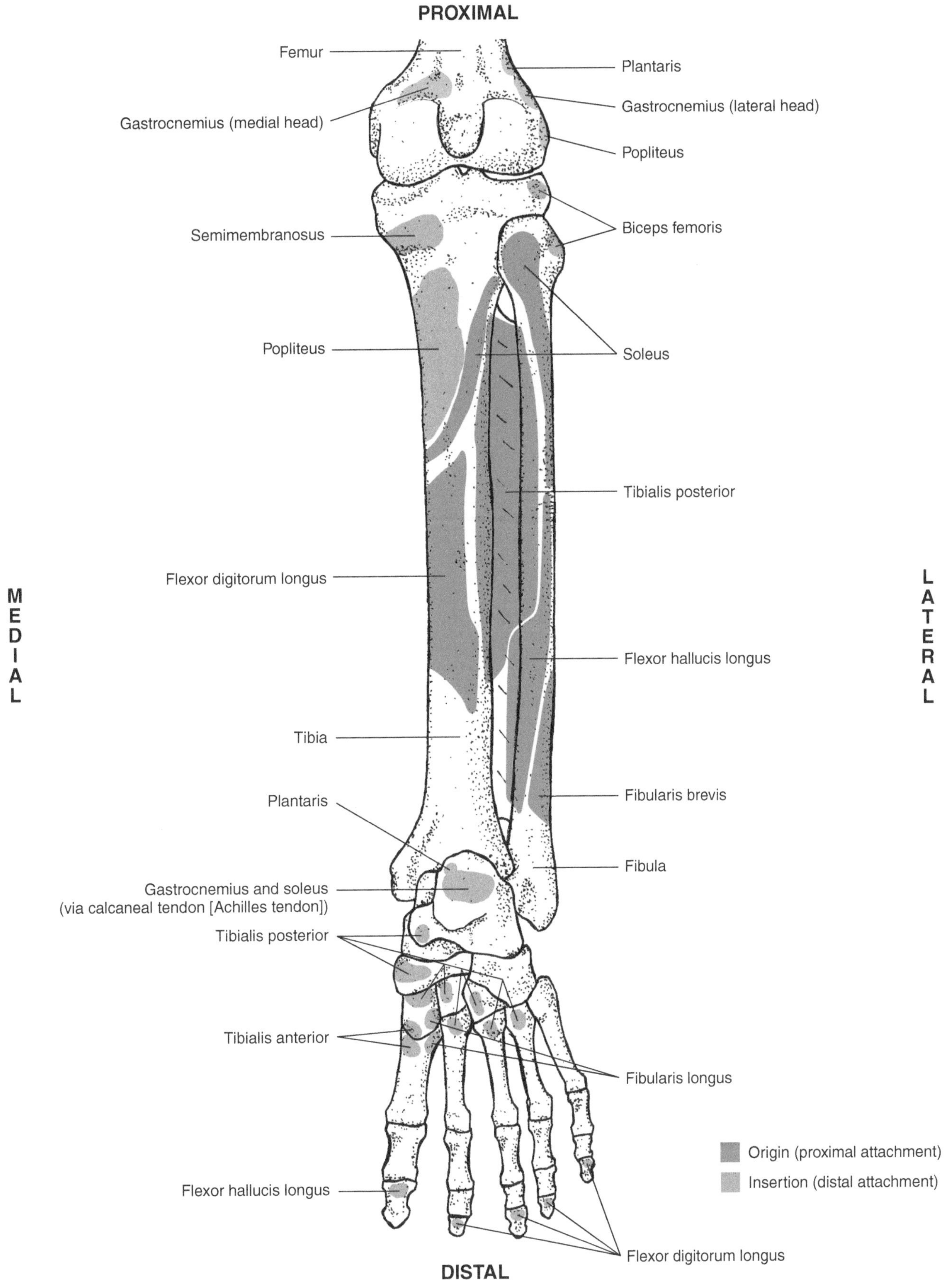

FIGURE 2-45 Posterior view of muscle attachment sites on the right leg.

2

PROXIMAL

LATERAL

MEDIAL

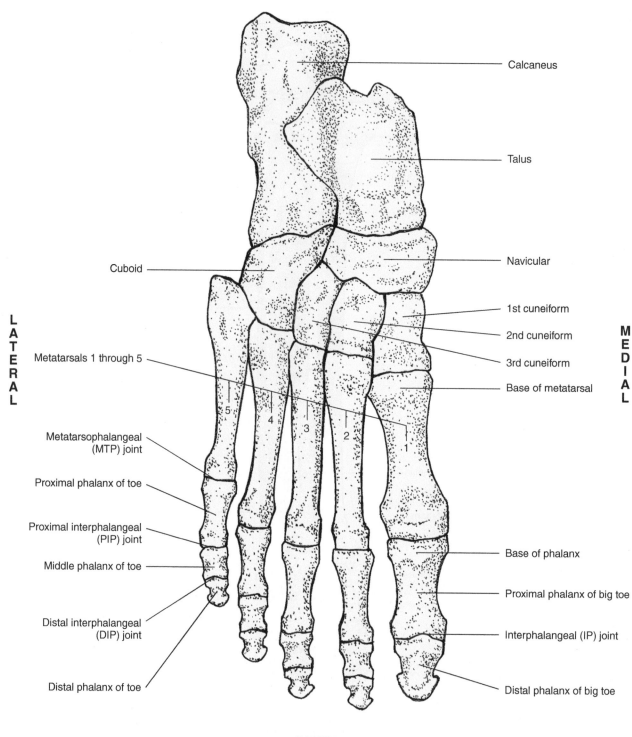

- Calcaneus
- Talus
- Navicular
- 1st cuneiform
- 2nd cuneiform
- 3rd cuneiform
- Base of metatarsal

Cuboid

Metatarsals 1 through 5

Metatarsophalangeal (MTP) joint

Proximal phalanx of toe

Proximal interphalangeal (PIP) joint

Middle phalanx of toe

Distal interphalangeal (DIP) joint

Distal phalanx of toe

- Base of phalanx
- Proximal phalanx of big toe
- Interphalangeal (IP) joint
- Distal phalanx of big toe

DISTAL

FIGURE 2-46 Dorsal view of bones and bony landmarks of the right foot.

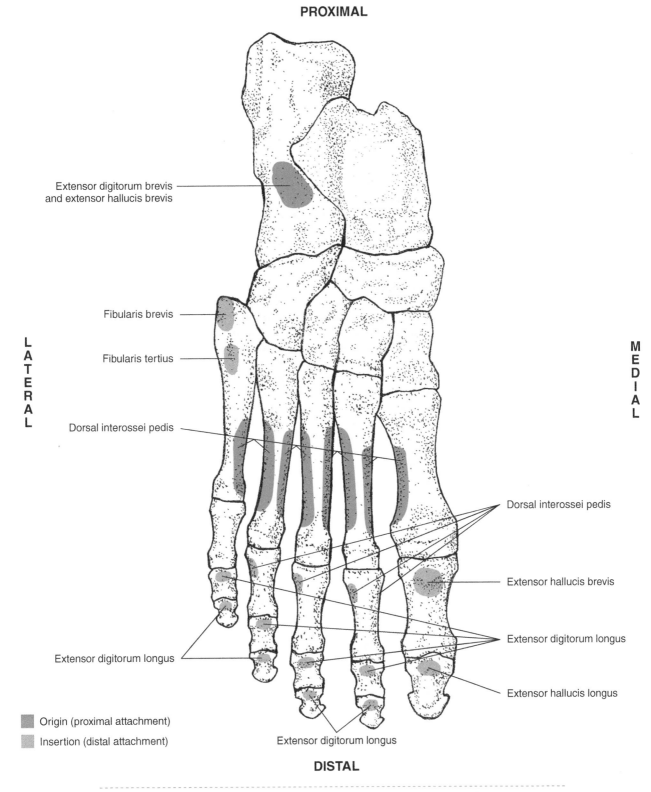

FIGURE 2-47 Dorsal view of muscle attachment sites on the right foot.

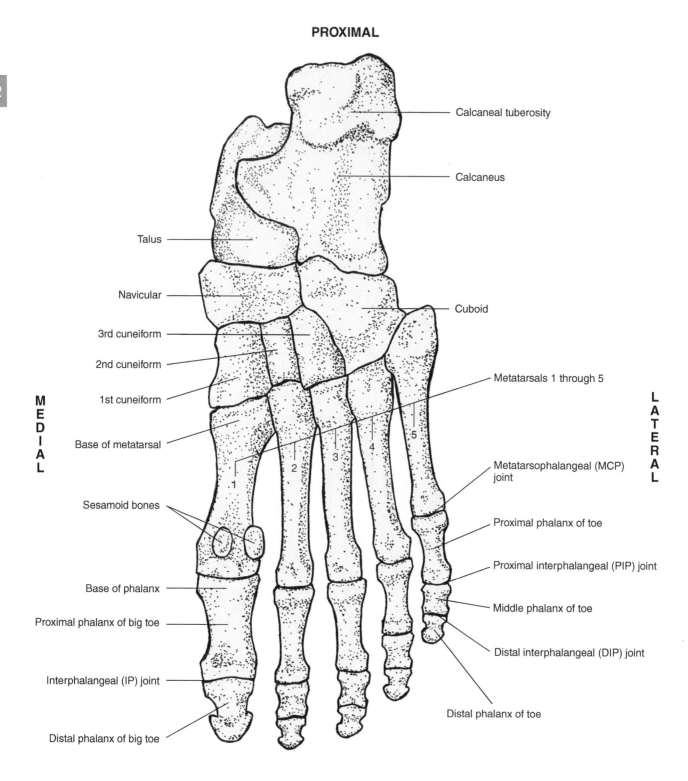

PROXIMAL

Calcaneal tuberosity

Calcaneus

Talus

Navicular

Cuboid

3rd cuneiform

2nd cuneiform

1st cuneiform

Metatarsals 1 through 5

Base of metatarsal

Metatarsophalangeal (MCP) joint

Sesamoid bones

Proximal phalanx of toe

Proximal interphalangeal (PIP) joint

Base of phalanx

Middle phalanx of toe

Proximal phalanx of big toe

Distal interphalangeal (DIP) joint

Interphalangeal (IP) joint

Distal phalanx of toe

Distal phalanx of big toe

MEDIAL

LATERAL

DISTAL

FIGURE 2-48 Plantar view of bones and bony landmarks of the right foot.

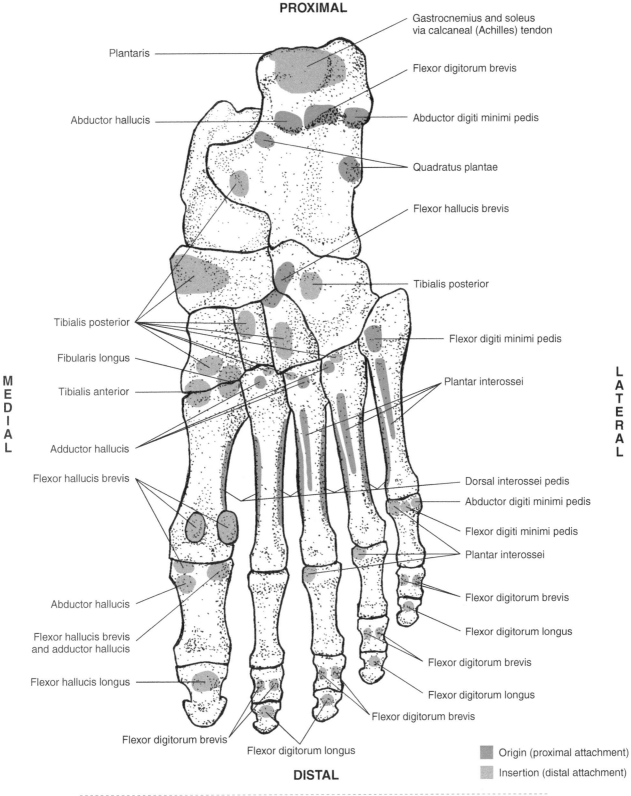

PROXIMAL

Plantaris

Abductor hallucis

Gastrocnemius and soleus
via calcaneal (Achilles) tendon

Flexor digitorum brevis

Abductor digiti minimi pedis

Quadratus plantae

Flexor hallucis brevis

Tibialis posterior

Tibialis posterior

Fibularis longus

Tibialis anterior

Flexor digiti minimi pedis

Plantar interossei

Adductor hallucis

Flexor hallucis brevis

Dorsal interossei pedis

Abductor digiti minimi pedis

Flexor digiti minimi pedis

Plantar interossei

Flexor digitorum brevis

Flexor digitorum longus

Abductor hallucis

Flexor hallucis brevis
and adductor hallucis

Flexor hallucis longus

Flexor digitorum brevis

Flexor digitorum longus

Flexor digitorum brevis

Flexor digitorum brevis

Flexor digitorum longus

**M
E
D
I
A
L**

**L
A
T
E
R
A
L**

Origin (proximal attachment)

Insertion (distal attachment)

DISTAL

FIGURE 2-49 Plantar view of muscle attachment sites on the right foot.

REVIEW QUESTIONS

Circle or fill in the correct answer for each of the following questions. More study resources are provided on the Evolve website at http://evolve.elsevier.com/Muscolino/knowthebody.

1. **What are the three major structural classifications of joints?**

   _____

   _____

   _____

2. **What are the three major functional classifications of joints?**

   _____

   _____

   _____

3. **Based on axial motion, what are the four major subdivisions of synovial joints?**

   _____

   _____

   _____

   _____

4. **Which of the following is a uniaxial joint?**
   a. Condyloid
   b. Saddle
   c. Pivot
   d. Ball-and-socket

5. **Which of the following is a biaxial joint?**
   a. Saddle
   b. Hinge
   c. Pivot
   d. Ball-and-socket

6. **Which of the following is a triaxial joint?**
   a. Saddle
   b. Condyloid
   c. Pivot
   d. Ball-and-socket

7. **If a joint is biaxial, in how many planes can motion be actively isolated?**
   a. 1
   b. 2
   c. 3
   d. 0

8. **Approximately how many bones are in the human body?**
   a. 53
   b. 145
   c. 206
   d. 312

9. **Which of the following types of joints only allows rotation motions?**
   a. Pivot
   b. Saddle
   c. Ball-and-socket
   d. Hinge

10. **Fibrous joints are generally considered to be**

    _____?
    a. Cartilaginous
    b. Synovial
    c. Synarthrotic
    d. Amphiarthrotic

How Muscles Function

MUSCLES CREATE PULLING FORCES

The essence of muscle function is that muscles create pulling forces. It is as simple as that. When a muscle contracts, it *attempts* to pull in toward its center. This action results in a pulling force being placed on its attachments. If this pulling force is sufficiently strong, the muscle will succeed in shortening and will move one or both of the body parts to which it is attached.

Realizing that this pulling force is equal on both of its attachments is also important. A muscle does not and cannot choose to pull on one of its attachments and not the other. In effect, a muscle is nothing more than a simple "pulling machine." When ordered to contract by the nervous system, it pulls on its attachments; when not ordered to contract, it relaxes and does not pull (Box 3-1).

Determining whether there is a cognate (i.e., a *similar term* in lay English) is usually extremely helpful when confronted with a new kinesiology term. This helps us understand the new kinesiology term intuitively instead of having to memorize its meaning. When it comes to the study of muscle function, the operative word is *contract* because that is what muscles do. However, in this case, it can be counterproductive to try to understand muscle contraction by relating it to how the term *contract* is defined in English. In English, the word "contract" means "to shorten." This leads many students to assume that when a muscle contracts, it shortens. This is not necessarily true, and making this assumption can limit our ability to truly grasp how the muscular system functions. In fact, most muscle contractions do not result in the muscle shortening; to examine the muscular system in this way is to overlook much of how the muscular system functions.

BOX 3-1

To call a muscle nothing more than a simple "pulling machine" does not lessen the amazing and awe-inspiring complexity of movement patterns that the muscular system produces. Any one muscle is a simple machine that pulls. However, when different aspects of various muscles are co-ordered to contract in concert with each other and in temporal sequence with one another, the sum of many "simple" pulling forces results in an amazingly fluid and complex array of movement patterns. The director of this symphony who coordinates these pulling forces is the nervous system.

WHAT IS A MUSCLE CONTRACTION?

When a muscle contracts, it *attempts* to shorten. Whether or not it succeeds in shortening is based on the strength of its contraction compared with the resistance force it encounters that opposes its shortening. For a muscle to shorten, it must move one or both of its attachments. Therefore the resistance to shortening is usually the weight of the body parts to which the muscle is attached. Let's look at the brachialis muscle that attaches from the humerus in the arm to the ulna in the forearm (Figure 3-1).

For the brachialis to contract and shorten, it must move the forearm toward the arm or move the arm toward the forearm or both. The resistance to moving the forearm is the weight of the forearm plus the weight of the hand that must move (*go along for the ride*) with the forearm. The resistance to moving the arm is the weight of the arm plus the weight of much of the upper part of the body that must move (*go along for the ride)* when the arm moves toward the forearm. Consequently, for the brachialis to contract and shorten, it must generate a force that is greater than the weight of the forearm (and hand) or the arm (and upper body). Because the forearm and hand weigh less than the arm and upper body, when the brachialis contracts and shortens, the forearm usually moves, not the arm. Thus the minimum force that the brachialis must generate if it is to contract and shorten is the weight of its lighter attachment—the forearm.

However, even if the brachialis contracts with insufficient strength to shorten, it is important to understand that it is still exerting a pulling force on its attachments. This pulling force can play an important role in musculoskeletal function. When a muscle's function is described, it is usually stated in terms of its joint actions, which are its shortening contractions. For this reason, the tendency is to focus on the shortening contraction of a muscle and overlook the importance of its contraction when it does not shorten.

Concentric Contraction

Let's first look at what happens when a muscle contracts and does shorten. A shortening contraction of a muscle is called a *concentric contraction*. The word "concentric" literally means "with center." In other words, when a concentric contraction occurs, the muscle moves toward its center. As we have said, for a muscle to contract and shorten, it must move at least one of its attachments. Let's explore the idea of concentric contraction by looking at a "typical" muscle (Figure 3-2).

A muscle attaches to two bones and, in doing so, crosses the joint that is located between them (Box 3-2). Let's call one of the attachments *A* and the other attachment *B*. When the muscle contracts, it creates

---

BOX 3-2

A typical muscle attaches to two bones and crosses the joint between them. However, some muscles have attachments to more than two bones and some muscles cross more than two joints. To help understand the underlying concept of a muscle's contraction, we will use a typical muscle that attaches to two bones and crosses one joint for our examples.

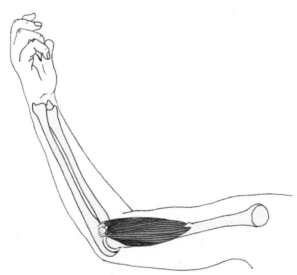

FIGURE 3-1 The brachialis muscle attaches from the humerus in the arm to the ulna in the forearm. For the brachialis to contract and shorten, it must move the forearm toward the arm or move the arm toward the forearm or both.

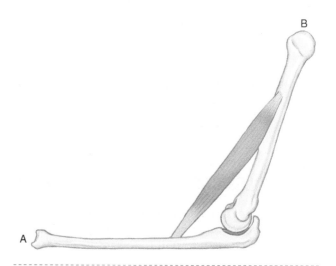

FIGURE 3-2 A "typical" muscle is shown. It attaches to bone *A* and bone *B* and crosses the joint that is located between them.

a pulling force on both bones. If this pulling force is strong enough, then a concentric contraction can occur in three possible ways: (1) the muscle can either succeed in pulling bone *A* toward bone *B*, (2) it can pull bone *B* toward bone *A*, or (3) it can pull both bones *A* and *B* toward each other (Figure 3-3). The bone that moves is described as the *mobile attachment*, and the bone that does not move is described as the *fixed attachment*. For a concentric contraction to occur, at least one of the attachments must be mobile and move. Regardless of which attachment moves, when a muscle contracts and does generate sufficient force to move one or both of its attachments, it is the mover of the joint action that is occurring and called the *mover* or *agonist*. By definition, when a mover muscle contracts, it contracts concentrically.

If we now explore concentric contraction a little further and ask which attachment will be the mobile one that does the moving, the answer will be the one that offers the least resistance to moving. That attachment will usually be the lighter attachment. When we are looking at muscles on the extremities of the body, the lighter attachment is usually the distal one. In the upper extremity, the hand is lighter than the forearm, the forearm is lighter than the arm, and the arm is lighter than the shoulder girdle/trunk. In the lower extremity, the foot is lighter than the leg, the leg is lighter than the thigh, and the thigh is lighter than the pelvis. Furthermore, as we have stated, for the more proximal attachment to move, the core of the body must usually move with it, which adds even more weight and resistance to moving. Consequently, when a muscle concentrically contracts, it usually moves its distal attachment. For this reason, when a muscle's

joint actions are learned, they are usually presented and demonstrated with the proximal attachment fixed and the distal attachment mobile. These actions are termed the *standard mover actions* of the muscle.

Reverse Actions

Although the more common and typically thought of muscle action (the standard action) is one in which the proximal attachment stays fixed and the distal attachment moves, this is not always the case. In fact, often it is not. Let's look at a concentric contraction of the brachialis muscle across the elbow joint. When the brachialis contracts, it would most likely move the distal attachment toward the proximal attachment, moving the forearm and hand toward the arm (Figure 3-4, *A*). However, if the hand holds onto an immovable object such as a pull-up bar, then because the hand is fixed, the forearm is also fixed and cannot move unless the pull-up bar is ripped off the wall. Therefore the arm will now offer less resistance to moving than the forearm, and if the brachialis contracts with sufficient force to move the arm (and the weight of the trunk that must move with it), the arm will be moved toward the forearm and the person will do a pull-up (Figure 3-4, *B*). When the proximal attachment moves toward the distal attachment instead of the distal one moving toward the proximal one, it is called a *reverse mover action*. In this scenario, therefore, flexing the forearm toward the arm at the elbow joint is the typically thought of standard action, and flexing the arm toward the forearm at the elbow joint is the reverse action. For every standard action of a muscle, a reverse action is always theoretically possible.

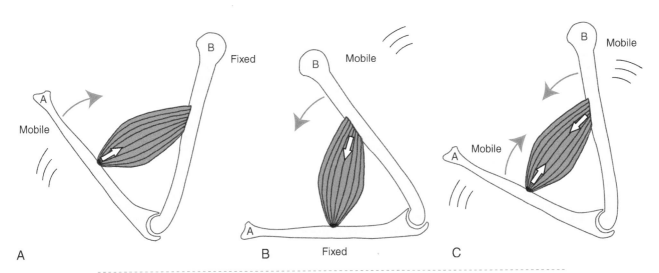

FIGURE 3-3 A muscle can concentrically contract and cause motion in one of three ways. By naming the muscle's attachments *A* and *B*, we can describe these three scenarios. **A,** Bone *A* moves toward bone *B*. **B,** Bone *B* moves toward bone *A*. **C,** Both bones *A* and *B* move toward each other.

3

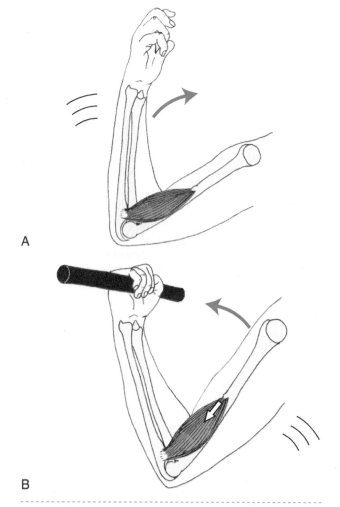

A

B

FIGURE 3-4 *A,* The standard mover action of the brachialis muscle in which the distal forearm moves toward the proximal arm. *B,* When the hand is fixed, the reverse mover action occurs; the proximal arm moves toward the distal forearm.

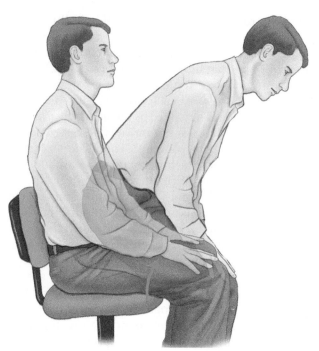

FIGURE 3-5 When we stand up from a seated position, the quadriceps femoris muscles create their reverse mover action, which is the extension of the thighs at the knee joints; in other words, extending the more proximal thighs toward the distal legs instead of extending the more distal legs toward the proximal thighs.

How often reverse actions occur varies across the body and is also based on what motions and activities are being performed. In the upper extremity, reverse actions usually occur whenever the hand is gripping an immovable object. A pull-up bar as illustrated in Figure 3-4, *B,* is one example of this. Many other examples in everyday life exist, such as using a banister when walking up the stairs, someone helping to pull you up from a seated to standing position, and a disabled person using a handicap bar.

In the lower extremity, reverse actions are extremely common because much of the time when we are standing, seated, or walking, our foot is planted on the ground. Unless we are on ice or some other slick surface, our foot is at least partially fixed and resistant to moving, resulting in our leg moving toward the foot. Similarly, with the distal end fixed, the thigh would have to move toward the leg and the pelvis would have to move toward the thigh.

An excellent example of this is when we use our quadriceps femoris muscle group to stand from a seated position (Figure 3-5). We usually think of the quadriceps femoris group as extending the leg at the knee joint. But in this case, it must perform the reverse action of extending the thigh at the knee joint. As the thighs extend at the knee joints, the rest of the body must also be lifted. If you palpate the quadriceps femoris in your anterior thighs as you stand up from a seated position, you will easily feel their contraction. In fact, it is because of this frequent activity of daily life that our quadriceps femoris group needs to be large and powerful.

In the axial body, we do not use the terms *proximal* and *distal.* Usually, standard muscle action moves the superior attachment toward the inferior one. This is because the upper axial body (head, neck, and upper trunk) is both lighter than the lower axial body (lower trunk) and because when we are sitting or standing, our lower body is more fixed and, consequently, more resistant to moving. Therefore when a muscle of the axial body moves the lower trunk toward the upper trunk, neck, and head, it is a reverse mover action. These reverse actions happen quite often when we are lying down, for example, when moving in bed, or when doing floor exercises.

When students first study muscle system function and the specific actions of muscles, it is extremely important not to develop a too rigid mindset and look only at a muscle as moving its distal (or superior) attachment when it concentrically contracts. Remember, a reverse mover action is always theoretically possible. Although some rarely occur, others occur frequently and play an integral part of everyday movement patterns and activities. In this text, when a muscle is discussed, both standard and reverse actions are presented.

NAMING A MUSCLE'S ATTACHMENTS: ORIGIN AND INSERTION VERSUS ATTACHMENTS

The classic method to name a muscle's attachments is to describe one attachment as the *origin* and the other as the *insertion*. Although the exact definitions have varied, the origin is usually defined as the more fixed attachment and the insertion as the more mobile attachment. Because the proximal attachment is usually the more fixed attachment and the distal attachment is usually the more mobile attachment, some medical dictionaries even define the origin as the more proximal attachment and the insertion as the more distal attachment.

In recent years, the use of the terms *origin* and *insertion* has been decreasing in favor. Perhaps the reason is that teaching students who are first learning muscles that one attachment of the muscle is usually fixed tends to promote the idea that it is always fixed. This belief can lead to less flexibility in how the students view muscular function because they tend to ignore the reverse actions of muscles wherein the insertion stays fixed and the origin moves. Given how often these reverse actions actually occur can handicap the student as he or she begins to use and apply muscle knowledge clinically with clients.

For these reasons, naming a muscle's attachments by simply describing their locations is gaining favor. After all, if the origin can also be defined as the proximal attachment and the insertion can also be defined as the distal attachment, why not skip use of the terms *origin* and *insertion* entirely and simply learn the names of the attachments as *proximal* and *distal*? Or, if the muscle is running superiorly and inferiorly or medially and laterally, simply naming the attachments using these locational terms is not only simpler, but it also has the advantage of pointing out to the student the fiber direction of the muscle. This helps the student see the muscle's line of pull, which is the most crucial step in figuring out its actions.

At present, both naming systems are used in the field of kinesiology, therefore being comfortable and conversant with both is important. For this reason, this text uses both origin/insertion (O and I) terminology and attachment terminology. Most importantly,

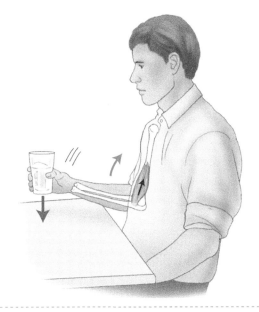

FIGURE 3-6 The right brachialis muscle eccentrically contracts to slow gravity's force of extension of the forearm at the elbow joint, allowing the glass to be safely lowered to the table top.

the student must learn that a muscle has two attachments; either one can potentially move, and what determines which one actually does move in any particular scenario depends on its relative resistance to being moved.

ECCENTRIC CONTRACTIONS

We have already discussed concentric contractions. They occur when a muscle contracts with a force that is greater than an attachment's resistance force to moving. Therefore the muscle moves the attachment and succeeds in shortening. As previously stated, a muscle does not always succeed in shortening when it contracts.

If a muscle contracts, attempting to pull in toward its center, but the resistance force is greater than the muscle's contraction force, not only will the muscle not succeed in shortening, but the muscle's attachment will actually be pulled farther away from the center of the muscle. A lengthening of the muscle as it contracts will be the result. A lengthening contraction is defined as an *eccentric contraction*.

Eccentric contractions happen most often when a muscle is working against gravity. For example, if I am holding an object and want to lower it down to a tabletop, I can let gravity bring my forearm and hand down. However, if the object is fragile, I need to lower it slowly so that it does not crash down onto the table and break. This requires me to contract musculature that opposes gravity so that the object can be lowered slowly and safely (Figure 3-6). In this example, the purpose of the muscle contraction is not to beat gravity and raise the object; rather, its purpose is to lose to gravity but to do so slowly so that the effect of the force of gravity is slowed and the object is lowered slowly. Therefore the purpose of an eccentric contraction is to slow or restrain a joint action that is caused by another force, usually gravity. Because the muscle that eccentrically contracts opposes the joint action movement that is occurring, it is called the *antagonist*. By definition, when an antagonist muscle contracts, it contracts eccentrically (Box 3-3).

> Note: Eccentric contractions are sometimes referred to as negative contractions.

ISOMETRIC CONTRACTIONS

A concentric contraction occurs when the force of the muscle's contraction is greater than the resistance force; an eccentric contraction occurs when the force

---

BOX 3-3

By definition, when a mover muscle contracts and shortens, it contracts concentrically; and when an antagonist muscle contracts and lengthens, it contracts eccentrically. This does not mean that every muscle that is shortening is concentrically contracting or that every muscle that is lengthening is eccentrically contracting. A muscle can be relaxed as it shortens or lengthens.

---

of the muscle's contraction is less than the resistance force. An isometric contraction occurs when the force of the muscle's contraction is equal to the resistance force. Because the two forces are equal, the muscle is neither able to win and shorten nor lose and lengthen. Instead, it stays the same length as it contracts. This is defined as an *isometric contraction*. In fact, the term *isometric* literally means *same length*. If the muscle stays the same length, then its attachments do not move. The function of an isometrically contracting muscle can be critically important because it fixes or, in other words, stabilizes its bony attachment (Figure 3-7).

ROLES OF MUSCLES

As we have seen, muscle function can be viewed very simply: muscles contract and create pulling forces. However, muscles can contract concentrically and shorten as movers, contract eccentrically and lengthen as antagonists, or contract isometrically and stay the same length as stabilizers. All too often, students who first learn muscle function focus only on the muscle's standard mover concentric contractions. For a deeper understanding of muscle function, we need to understand and appreciate all types of contractions and all roles that a muscle can play in our movement patterns. Only this deeper understanding will allow for the critical thinking necessary for clinical application when it comes to the assessment and treatment of clients.

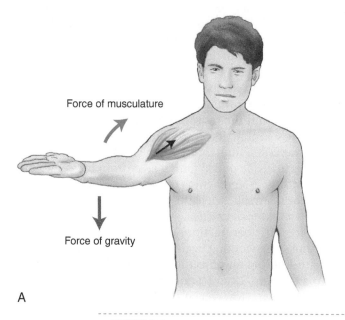

Force of musculature

Force of gravity

A

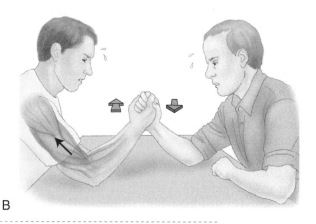

B

FIGURE 3-7 ***A,*** The person's deltoid muscle isometrically contracts with a force that is equal to the force of gravity so that the person's arm does not move. ***B,*** The musculature of the person arm wrestling is isometrically contracting because the resistance force from the opponent is exactly equal to the muscle's contraction force. Therefore no movement occurs.

SLIDING FILAMENT MECHANISM

To truly understand the bigger picture of concentric, eccentric, and isometric contractions, examining the actual mechanism that defines muscle contraction is helpful. This mechanism occurs on a microscopic level and is known as the *sliding filament mechanism.*

A muscle is made up of thousands of *muscle cells,* also known as *muscle fibers.* Within a muscle, these fibers are bundled together into groups called *fascicles.* A muscle also contains numerous layers of fibrous fascia that are identical to each other in structure but are given different names based on their location. *Endomysium* (plural: endomysia) surrounds each individual muscle fiber; *perimysium* (plural: perimysia) surrounds each fascicle; and *epimysium* surrounds the entire muscle (Figure 3-8). The endomysia, perimysia, and epimysium continue beyond each end of the muscle to create the fibrous tissue attachment of the muscle onto the bone. If this attachment is cordlike in shape,

it is called a *tendon.* If it is broad and flat, it is called an *aponeurosis.* The major purpose of the tendon/aponeurosis is to transmit the pulling force of the muscle belly to its bony attachment (Box 3-4).

If we look more closely at an individual muscle fiber, we see that it is filled with structures called *myofibrils.* Myofibrils run longitudinally within the muscle fiber and are composed of filaments (see Figure 3-8). These filaments are arranged into structures called *sarcomeres.* The term *sarcomere* literally means "unit of muscle." To truly understand how a muscle functions, understanding how a sarcomere functions is necessary.

> **BOX 3-4**
>
> Additional layers of fibrous fascia also envelop and surround groups of muscles within a region of the body. These layers are often called *intermuscular septa.*

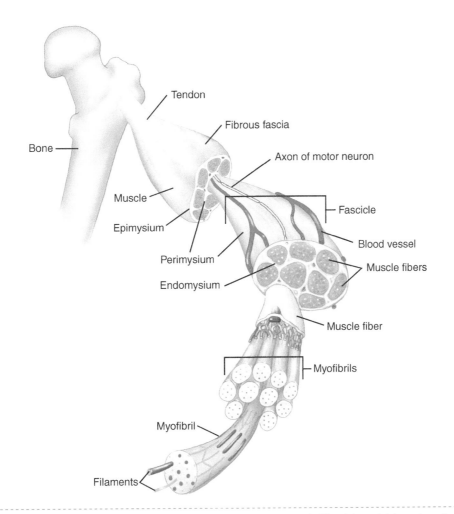

FIGURE 3-8 Cross sections of a muscle. A muscle is composed of fascicles, which are bundles of fibers. The fibers themselves are filled with myofibrils, which are composed of filaments. Fibrous fascial sheaths called endomysia, perimysia, and epimysium surround the fibers, fascicles, and entire muscle, respectively.

3

Sarcomeres are composed of thin and thick filaments. The thin filaments are *actin* and are arranged on both sides of the sarcomere and attach to the *Z-lines*, which are the borders of the sarcomere. The thick filament is a *myosin* filament and is located in the center and contains projections called heads. When a stimulus from the nervous system is sent to the muscle, binding sites on the actin filaments become exposed and the myosin heads attach onto them, creating *cross-bridges.* The myosin heads then attempt to bend in toward the center of the sarcomere, creating a pulling force on the actin filaments. If the pulling force is sufficiently strong, the actin filaments will be pulled in toward the center of the sarcomere, sliding along the myosin filament, hence the name *sliding filament mechanism.* This will cause the Z-lines to be pulled in toward the center and the sarcomere will shorten (Figure 3-9).

Whatever happens to one sarcomere happens to all the sarcomeres of all the myofibrils of the muscle fiber. If we extrapolate this concept, we see that if all the sarcomeres of a myofibril shorten, then the myofibril itself will shorten. If all the myofibrils of a muscle fiber shorten, then the muscle fiber will shorten. If

enough muscle fibers shorten, then the muscle itself will shorten, pulling one or both of its attachments in toward the center, causing motion of the body. This is how a concentric contraction occurs.

When a muscle's contraction is said to create a pulling force toward its center, that pulling force is the sum of the bending forces of all the myosin heads. If the sum of these forces is greater than the resistance to shortening, then the actin filaments will be pulled in toward the center of the sarcomere and a concentric contraction occurs. If the sum of these forces is less than the resistance to shortening, then the actin filaments will be pulled away from the center of the sarcomere and an eccentric contraction occurs. If the sum of the forces of the myosin heads is equal to the resistance force, then the actin filaments will not move and an isometric contraction occurs. Therefore the definition of muscle contraction is having myosin heads creating cross-bridges and pulling on actin filaments.

MUSCLE FIBER ARCHITECTURE

Not all muscles have their fibers arranged in the same manner. There are two major architectural types of muscle fiber arrangement: (1) longitudinal and (2) pennate. A longitudinal muscle has its fibers running along the length of the muscle. A pennate muscle has its fibers running obliquely to the length of the muscle. The major types of longitudinal muscles are demonstrated in Figure 3-10. The major types of pennate muscles are demonstrated in Figure 3-11.

LEARNING MUSCLES

- Essentially, when learning about muscles, two major aspects must be learned: (1) the attachments of the muscle and (2) the actions of the muscle.
- Generally speaking, the attachments of a muscle must be memorized. However, times exist when clues are given about the attachments of a muscle by the muscle's name.
  - For example, the name *coracobrachialis* tells us that the coracobrachialis muscle has one attachment on the coracoid process of the scapula and the other attachment on the brachium (i.e., the humerus).
  - Similarly, the name *zygomaticus major* tells us that this muscle attaches onto the zygomatic bone (and is bigger than another muscle called the *zygomaticus minor*).
- Unlike muscle attachments, muscle actions do not have to be memorized. Instead, by understanding the simple concept that a muscle pulls at its attachments to move a body part, the action or actions of a muscle can be reasoned out.

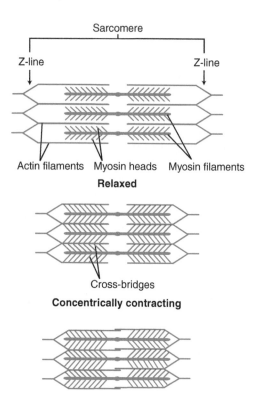

Relaxed

Concentrically contracting

Fully concentrically contracted

FIGURE 3-9 A sarcomere is composed of actin and myosin filaments. When the nervous system orders a muscle fiber to contract, myosin heads attach to actin filaments, attempting to pull them in toward the center of the sarcomere. If the pulling force is strong enough, the actin filaments will move and the sarcomere will shorten.

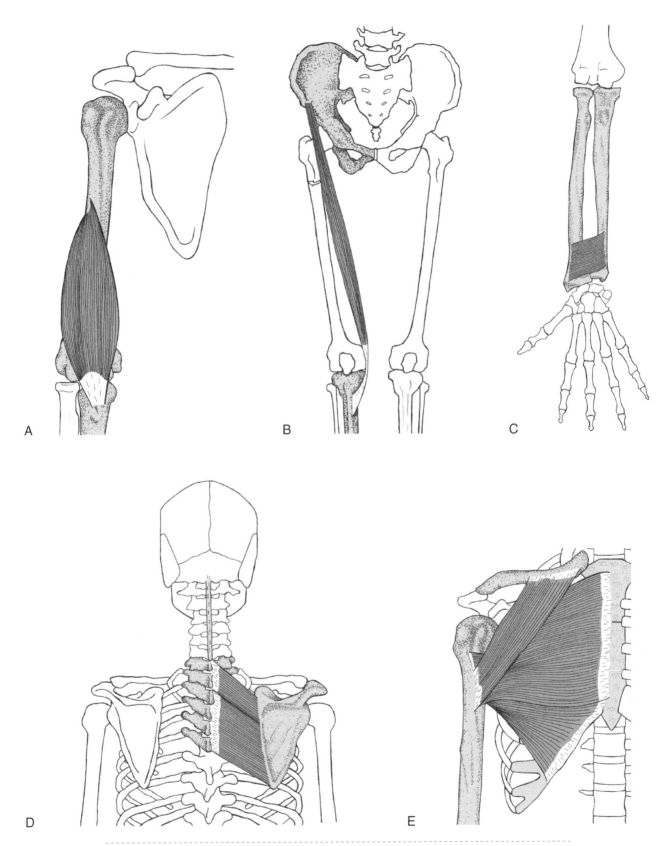

FIGURE 3-10 Various architectural types of longitudinal muscles. **A,** Brachialis demonstrates a fusiform-shaped (also known as spindle-shaped) muscle. **B,** Sartorius demonstrates a strap muscle. **C,** Pronator quadratus demonstrates a rectangular-shaped muscle. **D,** Rhomboid muscles demonstrate rhomboidal-shaped muscles. **E,** Pectoralis major demonstrates a triangular-shaped (also known as fan-shaped) muscle.

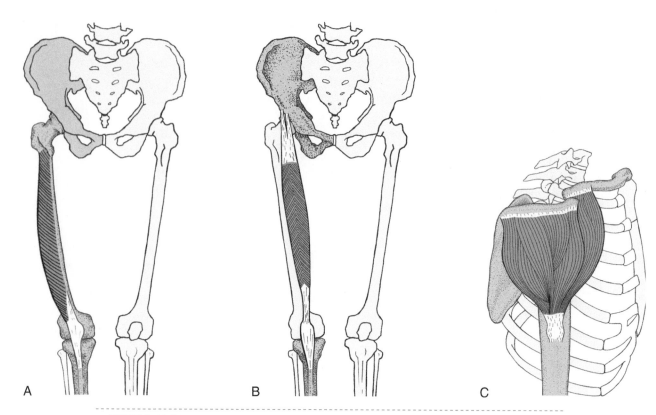

FIGURE 3-11 The three architectural types of pennate muscles. **A,** Vastus lateralis is a unipennate muscle. (Note: Central tendon is not visible in the anterior view.) **B,** Rectus femoris is a bipennate muscle. **C,** Deltoid is a multipennate muscle.

Five-Step Approach to Learning Muscles

When first confronted with having to study and learn about a muscle, the following five-step approach is recommended:

- Step 1: Look at the name of the muscle to see whether it gives you any "free information" that saves you from having to memorize attachments or actions of the muscle.
- Step 2: Learn the general location of the muscle well enough to be able to visualize the muscle on the body. At this point, you need only know it well enough to know the following:
  - What joint it crosses
  - Where it crosses the joint (e.g., anteriorly, medially)
  - How it crosses the joint (i.e., the direction in which its fibers are running—vertically or horizontally)
- Step 3: Use this general knowledge of the muscle's location (Step 2) to figure out the actions of the muscle.
- Step 4: Go back and learn (memorize, if necessary) the specific attachments of the muscle.

- Step 5: Now examine the relationship of this muscle to other muscles (and other soft-tissue structures) of the body. Look at the following:
  - Is this muscle superficial or deep?
  - What other muscles (and other soft tissue structures) are located near this muscle?

Figuring Out a Muscle's Actions (Step 3 in Detail)

- Once you have a general familiarity with a muscle's location on the body, it is time to begin the process of reasoning out the actions of the muscle. The most important thing that you must look at is the following:
  - The direction of the muscle fibers relative to the joint that it crosses
- By doing this, you can see the following:
  - The line of pull of the muscle relative to the joint
- This line of pull determines the actions of the muscle (i.e., how the contraction of the muscle causes the body parts to move at that joint).
- The best approach is to ask the following three questions:
  1. What joint does the muscle cross?
  2. Where does the muscle cross the joint?
  3. How does the muscle cross the joint?

3

Question 1—What Joint Does the Muscle Cross?

■ The first question to ask and answer in figuring out the action(s) of a muscle is to simply know what joint it crosses.
■ The following rule applies: If a muscle crosses a joint, it can have an action at that joint. (Note: *This, of course, assumes that the joint is healthy and allows movement to occur.*)
■ For example, if we look at the coracobrachialis (see Figure 6-26), knowing that it crosses the shoulder (glenohumeral [GH]) joint tells us that it must have an action at the GH joint.
■ We may not know what the exact action of the coracobrachialis is yet, but at least we now know at what joint it has its actions.
■ To figure out exactly what these actions are, we need to look at questions 2 and 3.

> Note: It is worth pointing out that the converse of the rule about a muscle having the ability to create movement (i.e., an action) at a joint that it crosses is also generally true. In other words, if a muscle does not cross a joint, it cannot have an action at that joint. (Exceptions to this rule exist.)

Questions 2 and 3—Where Does the Muscle Cross the Joint? How Does the Muscle Cross the Joint?

■ The above two questions must be examined together.
■ The *where* of a muscle crossing a joint is whether it crosses the joint anteriorly, posteriorly, medially, or laterally.
■ Placing a muscle into one of these broad groups is helpful because the following general rules apply:
  ■ Muscles that cross a joint anteriorly will usually flex a body part at that joint, and muscles that cross a joint posteriorly will usually extend a body part at that joint.
  ■ Muscles that cross a joint laterally will usually abduct or laterally flex a body part at that joint, and muscles that cross a joint medially will usually adduct a body part at that joint.
■ The *how* of a muscle crossing a joint is whether it crosses the joint with its fibers running vertically or horizontally, which is also important.
■ To illustrate this idea, we will look at the pectoralis major muscle (see Figure 6-12). The pectoralis major has two parts: (1) clavicular head and (2) sternocostal head. The *where* of these two heads of the pectoralis major crossing the GH joint is the same (i.e., they both cross the GH joint anteriorly). However, the *how* of these two heads crossing the GH joint is very different. The clavicular head crosses the GH joint with its fibers running primarily vertically; therefore it flexes the arm at the GH joint because it pulls the arm upward in the sagittal plane, which is termed *flexion*. However, the sternocostal head crosses the GH joint with its fibers running horizontally; therefore it adducts the arm at the GH joint because it pulls the arm from lateral to medial in the frontal plane, which is termed *adduction*.
■ With a muscle that has a horizontal direction to its fibers, another factor must be considered when looking at *how* this muscle crosses the joint; that is, whether the muscle attaches to the first place on the bone that it reaches or whether the muscle wraps around the bone before attaching to it. Muscles that run horizontally (in the transverse plane) and wrap around the bone before attaching to it create a rotation action when they contract and pull on the attachment.
■ For example, the sternocostal head of the pectoralis major does not attach to the first point on the humerus that it reaches. Rather, it continues to wrap around the shaft of the humerus to attach onto the lateral lip of the bicipital groove of the humerus. When the sternocostal head pulls, it medially rotates the arm at the GH joint (in addition to its other actions).
■ In essence, by asking the three questions of Step 3 of the five-step approach to learning muscles (What joint does a muscle cross? Where does the muscle cross the joint? How does the muscle cross the joint?), we are trying to determine the direction of the muscle fibers relative to the joint. Determining this will reveal the line of pull of the muscle, relative to the joint; that will give us the actions of the muscle—saving us the trouble of having to memorize this information!

Functional Group Approach to Learning Muscles

Once the five-step approach to learning muscles has been used a few times and learned, it is extremely helpful to begin to transition to the functional group approach to learning muscles. This approach places emphasis on seeing that muscles can be placed into a functional group, based on their common joint action. For example, if the biceps brachii has been studied and it is seen that it crosses the elbow joint anteriorly and flexes it, then it is easier to see and learn that the brachialis also flexes the elbow joint because it also crosses it anteriorly. In fact, all muscles that cross the elbow joint anteriorly belong to the functional group of elbow joint flexors. Similarly, all muscles that cross the elbow joint posteriorly belong to the functional group of elbow joint extensors.

Applying the functional group approach to the GH joint, it is seen that all muscles that cross it anteriorly with a vertical fiber direction (or at least a vertical component to their fiber direction) flex it. All muscles that cross it posteriorly with a vertical fiber direction extend it. All muscles that cross it laterally, abduct it; and all muscles that cross it medially adduct it. Functional groups of medial and lateral rotators are not as segregated location-wise; but, with closer inspection, it is seen that all medial rotators of the GH joint wrap in the same direction and all lateral rotators wrap in the other direction.

Visual and Kinesthetic Exercise for Learning a Muscle's Actions

Rubber Band Exercise

An excellent method for learning the actions of a muscle is to place a large, colorful rubber band (or large, colorful shoelace or string) on your body or on the body of a partner in the same place that the muscle you are studying is located.

- Hold one end of the rubber band at one of the attachment sites of the muscle, and hold the other end of the rubber band at the other attachment site of the muscle.
- Make sure that you have the rubber band running or oriented in the same direction as the direction of the fibers of the muscle. If it is not uncomfortable, you may even loop or tie the rubber band (or shoelace) around the body parts that are the attachments of the muscle.
- Once you have the rubber band in place, pull one of the ends of the rubber band toward the other attachment of the rubber band to observe the action that the rubber band/muscle has on that body part's attachment. Once done, return the attachment of the rubber band to where it began and repeat this exercise for the other end of the rubber band to see the action that the rubber band/muscle has on the other attachment of the muscle (Box 3-5).
- By placing the rubber band on your body or on your partner's body, you are simulating the direction of the muscle's fibers relative to the joint that it crosses.
- By pulling either end of the rubber band toward the center, you are simulating the line of pull of the muscle relative to the joint that it crosses. The resultant movements that occur are the mover actions that the muscle would have. This

BOX 3-5

When performing the rubber band exercise, it is extremely important that the attachment of the rubber band that you are pulling on is pulled exactly toward the other attachment and in no other direction. In other words, your line of pull should be exactly the same as the line of pull of the muscle (which is essentially determined by the direction of the fibers of the muscle). When performing the rubber band exercise, the attachment of the muscle that you are pulling on would be the mobile attachment in that scenario; the end that you do not move is the fixed attachment in that scenario. Further, by doing this exercise twice (i.e., by then repeating it by reversing which attachment you hold fixed and which one you pull on and move), you are simulating the standard mover action and the reverse mover action of the muscle.

is an excellent exercise both to see the actions of a muscle and to kinesthetically experience the actions of a muscle.

- This exercise can be used to learn all muscle actions and can be especially helpful for determining actions that may be a little more difficult to visualize, such as rotation actions.

Note: The use of a large, colorful rubber band is more helpful than a shoelace or string because when you stretch out a rubber band and place it in the location where a muscle would be, the natural elasticity of a rubber band creates a pull on the attachment sites that nicely simulates the pull of a muscle on its attachments when it contracts.

- If you can, you should work with a partner to perform this exercise. Have your partner hold one of the "attachments" of the rubber band while you hold the other "attachment." This leaves one of your hands free to pull the rubber band attachment sites (one at a time) toward the center.

Note of caution: If you are using a rubber band, be careful that you do not accidentally let go and have the rubber band hit you or your partner. For this reason, it would be preferable to use a shoelace or string instead of a rubber band when working near the face.

REVIEW QUESTIONS

Circle or fill in the correct answer for each of the following questions. More study resources are provided on the Evolve website at http://evolve.elsevier.com/Muscolino/knowthebody.

1. **What are the two types of filaments in a myofibril?**

   _____

   _____

2. **What are the three major fascial coverings of muscle tissue?**

   _____

   _____

   _____

3. **What three questions should be asked when trying to figure out the action(s) of a muscle?**

   _____

   _____

   _____

4. **Which of the following best describes the essence of muscle function?**
   a. Muscles shorten.
   b. Muscles move bones.
   c. Muscles stabilize.
   d. Muscles create pulling forces.

5. **What kind of contraction occurs when a muscle contracts and the attachments of the muscle move closer together?**
   a. Isometric
   b. Concentric
   c. Eccentric
   d. None of the above

6. **What kind of contraction occurs when a muscle contracts and the attachments of the muscle move farther apart?**
   a. Shortening
   b. Concentric
   c. Eccentric
   d. Isometric

7. **What body part can move when the elbow joint flexes?**
   a. Forearm
   b. Arm
   c. Choices a and b
   d. None of the above

8. **Which of the following terms best describes extension of the thigh at the knee joint?**
   a. Eccentric contraction
   b. Reverse action
   c. Negative contraction
   d. Standard action

9. **What type of muscle contraction tends to occur when gravity is the mover force?**
   a. Concentric
   b. Eccentric
   c. Shortening
   d. Isometric

10. **Which of the following is true regarding the origin of a muscle?**
    a. It is distal.
    b. It always stays fixed.
    c. It always moves.
    d. It can move toward the insertion.

3

How to Palpate

This chapter explains the science and art of palpation. In other words, it explains how to palpate. After an introduction to palpation, 20 guidelines of muscle palpation are discussed. The two most basic guidelines described as the *science of muscle palpation* are (1) know the attachments and (2) know the actions of the target muscle being palpated. The additional 18 guidelines describe how to begin and perfect the *art of muscle palpation*. In all, these guidelines can help increase palpatory literacy of the muscles of the body. Before beginning the muscle palpation protocols presented in Chapters 6 through 11, reading this chapter in its entirety is recommended.

Video segments showing how to palpate individual muscles are located on Evolve at http://evolve.elsevier.com/muscolino/knowthebody.

WHAT IS PALPATION?

Palpation may be defined in many ways. The word *palpation*, itself, derives from the Latin *palpatio*, which means "to touch." However, defining palpation as simply touching is too simplistic because more is involved. Inherent in the term *palpation* is not just touching but also the act of sensing or perceiving what is being touched. In this context, palpation involves more than just the fingers and hands. Palpation also involves the mind. Successful palpation requires us to feel with our brains, as well as with our fingers. When palpating, the therapist should be focused with a mindful intent; in other words, the therapist must be in his or her hands. All of the therapist's correlated knowledge of anatomy must be integrated into the sensations that the therapist's fingers are picking up from the client's body and sending to his or her brain. The therapist's mind must be open to the sensations that are coming in from the client, yet, at the same time, interpret these sensations with an informed mind (Figure 4-1). Incorporating mindful intent into examination and treatment sessions creates mindful touch.

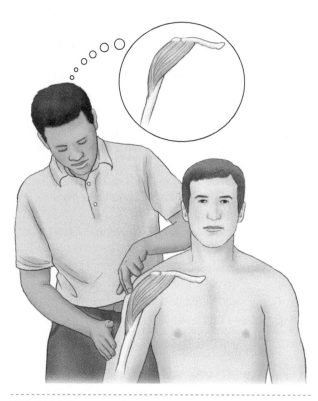

FIGURE 4-1 Palpation is as much an act of the mind as it is of the palpating fingers. Sensory stimuli entering through the therapist's hands must be correlated with a knowledge base of anatomy.

OBJECTIVES OF PALPATION: LOCATION AND ASSESSMENT

There are two main objectives when palpating. Objective 1 is locating the target structure. Objective 2 is assessing the target structure.

The first objective, and indeed perhaps the major objective of the novice therapist, is to locate the target structure being palpated. This feat is not easy to achieve. It is one thing to simply touch the tissues of the client. It is an entirely different matter to be able to touch the tissues and discern the target structure from all the adjacent tissues. This ability requires the therapist to locate all borders of the structure—superiorly, inferiorly, medially, laterally, and even superficially and deep. If the structure is immediately superficial to the skin, then this feat may not be very difficult. Indeed, the olecranon process of the ulna or a well-developed deltoid muscle may be visually obvious and located without even touching the client's body. However, if the target structure is deeper in the client's body, then locating the structure may present a great challenge.

As basic as palpation for the purpose of determining location may seem, it is a supremely important first objective because it follows that if a structure cannot be accurately located and discerned from adjacent tissues, then it cannot be accurately assessed. Once the target structure is located, then the process of assessment can begin. Assessment requires the interpretation of the sensations that the palpating fingers pick up from the target structure. It involves becoming aware of the qualities of the target structure—its size, shape, and other characteristics. Is it soft? Is it swollen? Is it tense or hard? All of these factors must be considered when assessing the health of the target structure.

It is worthy of note that as high-tech diagnostic and assessment equipment continues to be developed in Western medicine, palpating hands remain the primary assessment tool of a manual therapist. Indeed, for a manual therapist, palpation—the act of gathering information through touch—lies at the very heart of assessment. Armed with both an accurate location and an accurate assessment of the health of the target structure through careful palpation, the therapist can develop an effective treatment plan that can be confidently carried out.

Note: As crucial as palpation is to assessment, it is still only one piece of a successful assessment picture. Visual observation, history, findings from specific orthopedic assessment procedures, and the client's response to treatment approaches must also be considered when developing an accurate client assessment.

WHEN DO WE PALPATE?

Always. Whenever we are contacting the client, we should be palpating. This is true not only during the assessment phase of the session but also during the treatment phase. Too many therapists view palpation and treatment as separate entities that are compartmentalized within a session. A therapist often spends the first part of the session palpating and gathering sensory input for the sake of assessment and evaluation. Using the information gathered during this palpation assessment stage, a treatment plan is determined and the therapist then spends the rest of the session implementing the treatment plan by outputting pressure into the client's tissues. Rigidly seen in this manner, palpation and treatment might each be viewed as a one-way street: palpation is *sensory information in* from the client, and treatment is *motor pressure out* to the client. The problem with this view is that we can also glean valuable assessment information while we are treating.

Treatment should be a two-way street that involves not simply motor pressure out to the tissues of the client but also continued sensory information in from the tissues of the client's body (Figure 4-2). While we are exerting pressure on the client's tissue, we are also

sensing the quality of the tissue and its response to our pressure. This new information might guide us to alter or fine-tune our treatment for the client. Thus while we work, we continue to assess, gathering information that guides the pace, depth, or direction of the next strokes. Ideally, no stroke should be carried out in a cookbook manner, performed as if on autopilot. Treatment is a dynamic process. How the middle and end of each stroke are performed should be determined from the response of the client to that stroke as we perform it. This is the essence of mindful touch, having a fluid interplay between assessment and treatment; assessment informs treatment and treatment informs assessment, creating optimal therapeutic care for the client.

HOW TO LEARN PALPATION

A long-standing exercise to learn palpation is to take a hair and place it under a page of a textbook without seeing where you placed it. With your eyes closed, palpate for the hair until you find it and can trace its shape under the page. Once found, now replace the hair, this time under two pages, and palpate to locate and trace it. Continue to increase the number of pages placed over the hair until you cannot find it. If this exercise is repeated, the number of pages under which you can locate and trace the hair will gradually increase, and your sensitivity will improve.

Even more important than performing palpation exercises with textbooks, applying palpation directly to the client is imperative. When your hands are on your fellow students in school or on your clients if you are in professional practice, constantly try to feel for the structures about which you have learned in your anatomy, physiology, and kinesiology classes. As your hands are moving on the client's skin, close your eyes so that you block out extraneous sensory stimuli and try to picture all the subcutaneous structures over which your hands are passing. The better you can picture an underlying structure, the better you will be able to feel it with your palpating hands and with your mind. Once felt, you can focus on locating its precise location and assessing its tissue quality.

Given that the foundation of all manual skills rests on our palpatory ability to read the clues and signs that a client's body offers, the better we hone this skill, the greater palpatory literacy we gain. Perfecting our palpatory literacy is a work in progress—an endless journey. The more we polish and perfect this skill, the greater our therapeutic potential becomes, bringing greater benefit to our clients. However, written chapters can only provide guidelines and a framework for how to palpate. Ultimately, palpation is a kinesthetic skill and,

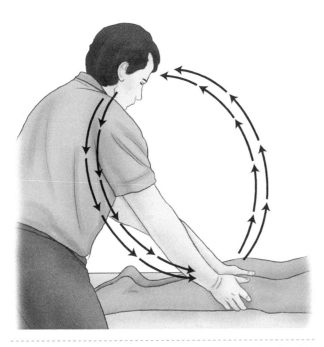

FIGURE 4-2 This figure illustrates the idea that palpation should be done whenever the therapist contacts the client, even when administering treatment strokes. As motor pressure is applied to the client's tissues, the hands should be picking up all palpatory sensory signals that help with assessment at the same time.

as such, can only be learned by kinesthetic means. In other words, "palpation cannot be learned by reading or listening; it can only be learned by palpation."*

PALPATION GUIDELINES

The following 20 guidelines are provided for successful muscle palpation. The first two guidelines make up the science of muscle palpation. The remaining guidelines begin and perfect the art of muscle palpation.

The Science of Muscle Palpation

Guideline 1: Know the Attachments of the Target Muscle

When a target muscle is superficial, it is usually not difficult to palpate. If we know where it is located, we can simply place our hands there and feel for it. Unless a great deal of subcutaneous fat is in that region of the body, apart from the client's skin, we will be directly on the muscle. Therefore the first step of muscle palpation

*Frymann VM: Palpation, its study in the workshop, *AAO Yearbook*, 16-31:1963.

is to know the attachments of the target muscle. For example, if we know that the deltoid is attached to the lateral clavicle, acromion process, spine of the scapula, and deltoid tuberosity of the humerus, then we need simply to place our palpating hand there to feel it (Figure 4-3).

Guideline 2: Know the Actions of the Target Muscle

Sometimes, even if a target muscle is superficial, it can be difficult to discern the borders of the muscle. If the target muscle is deep to another muscle, it can be that much harder to palpate and discern from more superficial and other nearby muscles. To better discern the target muscle from all adjacent musculature and other soft tissues, asking the client to contract the target muscle by performing one or more of its actions is helpful. If the target muscle contracts, it will become palpably harder. Assuming that all the adjacent muscles stay relaxed and therefore palpably soft, the difference in tissue texture between the hard target muscle and the soft adjacent muscles will be clear. This difference will allow an accurate determination of the location of the target muscle. Therefore the second step of muscle palpation is to know the actions of the target muscle (Figure 4-4).

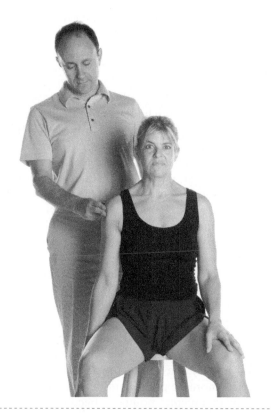

FIGURE 4-3 The deltoid is a superficial muscle and can be palpated by simply placing our palpating hand on the muscle between its attachments. Therefore knowing the attachments of the target muscle is the first necessary step when looking to palpate it.

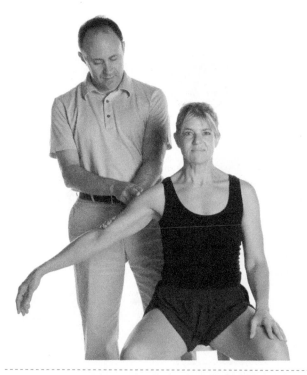

FIGURE 4-4 The precise location of the deltoid is more easily palpated if the deltoid is contracted. In this figure, the client is asked to abduct the arm at the shoulder against the force of gravity. When a muscle contracts, it becomes palpably harder and is easier to distinguish from the adjacent soft tissues. Therefore knowing the actions of the target muscle is the second necessary step when looking to palpate a muscle.

Guidelines 1 and 2 of muscle palpation involve knowing the "science" of the target muscle; in other words, knowing the attachments and actions of the muscle that were learned when the muscles of the body were first learned. Armed with this knowledge, the majority of muscle palpations can be *reasoned out* instead of memorized. Using the attachments and actions to palpate a target muscle can be thought of as the science of muscle palpation.

Beginning the Art of Muscle Palpation

Guideline 3: Choose the Best Action of the Target Muscle to Make it Contract

Applying knowledge of the attachments and actions of a target muscle to palpate it is a solid foundation for palpatory literacy. However, effective palpation requires not only that the target muscle contracts, but it also requires that an isolated contraction of the target muscle occurs. This means that the target muscle needs to be the only muscle that contracts, and all muscles near the target muscle must remain relaxed. Unfortunately, because adjacent muscles often share the same joint action with the target muscle, simply placing our hands on the location of the target muscle and then choosing any one of the target muscle's actions to contract it is usually not enough. If the action chosen is shared with an adjacent muscle, then the adjacent muscle will also contract, making it very difficult to discern the target muscle from it.

For this reason, knowing which joint action to ask the client to perform requires the therapist to be creative and to think critically. This knowledge is where the art of muscle palpation begins. It requires knowledge of not only of the actions of the target muscle, but also the actions of all adjacent muscles. With this knowledge, the client can be asked to perform the best joint action for the palpation of the target muscle.

For example, if the flexor carpi radialis of the wrist flexor group is the target muscle, then asking the client to flex the hand at the wrist joint will engage not only the flexor carpi radialis but also the other two wrist flexor group muscles—the palmaris longus and flexor carpi ulnaris. In this case, to palpate and discern the flexor carpi radialis from the adjacent palmaris longus and flexor carpi ulnaris, the client should be asked to perform radial deviation of the hand at the wrist joint instead of flexion of the hand at the wrist joint. This action will isolate the contraction to the flexor carpi radialis. It becomes palpably harder than the relaxed and palpably softer palmaris longus and flexor carpi ulnaris muscles, which facilitate palpating and locating the flexor carpi radialis (Figure 4-5).

Note: There are times when the client is not able to perform only the action that is being asked by the therapist; this is especially true with motions of the toes, because we do not usually develop the coordination necessary to isolate certain toe actions. In addition, if for any reason, a client contracts a muscle during a palpation protocol that he or she is not supposed to, preventing the body part from moving does not help the palpation. It is the *contraction* of any muscle other than the target muscle that is undesirable, not the movement of a client's body part.

Perfecting the Art of Muscle Palpation

Knowing the attachments and actions of the target muscle are the first two steps of learning the science of muscle palpation. Determining which joint action to ask the client to perform is the beginning of learning the art of muscle palpation. However, perfecting the art of muscle palpation involves the knowledge and

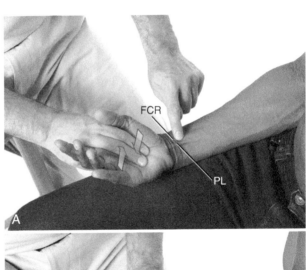

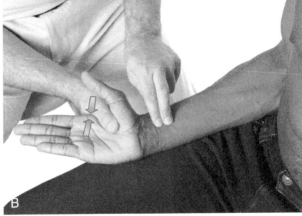

FIGURE 4-5 The flexor carpi radialis (FCR) muscle is engaged and palpated. *A,* If the client flexes the hand against resistance, the adjacent palmaris longus (PL) also contracts, making it difficult to discern the FCR. *B,* If the client, instead, radially deviates the hand against resistance, the PL remains relaxed, making it easier to discern the FCR.

4

application of many more guidelines. These additional guidelines are presented in the following pages. After discussing each of the guidelines, a summary list of all 20 muscle palpation guidelines is given. Memorizing a list this long is difficult, if not impossible; instead, these guidelines need to be learned by using them as the palpations of the skeletal muscles of the body are discussed in Chapters 6 through 11 of this book. With practice, these guidelines will become familiar and comfortable to you and will enhance the art and science of your muscle palpation technique.

Guideline 4: Add Resistance to the Contraction of the Target Muscle

When a client is asked to perform one of the joint actions of the target muscle to make it contract, harden, and stand out, there are times when this contraction is not forceful enough to make it easily palpable. This is especially true if the joint action does not require a large body part to be moved and/or if the body part that is moved is not moved against gravity. When the client's contraction of the target muscle is not forceful enough, it might be necessary for the therapist to add resistance so that the target muscle contracts harder and stands out more. A good example is when the target muscle is the pronator teres and the client is asked to pronate the forearm at the radioulnar joints. Because the forearm is not a very large body part and pronation does not occur against gravity, the pronator teres muscle will contract, but most likely not forcefully enough to make it stand out and be easily palpable. In this case, the

therapist can add resistance to the client's contraction by resisting the forearm during pronation. This will require a more forceful contraction of the pronator teres, making it easier to palpate and discern from the adjacent musculature (Figure 4-6). When palpating, the hand of the therapist that is doing the palpation is called the *palpation hand*. The other hand, in this case offering resistance, is called the *resistance hand*.

Resisting a client's target muscle contraction is not a battle between the therapist and client to see who is stronger. The role of the therapist is simply to oppose the force of the client's muscle contraction, not overpower the client. The degree that the client is asked to contract the target muscle can vary. Ideally, it should be the lightest amount necessary to bring out the target muscle's contraction so that it is palpable. However, a forceful contraction might be needed at times to achieve this. A good guideline is to begin with a gentle resistance as you try to palpate the target muscle. If it is not successful, then gradually increase the force of the resistance as necessary.

When you ask the client to contract the target muscle or to contract it against your resistance during palpation, remember to give the client a rest every few seconds or so. Holding a sustained isometric contraction can become uncomfortable and painful. It is more comfortable for the client and actually better for our palpation procedure if the client is asked to contract and relax the target muscle alternately instead of holding a sustained isometric contraction. (See Guideline 9 for additional text on alternately contracting and relaxing the target muscle.)

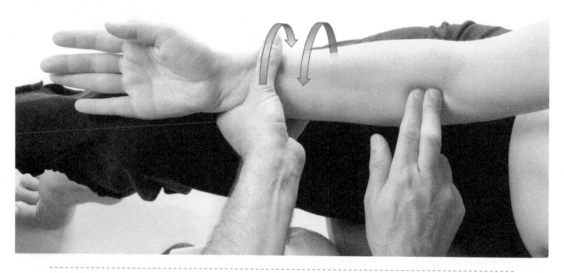

FIGURE 4-6 To create a more forceful contraction of the pronator teres muscle, the therapist can hold on to the client's distal forearm and resist forearm pronation at the radioulnar joints. Adding resistance increases the contraction force of the client's target muscle. The muscle "pops out" and is easier to palpate. Note that the stabilization hand resisting the client's forearm pronation is placed on the distal forearm and does not cross the wrist joint to hold the client's hand. Otherwise, additional muscles are likely to contract, and the target muscle contraction will not be isolated.

Further, whenever the therapist adds resistance to the contraction of the target muscle, it is extremely important not to cross any additional joints with the placement of the stabilization hand. The goal of having a client contract the target muscle during palpation is to limit contraction to the target muscle. This way, it will be the only muscle that is palpably hard and can be discerned from the adjacent relaxed and palpably soft muscles. However, if the therapist's stabilization hand does cross other joints, it is likely that muscles crossing these joints will also contract, which will defeat the purpose of having an isolated contraction of the target muscle.

For example, in the case of the pronator teres palpation, when resistance to forearm pronation is added, it is important that the therapist's stabilization hand does not cross the wrist joint and hold the client's hand. If the stabilization hand holds the client's hand, then other muscles that cross the client's wrist joint, such as the muscles of the wrist flexor group that move the hand at the wrist joint or flexor muscles of the fingers, will likely also contract, making it difficult to discern the pronator teres from these adjacent muscles. Therefore the resistance hand should be placed on the client's forearm (see Figure 4-6). Ideally, placing the resistance hand on the distal end of the forearm affords the best leverage force so that the therapist does not have to work as hard.

Generally, if the therapist is resisting an action of the arm at the glenohumeral joint, then the therapist's stabilization hand should be placed just proximal to the elbow joint and not cross the elbow joint to grasp the client's forearm. If the therapist is resisting an action of the forearm at the elbow joint, then the therapist's stabilization hand should be placed on the distal forearm and not cross the wrist joint to grasp the client's hand. If the therapist is resisting an action of the hand at the wrist joint, then the therapist's stabilization hand should be placed on the palm of the hand and not cross the metacarpophalangeal joints to grasp the client's fingers. The same reasoning can be applied to the lower extremity and the axial body.

Guideline 5: Look Before You Palpate

Although palpation is performed via touching, visual observation can be a valuable tool for locating a target muscle. This is especially true for muscles that are superficial and whose contours show through the skin. Very often, a target muscle visually screams, "Here I am!" yet the therapist does not see it because the palpating hand is in the way. This may be true when the target muscle is relaxed but is even more likely to be true when the target muscle is contracted (especially if it contracts harder from increased resistance); when it contracts and hardens, it often pops out visually. For this reason, whenever attempting to palpate a target muscle, look first; then place your palpating hand over the muscle to feel for it.

For example, when palpating the palmaris longus and flexor carpi radialis muscles of the wrist flexor group, before placing your palpating hand on the client's anterior forearm, first look for the distal tendons of these two muscles at the anterior distal forearm near the wrist joint. They may be fully visible, aiding you in finding and palpating them (Figure 4-7, A). If they are not visible, ask the client to flex the hand at the wrist joint and add resistance if needed. Now, look again before placing your palpating hand on the client. When contracted, these distal tendons will even more likely tense and visually pop out, helping you locate and palpate them (Figure 4-7, B). The visual information of many muscles can help with their palpation. For this reason, a good rule is to always "look before you touch."

Guideline 6: First Find and Palpate the Target Muscle in the Easiest Place Possible

Once a target muscle has been found, continuing to palpate along its course is much easier than it is to locate it in the first place. For this reason, a good palpation guideline is to always feel for the target muscle wherever it is easiest to first find. Once located, you can then continue to palpate it toward one or both of its attachments. For example, using the flexor carpi radialis as an example, if the distal tendon is visually apparent (see Figure 4-7), then begin your palpation there. Once it is clearly felt, then continue to palpate toward its proximal attachment on the medial epicondyle of the humerus.

Guideline 7: Strum Perpendicularly Across the Target Muscle

When first locating a target muscle or when following a target muscle that has already been found, strumming perpendicularly across its belly or tendon is best. Strumming perpendicularly across a muscle belly or its tendon is like strumming or twanging a guitar string; you begin on one side of the belly or tendon, then you rise up onto its prominence, and then fall off the other side of it. This change in contour is much more palpably noticeable than if your palpating fingers simply glide longitudinally along the muscle (which offers little change in contour and thus does not help define the location of the target muscle).

When strumming perpendicularly across a muscle's belly or tendon, it is important to note that the movement of your palpating fingers is not a short vibration motion; rather, it must be large enough to begin off one side of the target muscle, rise onto it, go all the way across it, and end off the other side of it. This means that the length of excursion of your strumming motion must be fairly long. Figure 4-8 illustrates the belly of the pronator teres being strummed perpendicularly.

4

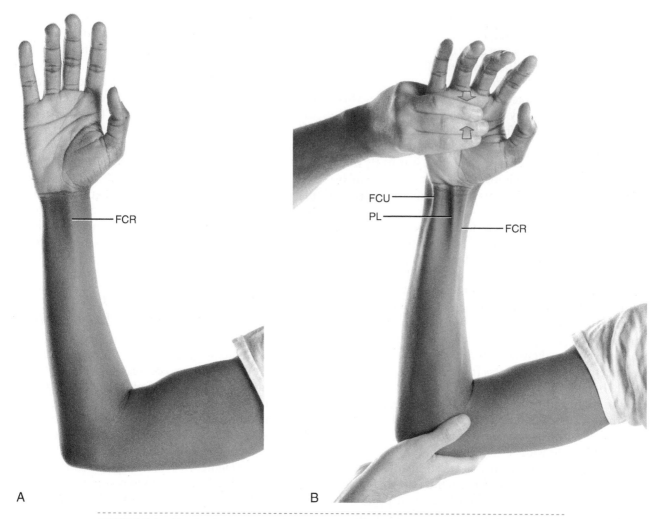

A   B

FIGURE 4-7 Looking for the presence of the target muscle is important before placing your palpating hand over the target muscle and blocking possibly useful visual information. **A,** The distal tendon of the flexor carpi radialis (FCR) muscle might be visible even when it is relaxed. **B,** When contracted (against resistance, in this case), the distal tendon tenses and becomes even more visually apparent. Note: the palmaris longus (PL) and flexor carpi ulnaris (FCU) tendons are also visible.

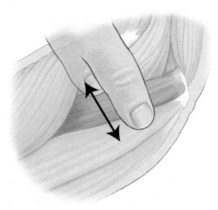

FIGURE 4-8 The pronator teres is being palpated by strumming perpendicularly across its belly. It is important that the excursion of the strumming motion is large enough to begin off the muscle on one side and end off the muscle on its other side.

Guideline 8: Use Baby Steps to Follow the Target Muscle

Once a target muscle has been found in the easiest place possible by strumming perpendicular to it, it should then be followed all the way to its attachments. This should be done in baby steps. Using baby steps to follow a muscle means that each successive "feel" of the muscle should be immediately after the previous feel so that no geography of the muscle's contour is skipped. If you feel the target muscle in one spot, then you should not skip a couple of inches down the muscle to feel it again. The farther down you skip, the more likely it is that you will no longer be on the muscle and will lose the course of its palpation. Figure 4-9 illustrates the idea that once a target muscle has been located, baby steps should be used to follow it toward its attachments.

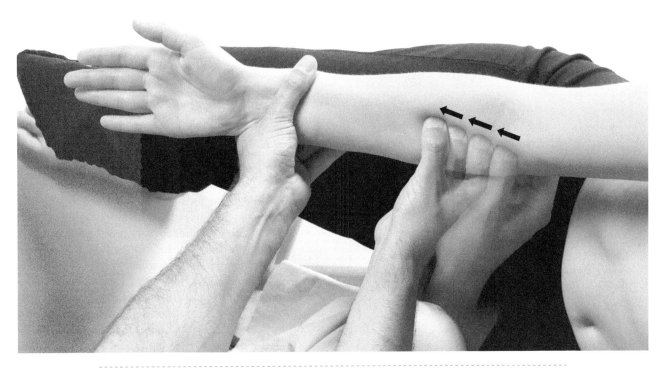

FIGURE 4-9 The pronator teres muscle is palpated in "baby steps" toward its distal attachment. Palpating in baby steps means that the muscle is palpated with successive feels, each one immediately after the previous one, which helps ensure that the therapist will successfully follow the course of the target muscle.

Guideline 9: Alternately Contract and Relax the Target Muscle

As previously stated, it can be uncomfortable for the client to hold a sustained isometric contraction of the target muscle while it is being palpated; therefore it is better for the client to alternately contract and relax it. In addition, having the client alternately contract and relax the target muscle while the therapist follows its course with baby steps aids in successful palpation. If the target muscle alternately contracts and then relaxes at each baby step of the palpation process, then the therapist can feel its change in texture from being soft when it is relaxed, to being hard when it is contracted, and to being soft when it is relaxed again. This assures the therapist that he or she is still on the target muscle. If the therapist does accidentally veer off the target muscle onto other tissue, then it will be evident because the tissue texture change from soft to hard to soft (as the target muscle contracts and then relaxes) will not be felt.

When the therapist does veer off course, the palpating fingers should be placed back at the last spot where the target muscle was clearly felt and then make the next baby step in a slightly different direction to relocate the course of the target muscle as the client is asked once again to contract and then relax the target muscle alternately.

Guideline 10: When Appropriate, Use Coupled Actions

Knowledge of coupled actions can help isolate contraction of a target muscle in certain instances to facilitate palpation. Most of these instances involve rotation of the scapula at the scapulocostal joint, because scapular rotation cannot occur on its own; rather, the scapula can only rotate when the arm is moved at the glenohumeral joint. For example, although it has a number of actions that could be used to make it contract, if the pectoralis minor is the target muscle to be palpated, most of these actions would also cause the pectoralis major to contract, which would block palpation of the pectoralis minor. The only effective action that would isolate contraction of the pectoralis minor in the anterior chest is downward rotation of the scapula. However, this rotation will occur only in conjunction with extension and/or adduction of the arm at the glenohumeral joint. Therefore to create downward rotation of the scapula to engage the pectoralis minor, ask the client to extend and adduct the arm at the glenohumeral joint. This action can be accomplished by first having the client rest the hand in the small of the back; then, to engage the pectoralis minor, have the client move the arm further into extension by moving the hand posteriorly away from the small of the back. This action will immediately engage the pectoralis minor, allowing it to be easily palpated through the pectoralis major (Figure 4-10). This same procedure can be used to palpate the rhomboid muscles through the middle trapezius (see Figure 6-7).

> Note: Knowledge of coupled actions can also be used with reciprocal inhibition to palpate a target muscle. For example, when palpating the levator scapulae, the client's arm is extended and adducted at the glenohumeral joint by placing the hand in the small of the back. This requires the coupled action of downward rotation of the scapula at the scapulocostal joint, which then reciprocally inhibits and relaxes the upper trapezius (because it is an upward rotator of the scapula). With the upper trapezius relaxed, the levator scapulae can be palpated through it. (For a fuller explanation of this, see the discussion on reciprocal inhibition, Guideline 11.)

Guideline 11: When Appropriate, Use Reciprocal Inhibition

Reciprocal inhibition is a neurologic reflex that causes inhibition of a muscle whenever an antagonist muscle is actively contracted. This neurologic reflex can be used to great advantage when palpating certain target muscles.

For example, if our target muscle is the brachialis and we want to make it contract so that it hardens and is easier to feel, we have no choice but to ask the client to flex the elbow joint because that is the only action of the brachialis. The problem with this action is that if the client flexes the forearm at the elbow joint to contract the brachialis, the biceps brachii will also contract. This contraction makes it difficult to palpate the brachialis because the biceps brachii overlies the brachialis in the anterior arm. Given that it is always the goal of a muscle palpation to have an isolated contraction of the target muscle (in this case, we want only the brachialis to contract), the biceps brachii needs to remain relaxed. Although the only action of the brachialis (elbow joint flexion) is an action of the biceps brachii, achieving isolated contraction is possible if we use the principle of reciprocal inhibition (Figure 4-11). To do this, we ask the client to flex the forearm at the elbow joint while the forearm is in a position of full pronation. Because

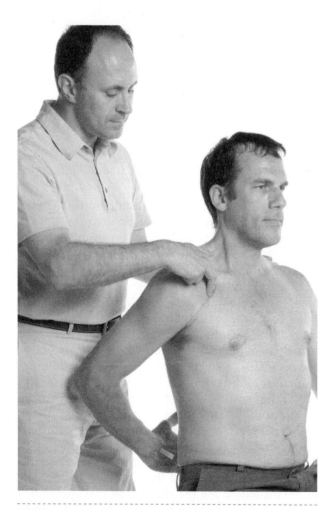

FIGURE 4-10 When the client moves the hand posteriorly away from the small of the back, extension of the arm occurs. This requires the coupled action of downward rotation of the scapula at the scapulocostal joint, which engages the pectoralis minor muscle so that it can be easily palpated through the pectoralis major muscle.

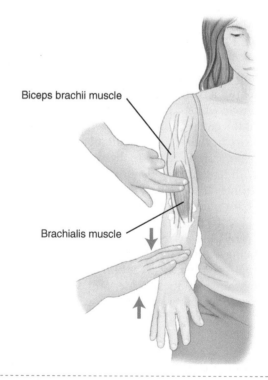

Biceps brachii muscle

Brachialis muscle

FIGURE 4-11 The principle of reciprocal inhibition is used to inhibit and relax the biceps brachii muscle as the brachialis muscle contracts to flex the forearm at the elbow joint. The biceps brachii, which is also a supinator of the forearm, is reciprocally inhibited because the forearm is pronated (as it is flexed).

the biceps brachii is also a supinator of the forearm, having the forearm pronated will reciprocally inhibit it from contracting; consequently, it will remain relaxed as the brachialis contracts to flex the forearm at the elbow joint. Thus we have achieved the goal of having an isolated contraction of our target muscle, the brachialis.

Another example of using the principle of reciprocal inhibition to isolate the contraction of a target muscle is palpating the scapular attachment of the levator scapulae. If we ask the client to elevate the scapula to contract and palpably harden the levator scapulae, the upper trapezius will also contract and harden, making it impossible to feel the levator scapulae at its scapular attachment deep to the upper trapezius. To stop the upper trapezius from contracting, ask the client to place the hand in the small of the back. This position of humeral extension and adduction requires downward rotation of the scapula at the scapulocostal joint. Because the upper trapezius is an upward rotator of the scapula, it will be reciprocally inhibited and stay relaxed. This position allows for an isolated contraction of and a successful palpation of the levator scapulae when the client is asked to elevate the scapula (Figure 4-12).

One important caution is provided when using the principle of reciprocal inhibition for a muscle palpation. When the client is asked to contract and engage the target muscle, the force of its contraction must be small. If the contraction is forceful, the client's brain will override the reciprocal inhibition reflex in an attempt to recruit as many muscles as possible for the joint action, and contraction of the muscle that was supposed to be reciprocally inhibited and relaxed will be the result. Once this other muscle contracts, it will likely block successful palpation of the target muscle. For example, when palpating for the brachialis, if flexion of the forearm at the elbow joint is performed forcefully, the biceps brachii will be recruited, making palpation of the brachialis difficult or impossible. Another example is palpating for the levator scapulae: if elevation of the scapula at the scapulocostal joint is performed forcefully, then the upper trapezius will be recruited, making palpation of the levator scapulae at its scapular attachment difficult or impossible.

Guideline 12: Use Appropriate Pressure

It is important to avoid being too heavy handed; sensitivity can be lost with excessive pressure. On the other hand, it is important to not be too light with your pressure either; some muscles are quite deep and require moderate-to-strong pressure to feel. Generally, when most new students have a difficult time palpating a target muscle, it is because their pressure is too light. Appropriate pressure means applying the optimal palpation pressure for each target muscle palpation (Figure 4-13).

Note: Occasionally, a deep muscle palpation is facilitated by extremely light pressure. If a muscle is so deep that its borders cannot be felt, then its location must be determined by feeling for the vibrations of its contraction through the tissues. This can only be felt with a very light touch.

Guideline 13: For Deep Palpations, Sink Slowly into the Tissue and Have the Client Breathe

All deep muscle palpations should be performed slowly. Although deep pressure can be uncomfortable for many clients, it is often accomplished quite easily if we work with the client as we palpate. Sinking slowly into the client's tissues and having

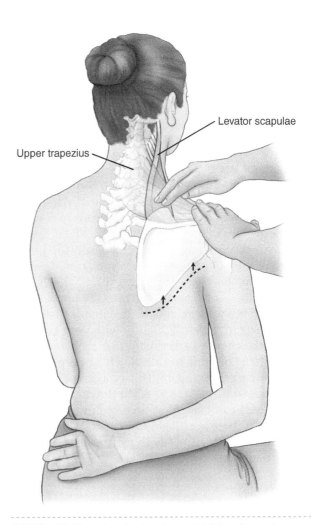

FIGURE 4-12 The principle of reciprocal inhibition is used to inhibit and relax the upper trapezius so that the scapular attachment of the levator scapulae can be more easily palpated as it contracts to elevate the scapula at the scapulocostal joint. The upper trapezius, which is also an upward rotator of the scapula, is reciprocally inhibited because the scapula is downwardly rotated (as it is elevated) because of the position of the hand in the small of the back.

4

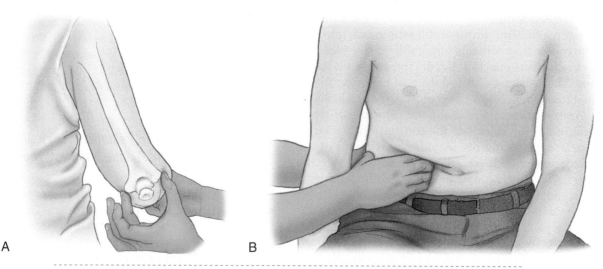

A   B

FIGURE 4-13 Use pressure that is appropriate to the structure being palpated. When the medial and lateral epicondyles of the humerus are being palpated, only light pressure is needed *(A)*. However, when the psoas major muscle is palpated, deeper pressure is required *(B)*.

the client breathe with the palpation process in a slow and rhythmic manner can accomplish this. An excellent example is palpating the psoas major in the abdominopelvic cavity. The psoas major must be palpated from the anterior perspective. Because the psoas major lies against the spinal column and forms part of the posterior abdominal wall, firm pressure is required to reach through the abdominal viscera. For the client to remain comfortable, the therapist needs to sink into the client's tissues very slowly as the client breathes slowly and evenly. To begin the palpation, ask the client to take in a moderate-to-deep breath; then, as the client slowly exhales, slowly sink in toward the psoas major. Reaching the psoas major is not necessary at the end of the client's first exhalation. Instead, ease off slightly with your pressure and ask the client to take in another moderate-sized breath; then continue to sink slowly in deeper as the client slowly exhales again. This process may need to be repeated a third time to reach the psoas major; a deep muscle can usually be accessed in this manner with two or three breaths by the client. What is most important to remember is that firm deep pressure must be applied slowly.

Note: When having a client breathe with your palpation as you sink slowly and deeply in the client's tissues to access a deep muscle, it is important that the client's breath is not quick and shallow. However, the breaths do not need to be very deep either; a very deep breath may push your palpating hands out, especially if you are palpating in the abdominal region. The pace of the breath is more important. The client's breathing should be slow, rhythmic, and relaxed. This type of breathing on the part of the client is facilitated if you breathe in a similar manner.

Guideline 14: Use Muscles as Landmarks

Once the bones and bony landmarks of the skeleton have been learned, using a bony landmark to help locate and palpate a target muscle is common. However, once the palpation of one muscle has been learned, it can also be a useful landmark for locating another adjacent muscle. For example, if palpation of the sternocleidomastoid (SCM) has been learned, then it is a simple matter to palpate the scalene muscles (see page 283). Locating the lateral border of the clavicular head of the SCM and then dropping off it immediately laterally are all that is required; you will be on the scalene group. This way is a much easier to locate the scalenes than to first try to palpate the anterior tubercles of the transverse processes of the cervical vertebrae. Similarly, the SCM can also be used to locate and palpate the longus colli muscle (see page 294). First locate the medial border of the sternal head of the SCM and then drop it off just medially and sink in toward the spinal column. Countless other examples exist wherein knowledge of one muscle's location can help the therapist locate another muscle that might otherwise be difficult to find.

Guideline 15: Relax and Passively Slacken the Target Muscle When Palpating its Bony Attachment

Palpating as much of a target muscle as possible is always desirable; preferably it should be palpated all the way from one bony attachment to its other bony attachment. However, following a target muscle all the way to its bony attachment is difficult at times. This is especially true if the client is contracting the target muscle, because this tenses and hardens its tendon, making it difficult to discern from its bony attachment.

Ironically, although contracting the target muscle helps us discern its belly from adjacent soft tissue because the muscle belly becomes hard, contracting the target muscle tenses and hardens the tendon of the muscle as well, which makes it harder to discern the hard tendon from the adjacent hard bony tissue of its attachment. In other words, contracting a target muscle helps discern it from adjacent soft tissue, but contracting it makes it more difficult to discern it from adjacent hard tissue, such as its bony attachments. Therefore having the client relax the target muscle and having the target muscle passively slackened as the therapist reaches its bony attachment is one guideline that can help the therapist follow a target muscle all the way to its bony attachment. Examples that use this guideline are palpating the proximal attachment of the rectus femoris muscle on the anterior inferior iliac spine (AIIS) of the pelvis (see Figure 10-26) and palpating the distal attachment of the subscapularis muscle on the lesser tubercle of the humerus (see Figure 6-23).

Guideline 16: Close Your Eyes When You Palpate

Although visually inspecting the palpation region is important when beginning palpation of the target muscle (see Guideline 5), once the visual inspection is done, it is often not necessary for a therapist to continue looking at the client's body as the palpation procedure continues. In fact, it can be greatly beneficial if the therapist closes his or her eyes when palpating. By closing the eyes, the therapist can block out extraneous sensory stimuli that might otherwise distract from what is being felt in the palpation finger pads. Closing the eyes allows the therapist to focus all attention on the palpating fingers, thereby increasing their sensory acuity.

Guideline 17: Construct a Mental Picture of the Client's Anatomy Under the Skin as You Palpate

As the therapist's eyes are closed during palpation, picturing the target muscle and other adjacent anatomic structures under the client's skin can also be beneficial. Creating this mental picture of the client's anatomy under the skin can facilitate correct initial location of the target muscle and facilitate the use of baby steps as the target muscle is followed toward its attachments.

Guideline 18: If a Client Is Ticklish, Have the Client Place a Hand Over Your Palpating Hand

Unfortunately, when clients are ticklish, palpating them is often difficult if not impossible because touching causes them to pull away. This is especially true if we touch the client lightly. Therefore using firm pressure is usually best to palpate ticklish clients. However, some clients are extremely ticklish whether we touch

them lightly or firmly, which can interfere with palpation assessment and also with treatment. Asking the client to place one of his or her hands over our palpating hand is one technique that can be done to help lessen the sensitivity of a ticklish client. Ticklishness is a perceived invasion of one's space by another individual, which is why a person cannot tickle him or herself. Therefore if the client's hand is placed over our palpating hand, the client will subconsciously have a sense that he or she is in control of this space and will tend to be less ticklish. Using this guideline does not work with everyone in every circumstance, but it is worth trying and often successful.

Guideline 19: Keep Fingernails Short and Smooth

For some muscle palpations, the therapist's fingernails need to be very short (Figure 4-14, *A*), especially when it comes to deep palpations such as when palpating the subscapularis muscle (see Figure 6-23), quadratus lumborum muscle (see Figure 8-16), or the vertebral attachments of the scalene muscles (see Figure 8-35). Unfortunately, everyone has a different sense of what short means when it comes to the length of fingernails. As a result, some therapists allow their nails to be too long. Consequently, they are unable to palpate some muscles comfortably and either cause pain and leave fingernail marks on the client or, just as bad, avoid adequately palpating or working musculature of the client that is in need of treatment because they are afraid of hurting the client with their nails. The exact fingernail length that is necessary will vary from one palpation to another. A good way to check for appropriate fingernail length is to place the pads of your palpating hand fingers away from you and try to catch the fingernails of your palpating hand with a fingernail of your other hand (Figure 4-14, *B*). If you can, then the fingernails are likely too long. If you cannot, then the length of your fingernails is short enough for deep palpations.

Just as important, fingernails must be smooth (i.e., their edges are not sharp). When filing fingernails, finishing with a fingernail file that buffs and smooths the edges of the nails is important. Short nails that are sharp can be just as uncomfortable or painful to the client as long fingernails.

Guideline 20: Use the Optimal Palpation Position

The optimal palpation position is simply the client position that is most effective for the palpation of a particular target muscle. It is important to realize that the optimal position in which to palpate a certain target muscle might not be the position that a client is usually in when that muscle is being treated. Clients are usually treated in the prone or supine position. However, some muscles are optimally palpated with the client side lying, standing, or seated. For example,

4

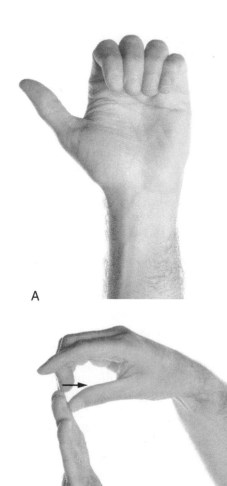

A

B

FIGURE 4-14 Fingernails need to be very short for muscle palpations, especially of deep muscles. **A,** The proper length for fingernails when palpating and working deeply is shown. **B,** An easy way to check whether fingernail length is short enough for deeper palpations is seen. See if you can catch the fingernails of your palpating hand (when the pads are oriented away from you) with a fingernail of your other hand. If you can, that fingernail may be too long.

the pectoralis minor is most often treated with the client supine. However, the optimal client position in which to palpate the pectoralis minor is probably seated. This is because the seated position better allows the client to first place the hand in the small of the back and then move the hand posteriorly away from the small of the back (creating downward rotation of the scapula to engage the pectoralis minor) (see Figure 6-14, *B*). For this reason, although it is usually preferred to not have the client change positions in the middle of a treatment session, if accurate palpation is critical

to the assessment and treatment of the client, it might be necessary to do so. To avoid this interruption to the flow of a treatment session, the therapist may choose to do all palpation assessments at the beginning of the session before commencing with treatment.

Apply Guidelines and Be Creative

Although the science of muscle palpation begins with a solid knowledge of the attachments and actions of the target muscle, turning palpation into an art requires much more. The art of muscle palpation involves weaving the knowledge of the attachments and actions of the target muscle and all adjacent musculature, as well as the many guidelines listed in this chapter, into a cohesive approach that allows the target muscle to be discerned from adjacent tissues. Overall, what are necessary are sensitive hands, critical thinking, and a willingness to be creative.

Summary List of Muscle Palpation Guidelines

Each of the following muscle palpation guidelines has already been discussed in this chapter. All 20 are summarized in the following list:

1. Know the attachments of the target muscle to know where to place your hands.
2. Know the actions of the target muscle. The client will most likely be asked to perform one of them to contract the target muscle so that it can be discerned from the adjacent musculature. (Make sure that the client is not asked to hold the contraction too long or the target muscle may fatigue and the client may become uncomfortable.)
3. Think critically to choose exactly which joint action of the target muscle will best isolate its contraction.
4. If necessary, add resistance to the client's contraction of the target muscle. (When resistance is added, do not cross any joints that do not need to be crossed; in other words, be sure to resist only the desired action of the target muscle
5. Look before placing your palpating hand on the client. (This is especially important with superficial muscles.)
6. First find and palpate the target muscle in the easiest place possible.
7. Strum perpendicularly across the belly or tendon of the target muscle.
8. Once located, follow the course of the target muscle in small successive baby steps.
9. At each baby step of palpation, have the client alternately contract and relax the target muscle and feel for this tissue texture change as the muscle goes from relaxed and soft, to contracted and hard, to relaxed and soft again.

10. Use your knowledge of coupled actions to palpate target muscles that are scapular rotators.
11. Use reciprocal inhibition whenever needed to aid palpation of the target muscle. (When reciprocal inhibition is used, do not have the client contract the target muscle too forcefully, or the muscle that is being reciprocally inhibited may be recruited anyway.)
12. Use appropriate pressure. Appropriate pressure is neither too heavy nor too light.
13. When using deep palpation pressure, sink slowly into the client's tissues as the client breathes slowly and evenly.
14. Once the palpation of one muscle is known, it can be used as a landmark to locate other muscles.
15. Relax and passively slacken the target muscle when palpating it at its bony attachment.
16. Close your eyes when you palpate to focus your attention on your palpating fingers.
17. Construct a mental picture of the client's anatomy under the skin as you palpate.
18. If the client is ticklish, use firm pressure and have the client place a hand over your palpating hand.
19. Fingernails need to be very short and smooth.
20. Place the client in a position that is optimal for the muscle palpation.

REVIEW QUESTIONS

Circle or fill in the correct answer for each of the following questions. More study resources are provided on the Evolve website at http://evolve.elsevier.com/Muscolino/knowthebody.

4

1. **What are the two major objectives of palpation?**

   _____

   _____

2. **When should we be palpating our clients?**
   a. At the beginning of the session
   b. At the end of the session
   c. When the client is in pain
   d. Whenever we are contacting them

3. **What two guidelines make up the "science of muscle palpation?"**

   _____

   _____

4. **When asking the client to contract to palpate the target muscle, which of the following is our goal?**
   a. Contraction of the target muscle and its synergists
   b. Contraction of the target muscle only
   c. Contraction of the target muscle and all nearby muscles
   d. Inhibition and relaxation of the target muscle

5. **Where on the client's body should the therapist's stabilization/resistance hand be placed when palpating and engaging the pronator teres?**
   a. Arm
   b. Forearm
   c. Palm of hand
   d. Fingers

6. **For what type of muscle is it important to look before you touch?**

   _____

7. **Where should a muscle be first palpated?**
   a. At its proximal attachment
   b. At its distal attachment
   c. At the mid belly
   d. At the easiest place possible to locate the muscle

8. **In what direction should we orient our palpating stroke relative to the target muscle?**

   _____

9. **What term describes that each successive "feel" of a muscle should be immediately after the previous one?**

   _____

10. **What reflex can be used to relax a muscle that has the same actions as the palpation target muscle?**

    _____

Bony Palpation

Chapter 5 offers a palpation tour of bones, bony landmarks, and joints of the human body. The tour begins with the upper extremity, then addresses the axial body, and concludes with the lower extremity. Although any one bone or bony landmark can be independently palpated, this chapter is set up sequentially to flow from one landmark to another; therefore following the order presented here is recommended.

UPPER EXTREMITY

ANTEROMEDIAL VIEW

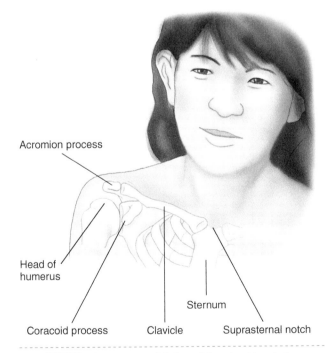

FIGURE 5-1 Anteromedial view of the shoulder girdle.

Acromion process

Head of humerus

Coracoid process

Clavicle

Sternum

Suprasternal notch

ANTEROMEDIAL VIEW

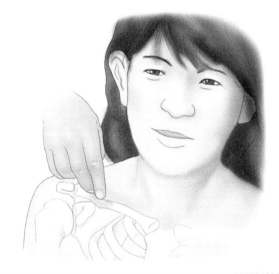

FIGURE 5-2 Clavicle: Find the notch at the superior border of the sternum and palpate laterally, feeling for the sternoclavicular joint. From there, slide along the shaft of the **clavicle** from medial to lateral (proximal to distal) to feel its entire length. Notice that the medial end of the clavicle is convex anteriorly and the lateral end of the clavicle is concave anteriorly.

ANTEROMEDIAL VIEW

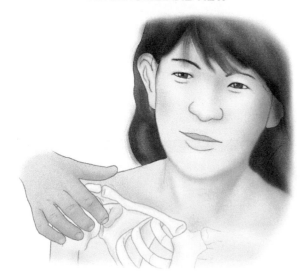

FIGURE 5-3 Coracoid process of the scapula: From the concavity at the lateral (distal) end of the clavicle, drop inferiorly off the clavicle to find the **coracoid process of the scapula** (located deep to the pectoralis major muscle). When palpating the coracoid process, notice that its apex (tip) points laterally.

ANTEROMEDIAL VIEW

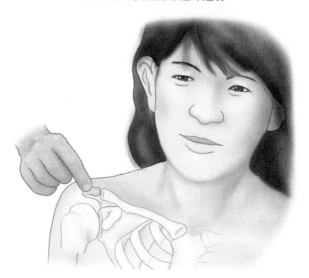

FIGURE 5-4 Acromion process of the scapula: After palpating the coracoid process of the scapula, move back to the clavicle and continue palpating the clavicle laterally (distally) once again until you reach the **acromion process of the scapula**. The acromion process of the scapula is at the far lateral end (i.e., the tip of the shoulder).

POSTEROLATERAL VIEW

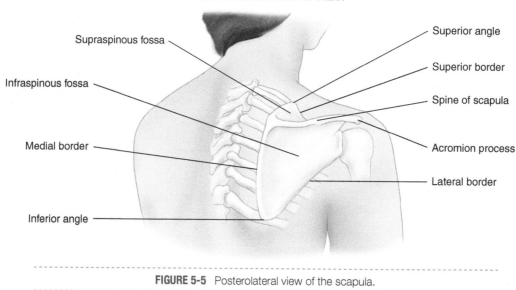

Supraspinous fossa

Infraspinous fossa

Medial border

Inferior angle

Superior angle

Superior border

Spine of scapula

Acromion process

Lateral border

FIGURE 5-5 Posterolateral view of the scapula.

POSTEROLATERAL VIEW

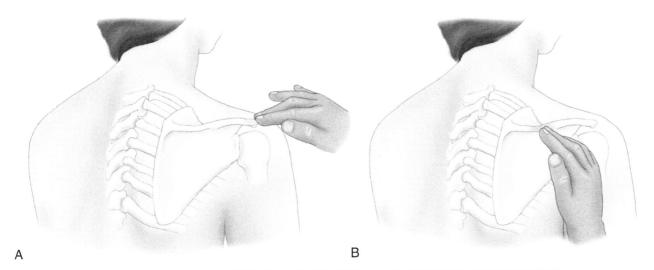

A

B

FIGURE 5-6 Acromion process and spine of the scapula: The **spine of the scapula** is the posterior continuation of the acromion process. To locate the spine of the scapula, begin on the acromion process **(A),** and continue palpating along it posteriorly. The spine of the scapula **(B)** can be palpated all the way to the medial border of the scapula. The spine of the scapula can be best palpated if you strum it perpendicularly by moving your palpating fingers up and down across it as you work your way posteriorly and then medially.

POSTEROLATERAL VIEW

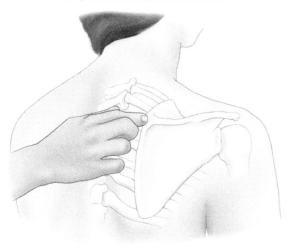

POSTEROLATERAL VIEW

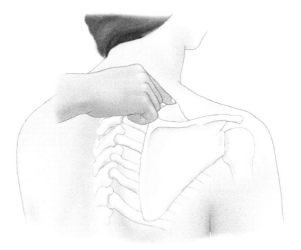

FIGURE 5-7 Medial border of the scapula (at the root of the spine of the scapula): Continue palpating along the spine of the scapula until you reach the **medial border of the scapula.** Where the spine of the scapula ends at the medial border is called the **root of the spine of the scapula.** Passively retracting the client's scapula makes it much easier to locate the medial border.

FIGURE 5-8 Superior angle of the scapula: Once the medial border of the scapula has been located, palpate along it superiorly until you reach the **superior angle of the scapula.** Having the client elevate and depress the scapula as you palpate for its superior angle can be helpful.

POSTEROLATERAL VIEW

POSTEROLATERAL VIEW

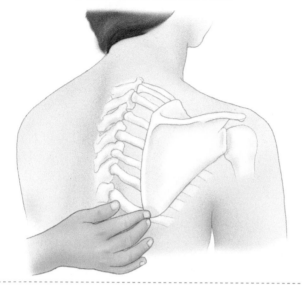

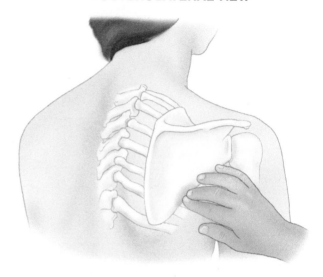

FIGURE 5-9 Inferior angle of the scapula: Palpate along the medial border of the scapula from the superior angle down to the **inferior angle of the scapula.**

FIGURE 5-10 Lateral border of the scapula: Once you are at the inferior angle of the scapula, continue palpating superiorly along the **lateral border of the scapula.** It is easiest to feel the lateral border if your pressure is directed medially. Although challenging, the lateral border of the scapula can usually be palpated all the way to the **infraglenoid tubercle of the scapula,** just inferior to the glenoid fossa of the scapula. To confirm that you are on the infraglenoid tubercle, ask the client to extend the forearm at the elbow joint against resistance to bring out the infraglenoid attachment of the long head of the triceps brachii (you can provide the resistance or the client can provide the resistance by pressing the forearm against his or her own thigh).

ANTEROLATERAL VIEW

SUPERIOR VIEW

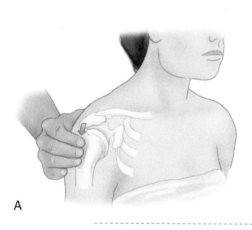

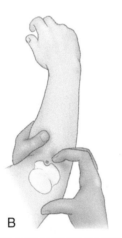

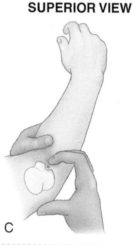

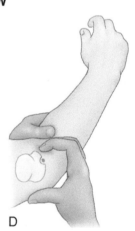

A

B

C

D

FIGURE 5-11 Greater tubercle, bicipital groove, and lesser tubercle of the humerus: The **greater tubercle** is located on the lateral side of the **bicipital groove;** the **lesser tubercle** is located on the medial side. First locate the anterolateral margin of the acromion process of the scapula and then immediately drop off it onto the head of the humerus; you should be on the greater tubercle of the humerus (**A** and **B**). Now, with a flat finger pad palpation across the anterior surface of the head of the humerus, passively move the client's arm into lateral rotation at the glenohumeral joint. You should be able to feel your palpating finger dropping into the bicipital groove as it passes under your finger pads **(C).** As you continue to move the client's arm passively into lateral rotation, you will then feel the lesser tubercle under your fingers, just medial to the bicipital groove **(D).** If you do not successfully feel the tubercles and bicipital groove, alternately move the client's arm through medial and lateral rotation, feeling for them.

POSTERIOR VIEW

POSTERIOR VIEW

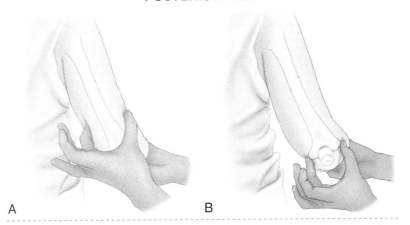

A

B

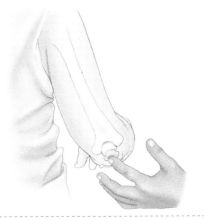

5

FIGURE 5-12 Medial and lateral epicondyles of the humerus: To locate the **medial and lateral epicondyles of the humerus,** ask the client to flex the forearm at the elbow joint to approximately 90 degrees; place your palpating fingers on the medial and lateral sides of the client's arm **(A)** and move distally down the client's arm. Your palpating fingers will clearly run into the medial and lateral epicondyles of the humerus; they will prominently be the widest points along the sides of the humerus near the elbow joint **(B).**

FIGURE 5-13 Olecranon process of the ulna: The **olecranon process of the ulna** is extremely easy to locate. With the thumb and middle finger on the medial and lateral epicondyles of the humerus, place your index finger on the olecranon process, located halfway between the two epicondyles.

NOTES: (1) If the client's elbow joint is flexed, the olecranon process will be located farther distally than the two epicondyles of the humerus. (2) Because of the presence of the ulnar nerve, known in lay terms as the "funny bone," be careful with palpatory pressure between the medial epicondyle of the humerus and the olecranon process of the ulna.

LATERAL VIEW

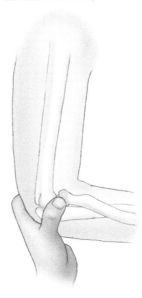

FIGURE 5-14 Radial head: The **radial head** lies at the proximal end of the radius. To palpate it, begin at the lateral epicondyle of the humerus and drop immediately distal to it. Feeling the joint space between the head of the radius and the humerus is possible. To bring out the radial head, place two fingers on either side (proximal and distal) of it and ask the client to alternately pronate and supinate the forearm at the radioulnar joints; the spinning of the head of the radius can be felt under your fingers.

5

LATERAL VIEW

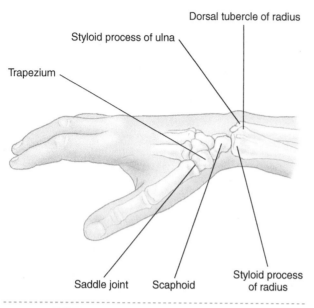

Dorsal tubercle of radius

Styloid process of ulna

Trapezium

Saddle joint   Scaphoid   Styloid process of radius

FIGURE 5-15 Lateral view of the wrist/hand.

LATERAL VIEW

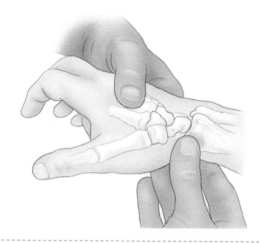

FIGURE 5-16 Styloid process of the radius: Find the lateral shaft of the radius and continue palpating it distally until you reach the **styloid process of the radius** located at the distal end.

NOTE: A small portion of the distal lateral radial shaft is not directly palpable because it is deep to three deep thumb muscles of the posterior forearm.

LATERAL VIEW

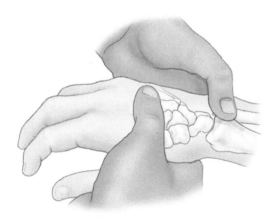

FIGURE 5-17 Dorsal (Lister's) tubercle: The **dorsal tubercle** (also known as **Lister's tubercle**) is located on the posterior side of the distal end of the radius. From the styloid process of the radius, palpate posteriorly onto the radius; the dorsal tubercle will be a prominence located in the middle of the distal posterior radial shaft.

LATERAL VIEW

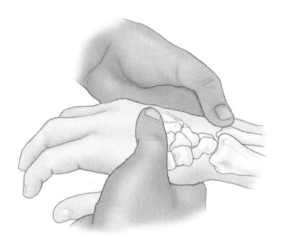

FIGURE 5-18 Styloid process of the ulna: The **styloid process of the ulna** is located at the distal end of the ulna on the posterior side. From the dorsal tubercle of the radius, move medially onto the posterior surface of the distal ulna and feel for the prominence of the ulnar styloid.

ANTERIOR (PALMAR) VIEW

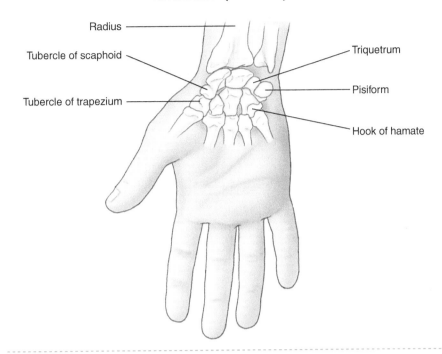

FIGURE 5-19 Anterior (palmar) view of the wrist.

ANTERIOR (PALMAR) VIEW

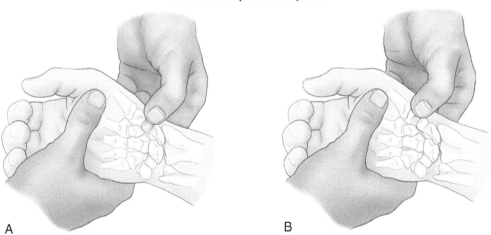

A   B

FIGURE 5-20 Tubercles of scaphoid and trapezium: The tubercles of the scaphoid and trapezium are prominent and palpable anteriorly on the hand. To locate them, palpate the lateral (radial) surface of the anterior hand and feel for two bony prominences. *A,* The **tubercle of the scaphoid** is the smaller, more proximal one of the two. *B,* The **tubercle of the trapezium** is the larger, more distal bony prominence.
   NOTE: The tubercle of the trapezium is located approximately ½ inch distal to the tubercle of the scaphoid.

ANTERIOR (PALMAR) VIEW

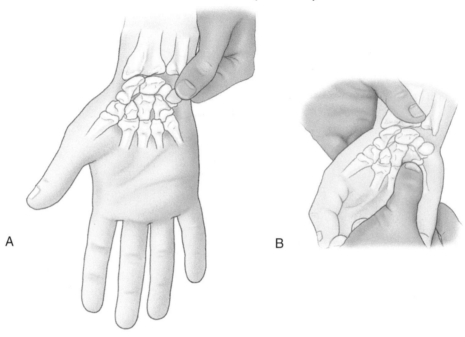

A

B

FIGURE 5-21 Pisiform and hook of the hamate: The **pisiform** is a carpal bone located anteriorly on top of the triquetrum in the proximal row of carpals on the ulnar side. The pisiform is prominent and easily palpated on the anterior side of the wrist, just distal to the ulna **(A)**. The hamate is also easily palpated anteriorly in the palm. Specifically, the **hook of the hamate** is palpable here. Begin by locating the pisiform; then palpate approximately ½ to ¾ inch distal and lateral (i.e., toward the midline of the hand) from the pisiform **(B)**.

NOTE: The hook of the hamate is fairly pointy and can be somewhat tender to palpation.

AXIAL BODY

INFEROLATERAL VIEW

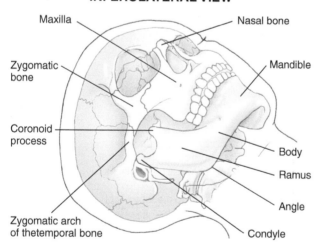

Maxilla

Nasal bone

Zygomatic bone

Mandible

Coronoid process

Body

Ramus

Angle

Zygomatic arch of thetemporal bone

Condyle

FIGURE 5-22 An oblique (inferolateral) view of the face.

INFEROLATERAL VIEW

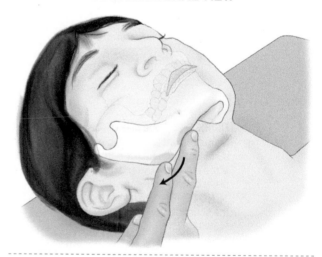

FIGURE 5-23 Body and angle of the mandible: The **body of the mandible** is subcutaneous and easily palpable. Begin palpating the inferior border of the body of the mandible anteriorly and continue palpating it laterally and posteriorly until the **angle of the mandible** is reached. The angle of the mandible is the transition area where the body of the mandible becomes the ramus of the mandible.

INFEROLATERAL VIEW

INFEROLATERAL VIEW

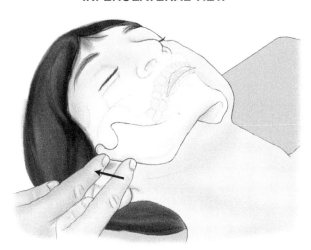

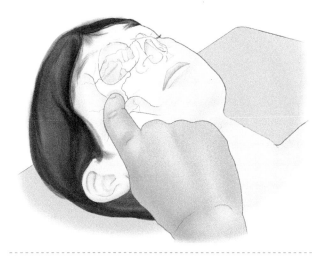

FIGURE 5-24 Ramus (posterior border) and condyle of the mandible: The **ramus of the mandible** branches off from the body of the mandible at the angle of the mandible. The posterior border of the ramus is fairly easy to palpate for its entire course and gives rise to the **condyle (of the ramus) of the mandible.** To palpate the ramus, begin at the angle of the mandible and palpate superiorly along the posterior border until the condyle is reached, anterior to the ear. To bring out the condyle, ask the client to alternately open and close the mouth. This allows one to feel the movement of the condyle of the mandible at the **temporomandibular joint (TMJ).**

NOTE: The condyle can also be palpated from within the ear. Wearing a finger cot or glove, gently place your palpating finger inside the client's ear, press anteromedially, and ask the client to alternately open and close the mouth. The movement of the condyle of the mandible at the TMJ will be clearly palpable.

FIGURE 5-25 Zygomatic bone: The **zygomatic bone,** commonly referred to as the *cheekbone*, is easily palpated inferolateral to the eye. Once located, explore the zygomatic bone to its borders with the maxilla, frontal bone, and temporal bone.

LATERAL VIEW

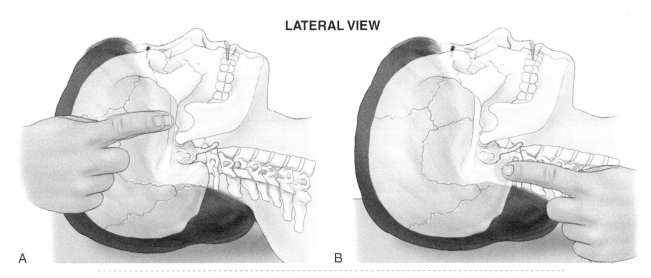

A

B

FIGURE 5-26 Temporal bone: To palpate the zygomatic arch of the temporal bone, first find the zygomatic bone (see Figure 5-25). Once located, continue palpating the zygomatic bone posteriorly until you reach the **zygomatic arch of the temporal bone (A).** Strumming your fingers vertically over the zygomatic arch can be helpful. The entire length of the zygomatic arch of the temporal bone can be palpated.

To palpate the **mastoid process of the temporal bone,** palpate just posterior to the earlobe, then press medially and strum over the mastoid process by moving your palpating finger anteriorly and posteriorly *(B).*

LATERAL VIEW

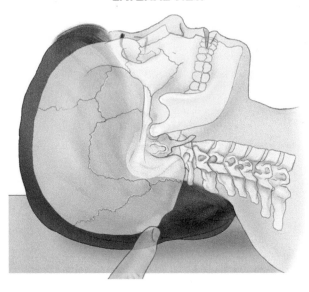

FIGURE 5-27 External occipital protuberance (EOP): The EOP is a midline bump on the superior nuchal line of the occiput at the back of the head. The EOP is usually fairly large and prominent and therefore readily palpable.

LATERAL VIEW

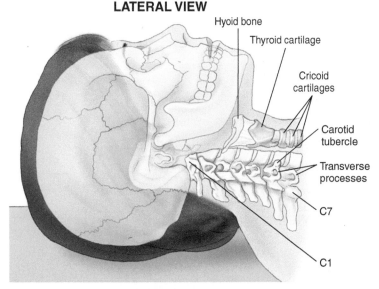

Hyoid bone
Thyroid cartilage
Cricoid cartilages
Carotid tubercle
Transverse processes
C7
C1

FIGURE 5-28 A lateral view of the neck.

NOTE: With all palpations in the anterior neck, a careful and sensitive touch is necessary and palpatory pressure must be applied gradually. Many structures in the anterior neck are very sensitive and can be tender. Furthermore, the carotid arteries are found in the anterior neck; pressure on them cannot only potentially restrict blood flow within them to the anterior brain, but it can also trigger a neurologic reflex (the carotid reflex) that can lower blood pressure. For this reason, palpating the anterior neck unilaterally (i.e., one side at a time) is best. If you feel that your palpating fingers are on the carotid artery, either move slightly off it or gently displace it from your palpating fingers. Generally, palpation of the structures of the anterior neck is best accomplished if the client's neck is relaxed and either in a neutral position or a position of slight passive flexion. Some of the following palpations are cartilage structures, not bony landmarks.

LATERAL VIEW

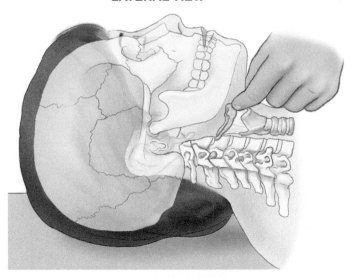

FIGURE 5-29 Hyoid bone: The **hyoid bone** is found in the anterior neck, inferior to the mandible (located at the level of the third cervical vertebra). To find the hyoid bone, begin at the mandible and move inferiorly in the anterior neck until you feel hard bony tissue. Once on the hyoid bone, ask the client to swallow, and movement of the hyoid bone will be felt. The hyoid bone is very mobile, and passively moving it from side to side is possible.

NOTE OF TRIVIA: The hyoid bone is the only bone in the human body that does not articulate (form a joint) with another bone.

LATERAL VIEW

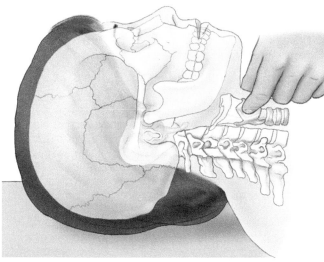

FIGURE 5-30 Thyroid cartilage: The **thyroid cartilage** is located in the anterior neck, inferior to the hyoid bone (the thyroid cartilage is located at the level of the fourth and fifth cervical vertebrae). Once the hyoid bone has been located, drop off it inferiorly; you will feel a joint space and then the thyroid cartilage will be felt. Palpate the small midline superior notch; then gently palpate both sides of the thyroid cartilage. Movement of the thyroid cartilage will be clearly felt if the client is asked to swallow. Palpation of the thyroid cartilage must be done gently and carefully because the thyroid gland often overlies part of the thyroid cartilage.

LATERAL VIEW

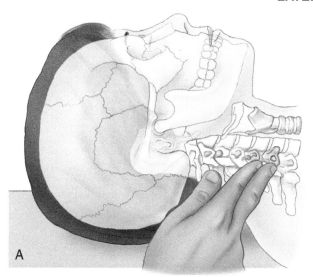

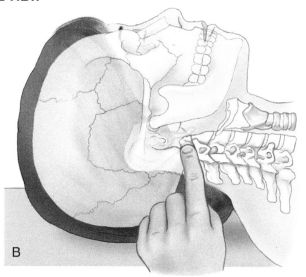

A

B

FIGURE 5-31 Transverse processes of C1 through C7: The **transverse processes (TPs)** of C2 through C7 are bifid (i.e., each TP has two points instead of one) and have **anterior tubercles** and **posterior tubercles.** These TPs may be palpated but must be palpated with gentle pressure because their tubercles are pointy; pressing the overlying musculature into them can be tender for the client. Begin by finding the carotid tubercle (anterior tubercle of the TP of C6); then palpate inferiorly and superiorly to find the other TPs. The direction of your pressure should be posterior and/or posteromedial *(A).*

The **TP of C1** (the atlas) has the widest transverse process of the cervical spine. The TP of C1 can be palpated at a point that is directly posterior to the posterior border of the ramus of the mandible, directly anterior to the mastoid process of the temporal bone, and directly inferior to the ear. In this depression of surrounding soft tissue, the hard TP of C1 will be readily palpable *(B).*

NOTES: (1) Pressure on the TP of C1 should be gentle because this landmark is often sensitive and tender to pressure, and the facial nerve (CN VII) is located nearby. (2) The TP of C1 is much more anterior than most therapists expect.

5

LATERAL VIEW

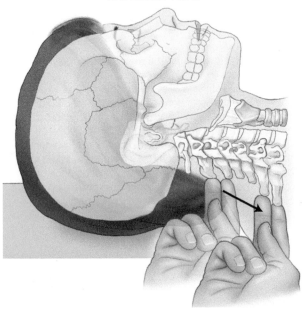

FIGURE 5-32 Spinous processes of C2 through C7: The **spinous processes (SPs)** of the cervical spine are palpated in the midline of the posterior neck. There are seven cervical vertebrae; however, not all of the cervical SPs are always palpable. Because of the lordotic curve of the spine of the neck (concave posteriorly), the SPs are often deep in the concavity and therefore difficult to palpate. The exact number of cervical SPs that can be palpated is primarily determined by the degree of the lordotic cervical curve of the client. The most prominent cervical SPs are those of C2 and C7; these two are always palpable.

Begin by finding the external occipital protuberance in the midline of the occiput. From there, drop inferiorly off the occiput onto the cervical spine; the first cervical SP that will be palpable will be the SP of C2. As with most cervical SPs, the C2 SP is bifid. It should be noted that these bifid points are not always symmetrical; one may be larger than the other. From C2, continue palpating inferiorly, feeling for additional cervical SPs.

In some individuals, the next SP that will be readily palpable will be the one on C7 at the inferior end of the cervical spine. The SP of C7 is clearly larger than the other lower cervical SPs, giving C7 the name **vertebra prominens.** In other individuals who have a decreased cervical spinal curve, palpating and counting all the SPs from C2 to C7 may be possible.

NOTE: C1 (the atlas) does not have an SP; it has what is called a posterior tubercle. To palpate the **posterior tubercle of C1**, palpate between the SP of C2 and the occiput, pressing anteriorly into the soft tissue.

LATERAL VIEW

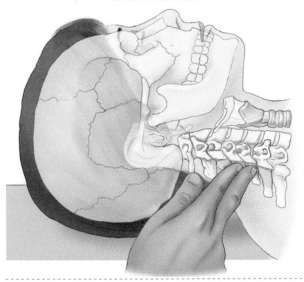

FIGURE 5-33 Laminar groove of the cervical spine: The **laminar groove** of the cervical spine is the groove that is found between the spinous processes medially and the articular processes laterally (i.e., the laminar groove overlies the laminae of the vertebrae). A number of muscles lie in the laminar groove; consequently, direct palpation of the laminae at the floor of the laminar groove is difficult. Palpate just lateral to the spinous processes and you will be in the laminar groove.

LATERAL VIEW

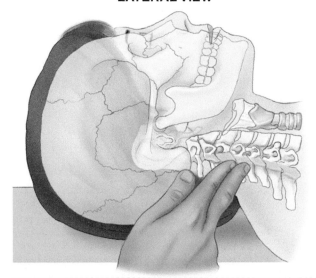

FIGURE 5-34 Articular processes (facets) of the cervical spine: The inferior and superior **articular processes** that create the **facet joints** of the cervical spine also create what is called the **articular pillar** or the **cervical pillar** because of the way they are stacked. They are easily palpable at the lateral side of the laminar groove (approximately 1 inch lateral to the spinous processes). The client must be supine and relaxed for palpation to be successful. Begin palpation at the spinous process of C2 and palpate laterally past the laminar groove and feel for the articular process of C2. Continue to palpate inferiorly until you reach the bottom of the neck.

NOTE: The articular processes of the cervical spine are an excellent contact point when performing joint mobilizations to the cervical spine.

SUPEROLATERAL VIEW

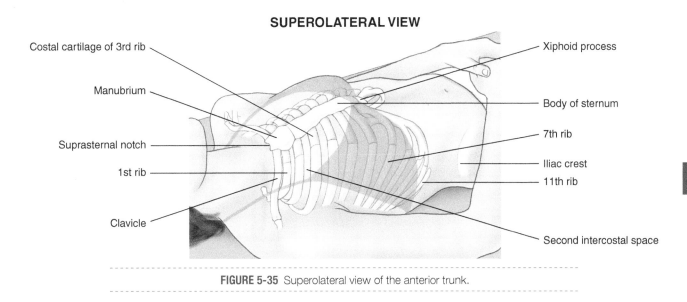

Costal cartilage of 3rd rib

Manubrium

Suprasternal notch

1st rib

Clavicle

Xiphoid process

Body of sternum

7th rib

Iliac crest

11th rib

Second intercostal space

FIGURE 5-35 Superolateral view of the anterior trunk.

SUPEROLATERAL VIEW

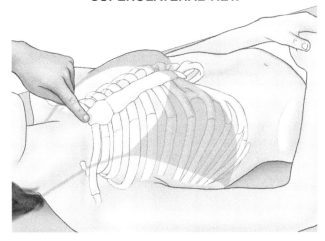

FIGURE 5-36 Suprasternal notch of the sternum: The **suprasternal notch of the manubrium of the sternum** is subcutaneous and easily palpable. Simply palpate at the superior border of the sternum, and the depression of the suprasternal notch will be readily felt between the medial ends of the two clavicles.

NOTE: The suprasternal notch is also known as the **jugular notch.**

SUPEROLATERAL VIEW

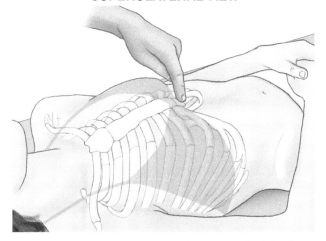

FIGURE 5-37 Xiphoid process of the sternum: The **xiphoid process of the sternum** is at the inferior end of the sternum. The xiphoid process is cartilaginous but may calcify into bone as a person ages. To locate the xiphoid process, continue palpating inferiorly along the anterior surface of the sternum until you feel the small, pointy xiphoid process at the inferior end. Because the xiphoid process is made of cartilage, exerting mild pressure on it and feeling it move are possible.

NOTE: The xiphoid process is a landmark often used to find the proper hand position to administer cardiopulmonary resuscitation (CPR).

5

SUPEROLATERAL VIEW   ANTEROLATERAL VIEW

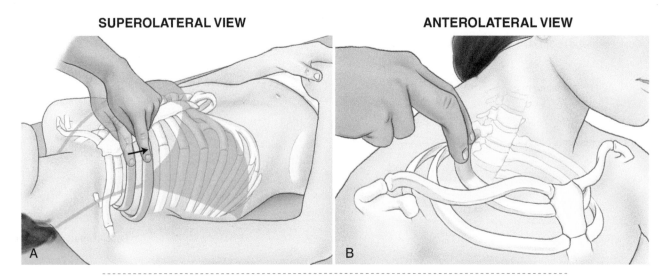

A   B

FIGURE 5-38 Anterior rib cage: The anterior side of the **rib cage** is composed of 12 **ribs,** 7 **costal cartilages** that join the ribs to the sternum, and the 11 **intercostal spaces** located between the adjacent ribs and/or costal cartilages. All ribs, costal cartilages, and intercostal spaces can be palpated anteriorly and anterolaterally (except where the breast tissue of female clients interferes with palpation). The ribs and/or costal cartilages will be sensed as hard bony/cartilaginous tissue located subcutaneously, and the intercostal spaces will be sensed as depressions of soft tissue located between the ribs and/or the costal cartilages. Once each rib has been successfully palpated, try to follow it medially and laterally for its entire course, as far as possible.

To palpate ribs 2 through 10: Palpate the anterior rib cage lateral to the sternum. Generally, for ribs 2 through 10, identifying them by strumming across them in a superior to inferior manner is easiest. The first intercostal space is inferior to the medial end of the clavicle and between the first and second ribs. From there, palpate inferiorly and count the intercostal spaces and ribs until you find the seventh costal cartilage *(A).* Because of the contour of the rib cage, continuing to palpate ribs 7 through 10 and their costal cartilages more laterally in the anterior trunk is best.

To palpate ribs 11 and 12: Ribs 11 and 12 are called *floating ribs* because they do not articulate with the sternum. They must be palpated at the bottom of the rib cage, superior to the iliac crest, in the lateral and/or posterolateral trunk. Palpating ribs 11 and 12 is easiest by pressing directly into and feeling for their pointy ends.

NOTE: This pressure should be firm but gentle because you are pressing soft tissue into the hard pointy end of a bone.

To palpate the first rib: The first rib is probably the most challenging to palpate, but it can be felt. To palpate the first rib, find the superior border of the upper trapezius muscle and then drop off it anteriorly and direct your palpatory pressure inferiorly against the first rib *(B).* Asking the client to take in a deep breath will elevate the first rib up against your palpating fingers and make palpation easier.

POSTEROLATERAL VIEW

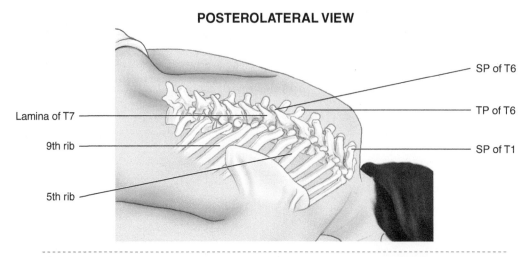

SP of T6

TP of T6

Lamina of T7

9th rib

SP of T1

5th rib

FIGURE 5-39 Superolateral view of the posterior trunk. *SP,* Sinous process; *TP,* transverse process.

POSTEROLATERAL VIEW

POSTEROLATERAL VIEW

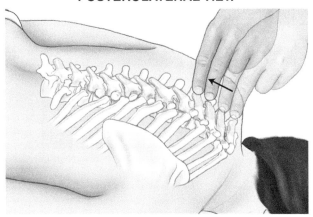

FIGURE 5-40 Spinous processes of the trunk: The spinous processes (SPs) of the 12 thoracic and 5 lumbar vertebrae are all palpable. Begin by locating the SP of C7 (also known as the *vertebra prominens*). It will usually be the first very prominent SP inferior to the SP of C2.

When the client is prone, if confusion exists as to which SP is C7, the following method will determine it. Palpate the SPs of the lower cervical spine with fingers on two or three of the prominent ones. Then passively flex and extend the client's head and neck. The SP of C6 will disappear from palpation with extension; the SP of C7 will not (i.e., the SP of C7 will be the highest SP palpable during flexion and extension).

Once the SP of C7 has been located, palpate each vertebral SP by placing your middle finger on the SP of that vertebra and your index finger in the **interspinous space** between that vertebra and the vertebra below. Continue palpating down the spine in this manner. Counting the SPs from C7 to L5 is usually possible.

NOTE: The SPs of the thoracic region are usually easily palpable because of the kyphotic thoracic spinal curve. However, palpating the lumbar SPs is a bit more challenging because of the lordotic lumbar spinal curve; to accomplish this, deeper pressure may be needed.

FIGURE 5-41 Transverse processes (TPs) of the trunk: The TPs of the trunk can be challenging to discern, but many of them can be palpated. Usually the TPs of the thoracic region can be felt approximately 1 inch lateral to the spinous processes (SPs). However, to determine the exact vertebral level of a TP can be difficult, because it is not located at the same level as the SP of the same vertebra. To determine the level of the TP that is being palpated, use the following method. Place one palpating finger on an SP, then press down onto the TPs nearby one at a time until you feel the pressure upon a TP move the SP that is under the palpating finger. The vertebral level of that TP will be the same as that of the SP that moved. This method is usually successful for the thoracic spine; palpation of the TPs of the lumbar spine is much more challenging.

LOWER EXTREMITY

OBLIQUE VIEW

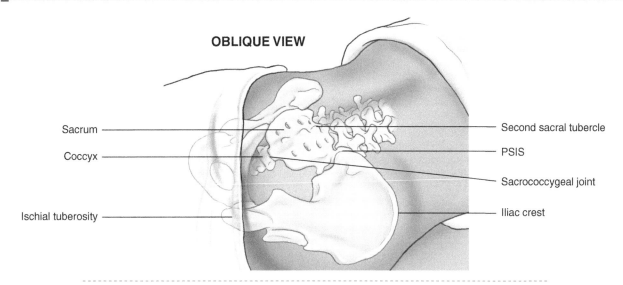

Sacrum

Coccyx

Ischial tuberosity

Second sacral tubercle

PSIS

Sacrococcygeal joint

Iliac crest

FIGURE 5-42 An inferolateral oblique view of the posterior pelvis. *PSIS,* Posterior superior iliac spine.

SUPEROLATERAL VIEW

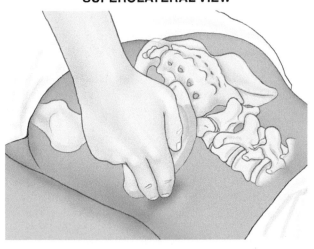

FIGURE 5-43 Iliac crest: The **iliac crest** is subcutaneous and easily palpable. With the client prone, place your palpating fingers on the iliac crest and follow it as far anterior as possible. It ends at the anterior superior iliac spine (ASIS). Then follow the iliac crest posteriorly to the posterior superior iliac spine (PSIS).

SUPEROLATERAL VIEW

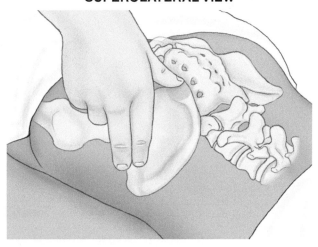

FIGURE 5-44 The posterior superior iliac spine: The **posterior superior iliac spine (PSIS)** is the most posterior aspect of the iliac crest and is usually visually prominent and easily palpable. It is located approximately 2 inches from the midline of the superior aspect (the base) of the sacrum. The PSIS is easily located because the skin drops in around the medial side of it, forming a dimple in most individuals. Visually locate the dimple first; then palpate into it, pressing slightly laterally against the PSIS.

INFEROLATERAL VIEW

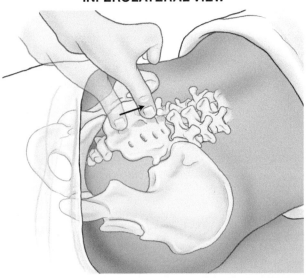

FIGURE 5-45 Sacrum: From the posterior superior iliac spine (PSIS), palpate the midline of the **sacrum**, feeling for the **sacral tubercles.** Once a sacral tubercle is located, continue palpating superiorly and inferiorly for the other sacral tubercles. The second sacral tubercle is usually at the level of the PSIS.

   NOTE: The **sacroiliac (SI) joint,** located between the sacrum and ilium on each side, is not directly palpable because of the overhang of the PSIS and the presence of the joint ligaments.

INFEROLATERAL VIEW

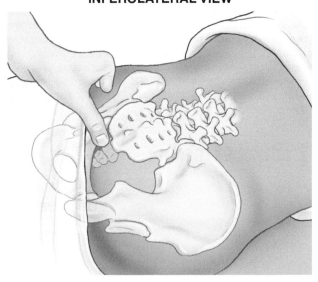

FIGURE 5-46 Coccyx: The **coccyx** is located directly inferior to the sacrum. It is subcutaneous and usually easily palpable. At the most superior aspect of the coccyx, the **sacrococcygeal joint** can usually be palpated.

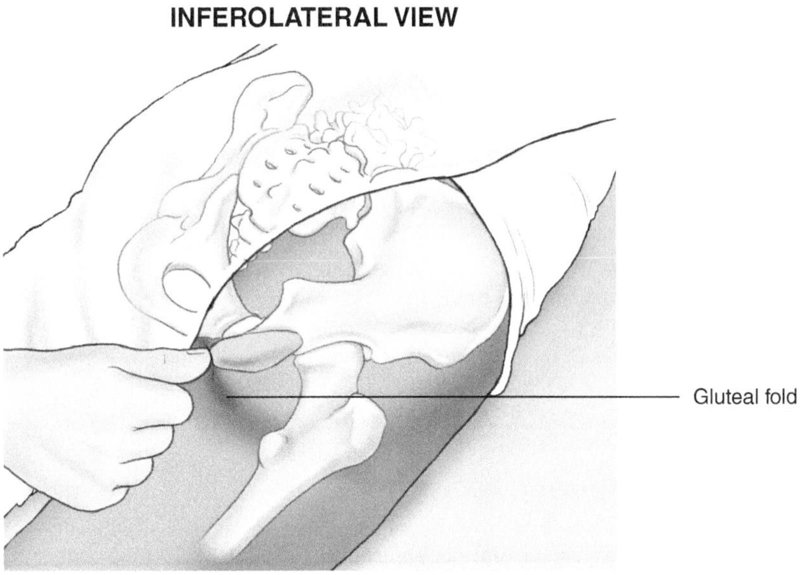

INFEROLATERAL VIEW

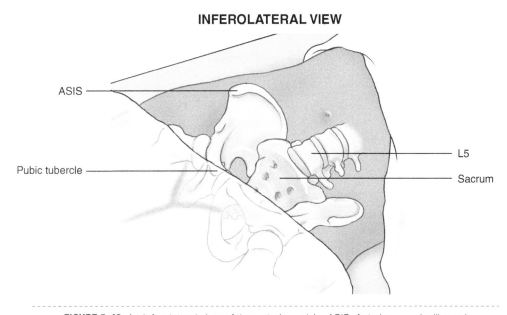

Gluteal fold

FIGURE 5-47 Ischial tuberosity: The **ischial tuberosity** is located deep to the **gluteal fold,** slightly medial to the midpoint of the buttock. Palpating it from the inferior perspective is best so that the palpating fingers do not have to palpate through the gluteus maximus. Moderate-to-deep pressure is necessary to palpate the ischial tuberosity; however, its palpation is not difficult and is usually not tender for the client. Once located, strum across the ischial tuberosity both horizontally and vertically to palpate it in its entirety.

INFEROLATERAL VIEW

ASIS

Pubic tubercle

L5

Sacrum

FIGURE 5-48 An inferolateral view of the anterior pelvis. *ASIS,* Anterior superior iliac spine.

5

INFEROLATERAL VIEW

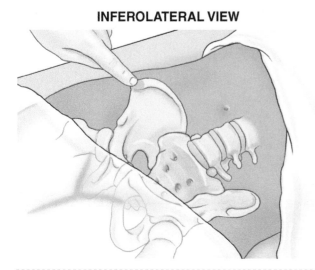

FIGURE 5-49 Anterior superior iliac spine: The **anterior superior iliac spine (ASIS)** is the most anterior aspect of the iliac crest. It is usually visually prominent and easily palpable. From the iliac crest (see Figure 5-43), continue palpating anteriorly until you reach the ASIS.

INFEROLATERAL VIEW

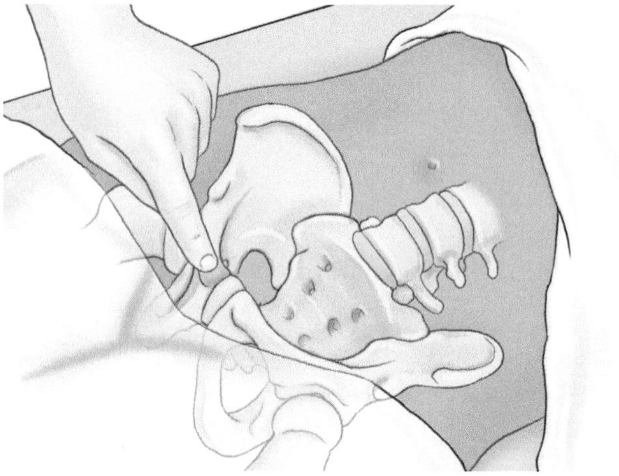

FIGURE 5-50 Pubic bone and pubic tubercle: The **pubic bone** is located at the most inferior aspect of the anterior abdomen. The **pubic tubercle** is on the anterior surface of the body of the pubic bone near the pubic symphysis joint and is at approximately the same level as the superior aspect of the greater trochanter of the femur. To locate the pubic bone, begin by palpating more superiorly on the anterior abdominal wall, then carefully and gradually palpate farther inferiorly, pressing gently into the abdominal wall until the pubic bone is felt. It helps to use the ulnar side of the hand and direct the pressure posteriorly and inferiorly. It is important that the abdominal wall muscles are relaxed so that when the pubic bone is reached, it will be readily felt.

DISTAL VIEW

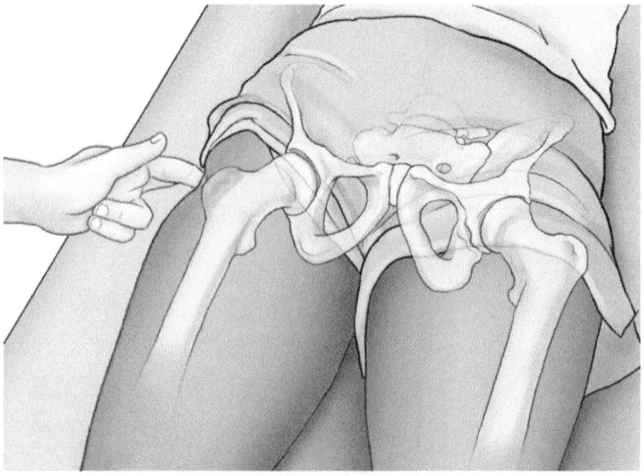

FIGURE 5-51 Greater trochanter: Begin palpation of the thigh by locating the **greater trochanter of the femur.** The greater trochanter is located in the proximal lateral thigh at approximately the same level as the public tubercle. It is fairly large (approximately 1½ × 1½ inches) and subcutaneous; hence, it is fairly easy to palpate; strum along the greater trochanter vertically and horizontally to feel the entire landmark.

DISTAL AND MEDIAL VIEW

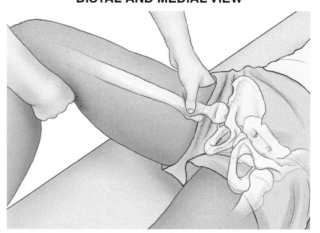

FIGURE 5-52 Lesser trochanter: The **lesser trochanter of the femur** is located in the proximal medial thigh. It is a palpable landmark but is appreciably more challenging to discern; palpating it with certainty requires more advanced palpation skills and knowledge of the psoas major muscle. To locate the lesser trochanter of the femur, the distal aspect of the psoas major muscle must be located (see page 360). Once located, follow the psoas major distally as far as possible. Then have the client relax his or her thigh in a position of flexion and lateral rotation of the thigh at the hip joint to relax and slacken the psoas major; then press in against the femur, feeling for the lesser trochanter.

DISTAL AND ANTERIOR VIEW

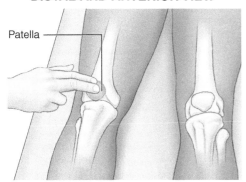

Patella

FIGURE 5-53 Patella: The **patella** (kneecap) is a prominent sesamoid bone located anterior to the distal femur. To best palpate the patella, have the client supine with the lower extremity relaxed. Palpate the entire patella, gently gliding along the patella horizontally and vertically.

ANTEROLATERAL VIEW

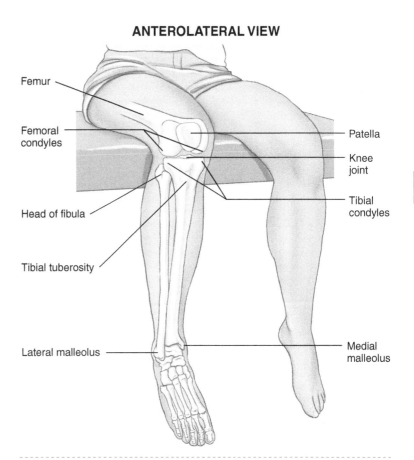

Femur

Femoral condyles

Head of fibula

Tibial tuberosity

Lateral malleolus

Patella

Knee joint

Tibial condyles

Medial malleolus

5

FIGURE 5-54 Anterolateral view of the leg with the knee joint flexed to 90 degrees.

ANTEROLATERAL VIEW

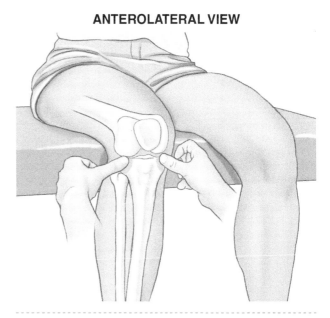

FIGURE 5-55 Femoral condyles: The inferior margins of the **medial femoral condyle** and **lateral femoral condyle** are palpable by pressing proximally up against the femur from the joint line of the knee on both sides of the patella. Once located, palpate farther proximally onto the medial and lateral **femoral condyles.**

ANTEROLATERAL VIEW

FIGURE 5-56 Tibial condyles: The superior margins of the **medial tibial condyle** and **lateral tibial condyle** are palpable by pressing distally down against the tibia from the joint line of the knee on both sides of the patella. Once located, palpate farther distally onto the medial and lateral **tibial condyles.**

5

ANTEROLATERAL VIEW

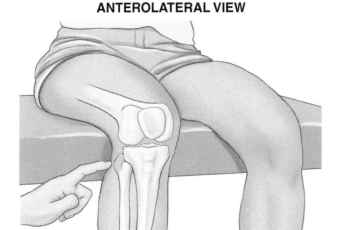

FIGURE 5-57 Head of the fibula: As you continue palpating along the superior margin of the lateral condyle of the tibia, you will reach the head of the fibula. The **head of the fibula** is the most proximal landmark of the fibula, is located on the posterolateral side of the knee, and can be palpated anteriorly, laterally, and posteriorly.

NOTE: The common fibular nerve is superficial near the head of the fibula; therefore care should be taken when palpating here.

ANTEROLATERAL VIEW

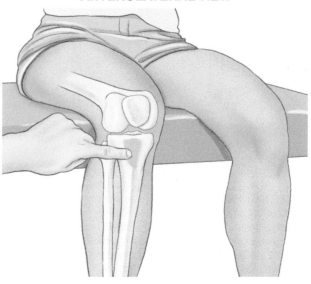

FIGURE 5-58 Tibial tuberosity: The **tibial tuberosity** is a prominent landmark located at the center of the proximal shaft of the anterior tibia, approximately 1 to 2 inches distal to the inferior margin of the patella. The quadriceps femoris muscle group attaches onto the tibial tuberosity.

ANTEROLATERAL VIEW

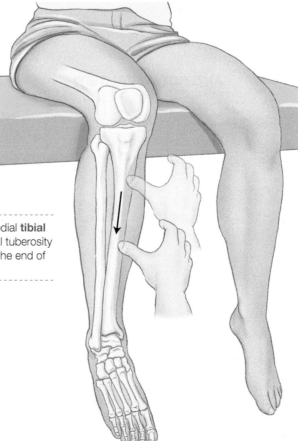

FIGURE 5-59 Tibial shaft: From the tibial tuberosity, the entire anteromedial **tibial shaft** is subcutaneous and easily palpable. Begin palpating at the tibial tuberosity and continue palpating distally until you reach the medial malleolus at the end of the anteromedial tibial shaft.

ANTEROLATERAL VIEW

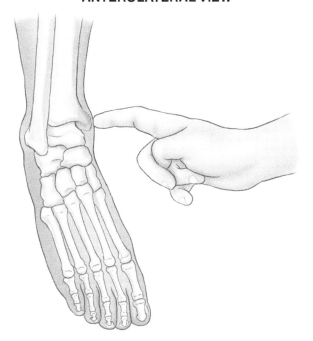

FIGURE 5-60 Medial malleolus: The **medial malleolus of the tibia** is the very prominent bony landmark at the ankle region that is located on the medial side. As you palpate down the shaft of the tibia, you will reach the medial malleolus. Palpate the circumference of this large bony landmark.

ANTEROLATERAL VIEW

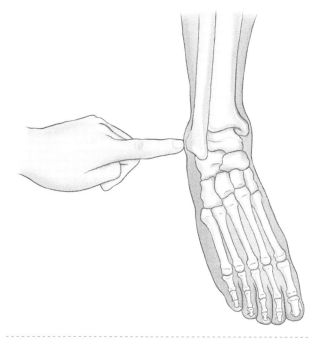

FIGURE 5-61 Lateral malleolus: The **lateral malleolus of the fibula** is the very prominent bony landmark that is located at the lateral side of the ankle region. The lateral malleolus is the distal expanded end of the fibula. Notice that the lateral malleolus of the fibula is located somewhat farther distal than is the medial malleolus of the tibia.

MEDIAL VIEW

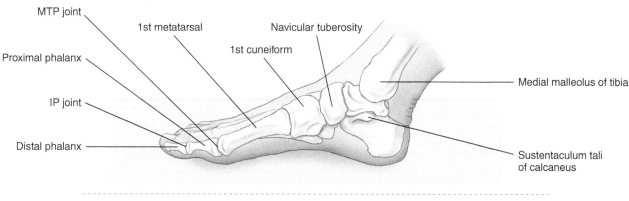

MTP joint

1st metatarsal

Navicular tuberosity

Proximal phalanx

1st cuneiform

IP joint

Distal phalanx

Medial malleolus of tibia

Sustentaculum tali of calcaneus

FIGURE 5-62 Medial view of the foot. *IP,* Interphalangeal; *MTP,* metatarsophalangeal.

5

MEDIAL VIEW

MEDIAL VIEW

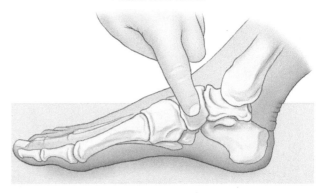

FIGURE 5-63 Sustentaculum tali of the calcaneus: From the medial malleolus of the tibia, drop your palpating finger approximately 1 inch distally; the **sustentaculum tali of the calcaneus** should be palpable. The sustentaculum tali forms a shelf upon which the talus sits. The joint line between the sustentaculum tali and the talus above is often palpable.

FIGURE 5-64 Navicular tuberosity: From the sustentaculum tali, move your palpating fingers approximately 1 inch anteriorly and the **navicular tuberosity** is quite prominent and palpable.

LATERAL VIEW

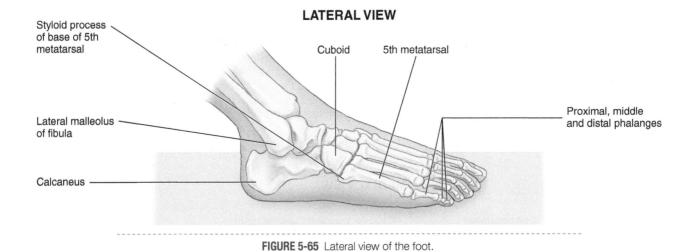

Styloid process of base of 5th metatarsal

Cuboid   5th metatarsal

Lateral malleolus of fibula

Proximal, middle and distal phalanges

Calcaneus

FIGURE 5-65 Lateral view of the foot.

LATERAL VIEW

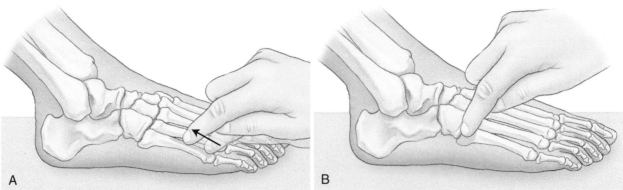

A

B

FIGURE 5-66 Fifth metatarsal: Palpate the lateral border of the foot and feel for the fifth metatarsal. The dorsal and lateral surfaces of the fifth metatarsal are readily palpable. Palpate from the expanded distal head to the middle of the shaft of the fifth metatarsal **(A).** Continue palpating proximally until you reach the large expanded proximal base **(B).** The base of the fifth metatarsal flares out and is called the **styloid process of the fifth metatarsal.**

LATERAL VIEW

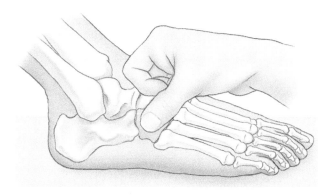

FIGURE 5-67 Cuboid: Just proximal to the fifth metatarsal along the lateral side of the foot is a depression where the **cuboid** lies. The depression is created by a combination of the flaring of the base of the fifth metatarsal (the styloid process of the fifth metatarsal) and the concave shape of the lateral border of the cuboid. Palpate with firm pressure medially into this depression and the cuboid can be felt.

PLANTAR VIEW

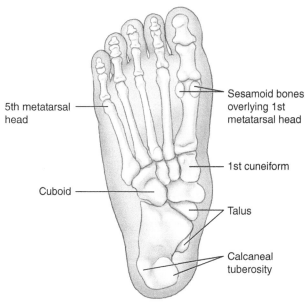

5th metatarsal head

Sesamoid bones overlying 1st metatarsal head

1st cuneiform

Cuboid

Talus

Calcaneal tuberosity

FIGURE 5-68 Plantar view of the foot.

PLANTAR VIEW

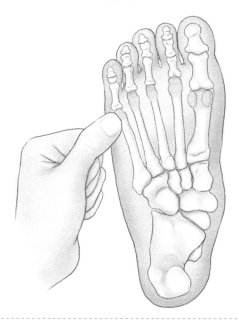

FIGURE 5-69 Metatarsal heads of toes one through five: The heads of all five metatarsals are palpable on the plantar surface of the foot. Although all five metatarsals are palpable, because of the concavity of the transverse arch of the foot, the heads of the first and fifth metatarsals are most prominent. Begin by palpating the head of the fifth metatarsal and then continue medially, palpating each of the other four metatarsal heads. Overlying the plantar surface of the head of the first metatarsal are two small **sesamoid bones.** When palpating the head of the first metatarsal on the plantar side, it is actually the two sesamoids that are felt.

PLANTAR VIEW

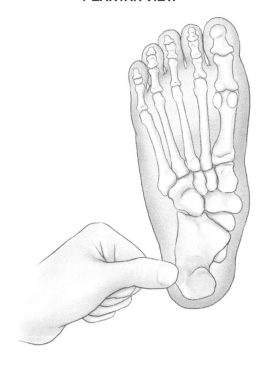

FIGURE 5-70 Calcaneal tuberosity: The **calcaneal tuberosity** can often be palpated on the plantar side of the foot. With the client's foot relaxed, palpate with firm pressure on either side of the midline of the plantar side of the calcaneus. The medial aspect of the calcaneal tuberosity is usually more prominent than the lateral aspect.

REVIEW QUESTIONS

Fill in the correct answer for each of the following questions. More study resources are provided on the Evolve website at http://evolve.elsevier.com/Muscolino/knowthebody.

1. What bony landmark of the scapula is found by dropping inferiorly off the lateral clavicle?

_____

2. What bony landmark is found at the "tip of the shoulder?"

_____

3. What bony landmarks are found at the widest points of the distal humerus near the elbow joint?

_____

_____

4. What are the two most prominent bony landmarks found on the medial side of the anterior hand?

_____

_____

5. What landmark of the temporal bone is found directly posterior to the earlobe?

_____

6. What are the two most prominent spinous processes of the cervical spine?

_____

_____

7. What bony landmark of the spine is found between the spinous processes medially and the articular processes laterally?

_____

8. What is the most posterior aspect of the iliac crest?

_____

9. What is the prominent bony landmark found at the midline of the proximal anterior tibia?

_____

10. What is the prominent bony landmark found approximately 1 inch distal to the medial malleolus of the tibia?

_____

Muscles of the Shoulder Girdle and Arm

The muscles of this chapter are involved with the motions of the shoulder girdle (scapula and clavicle), arm (humerus), and forearm (radius and ulna). The bellies of these muscles are located on the trunk, over the scapula, and on the arm. Trapezius, latissimus dorsi, and pectoralis major are large superficial muscles located on the trunk. Deltoid, triceps brachii, and biceps brachii (and to some degree the brachialis) are large superficial muscles located on the scapula and arm.

As a general rule, muscles that move the shoulder girdle have their origin (proximal attachment) on the trunk and their insertion (distal attachment) on the scapula or clavicle or both. These muscles move the scapula relative to the rib cage wall (trunk) at the scapulocostal joint and/or the clavicle at the sternoclavicular joint.

Muscles that move the arm have their origin (proximal attachment) on the trunk, clavicle, or scapula and their insertion (distal attachment) on the humerus. These muscles move the arm relative to the scapula at the glenohumeral joint.

Muscles that move the forearm have their origin (proximal attachment) on the scapula or humerus and their insertion (distal attachment) on the radius or ulna.

The companion CD at the back of this book allows you to examine the muscles of this body region, layer by layer, and individual muscle palpation technique videos are available in the Chapter 6 folder on the Evolve website.

OVERVIEW OF FUNCTION: MUSCLES OF THE SHOULDER GIRDLE

The following general rules regarding actions can be stated for the functional groups of muscles of the shoulder girdle:
- If a muscle attaches to the scapula and its other attachment is superior to the scapula, it can elevate the scapula at the scapulocostal joint.
- If a muscle attaches to the scapula and its other attachment is inferior to the scapula, it can depress the scapula at the scapulocostal joint.
- If a muscle attaches to the scapula and its other attachment is medial to the scapula on the posterior side (i.e., closer to the spine), it can retract (adduct) the scapula at the scapulocostal joint.

■ If a muscle attaches to the scapula and its other attachment is lateral to the scapula (i.e., closer to the anterior surface of the body), it can protract (abduct) the scapula at the scapulocostal joint. If a muscle attaches to the scapula away from the axis of scapular rotation (i.e., off axis), it can rotate the scapula either upwardly or downwardly at the scapulocostal joint. The rotation that the scapula performs depends on where it attaches.

■ Any muscle that moves the scapula at the scapulocostal joint can do the same motion of the clavicle at the sternoclavicular joint (and vice versa).

■ Reverse actions of these standard (typical) mover actions involve the scapula being fixed and the other attachment moving toward the scapula at the scapulocostal joint.*

OVERVIEW OF FUNCTION: MUSCLES OF THE GLENOHUMERAL JOINT

The following general rules regarding actions can be stated for the functional groups of muscles of the glenohumeral joint:

■ If a muscle crosses the glenohumeral joint anteriorly with a vertical direction to its fibers, it can flex the arm at the glenohumeral joint by moving the anterior surface of the arm toward the scapula.

■ If a muscle crosses the glenohumeral joint posteriorly with a vertical direction to its fibers, it can extend the arm at the glenohumeral joint by moving the posterior surface of the arm toward the scapula.

■ If a muscle crosses the glenohumeral joint laterally (superiorly, over the top of the joint), it can abduct the arm at the glenohumeral joint by moving the lateral surface of the arm toward the scapula.

■ If a muscle crosses the glenohumeral joint medially (inferiorly, below the center of the joint), it can adduct the arm at the glenohumeral joint by moving the medial surface of the arm toward the scapula.

■ Medial rotators of the arm wrap around the humerus from medial to lateral, anterior to the glenohumeral joint.

■ Lateral rotators of the arm wrap around the humerus from medial to lateral, posterior to the glenohumeral joint.

■ Reverse actions of these standard (typical) mover actions involve the scapula being moved relative to the humerus at the glenohumeral joint (the scapula will also be moved relative to the rib cage at the scapulocostal joint). These reverse actions are usually either rotation or tilt actions of the scapula.*

OVERVIEW OF FUNCTION: MUSCLES OF THE ELBOW AND RADIOULNAR JOINTS

The following general rules regarding actions can be stated for the functional groups of muscles of the elbow and radioulnar joints:

■ If a muscle crosses the elbow joint anteriorly with a vertical direction to its fibers, it can flex the forearm at the elbow joint by moving the anterior surface of the forearm toward the anterior surface of the arm.

■ If a muscle crosses the elbow joint posteriorly with a vertical direction to its fibers, it can extend the forearm at the elbow joint by moving the posterior surface of the forearm toward the posterior surface of the arm.

■ Reverse actions at the elbow joint involve moving the arm toward the forearm at the elbow joint. This movement usually occurs when the hand (and therefore the forearm) is fixed by holding onto an immovable object.*

■ If a muscle crosses the radioulnar joints anteriorly with a horizontal orientation to its fibers, it will pronate the forearm at the radioulnar joints by crossing the radius over the ulna.

■ If a muscle crosses the radioulnar joints posteriorly with a horizontal direction to its fibers, it will supinate the forearm at the radioulnar joints by moving the radius to be parallel with the ulna.

■ Reverse actions of these standard (typical) mover actions at the radioulnar joints involve moving the ulna toward the radius at the radioulnar joints. This movement usually occurs when the hand (and therefore the radius) is fixed by holding onto an immovable object.*

---

*A standard (typical) mover action is when the insertion (distal attachment) moves toward the origin (proximal attachment). A reverse mover action occurs when the origin moves toward the insertion.

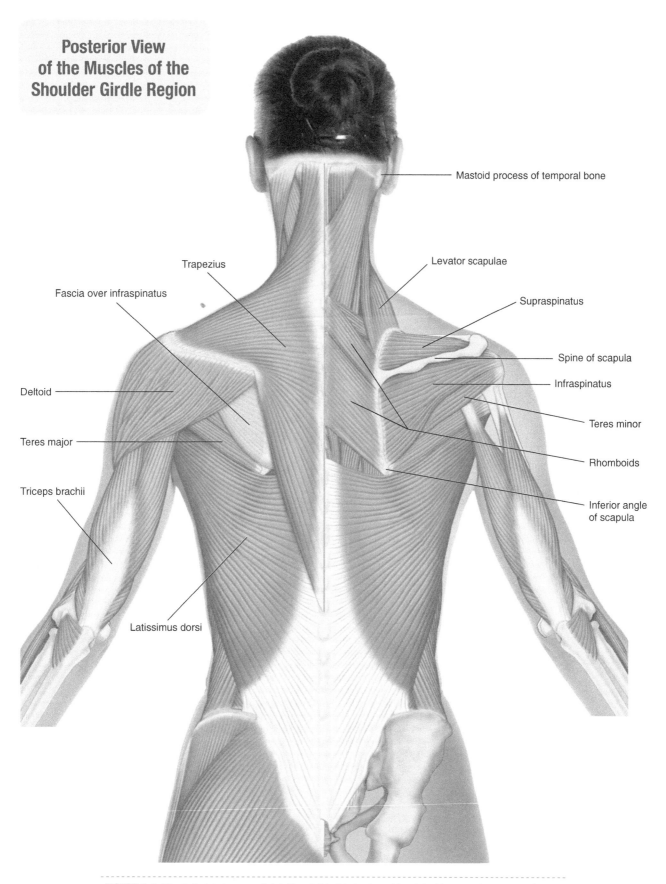

Posterior View of the Muscles of the Shoulder Girdle Region

Mastoid process of temporal bone

Trapezius

Levator scapulae

Fascia over infraspinatus

Supraspinatus

Spine of scapula

Deltoid

Infraspinatus

Teres major

Teres minor

Rhomboids

Triceps brachii

Inferior angle of scapula

Latissimus dorsi

FIGURE 6-1 The left side is superficial. The right side is deep (the deltoid, trapezius, sternocleido-mastoid, and infraspinatus fascia have been removed).

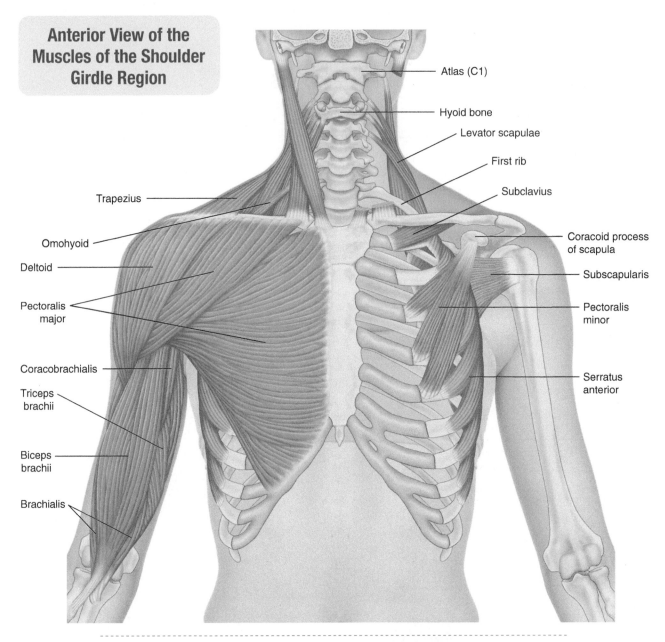

Anterior View of the Muscles of the Shoulder Girdle Region

Atlas (C1)

Hyoid bone

Levator scapulae

First rib

Subclavius

Coracoid process of scapula

Subscapularis

Pectoralis minor

Serratus anterior

Trapezius

Omohyoid

Deltoid

Pectoralis major

Coracobrachialis

Triceps brachii

Biceps brachii

Brachialis

FIGURE 6-2 The right side is superficial. The left side is deep (the deltoid, pectoralis major, trapezius, scalenes, omohyoid, and muscles of the arm have been removed; the sternocleidomastoid has been cut).

6

Right Lateral View of the Muscles of the Shoulder Girdle Region

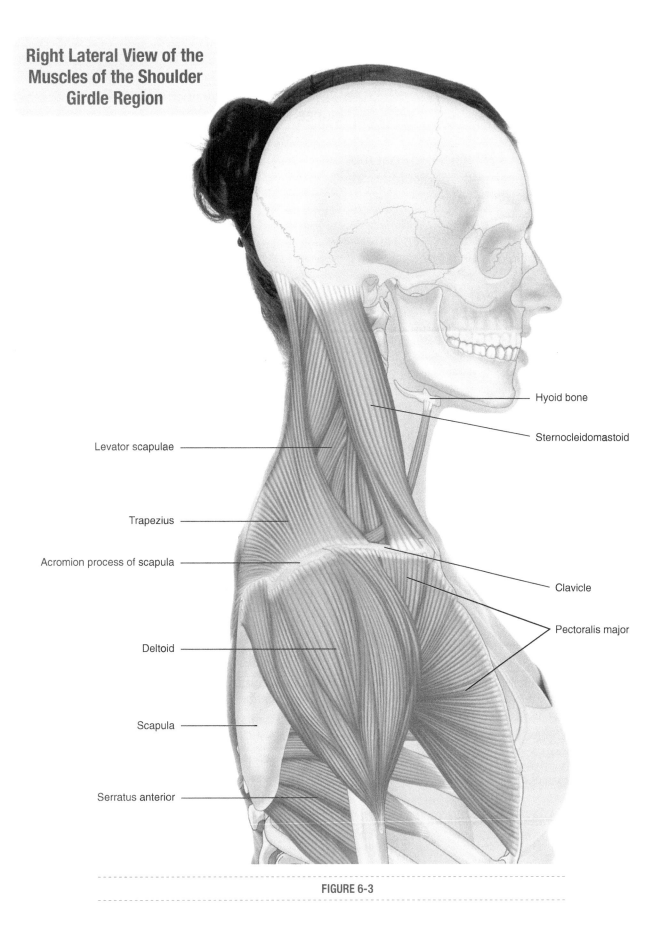

Hyoid bone

Sternocleidomastoid

Levator scapulae

Trapezius

Acromion process of scapula

Clavicle

Deltoid

Pectoralis major

Scapula

Serratus anterior

FIGURE 6-3

SHOULDER GIRDLE AND ARM
Trapezius

Pronunciation **tra-PEE-zee-us**

The trapezius is a broad flat superficial muscle that overlies the neck and middle and upper back. It is considered to have three parts: upper, middle, and lower. The trapezius is functionally important for neck and shoulder girdle motions (Figure 6-4).

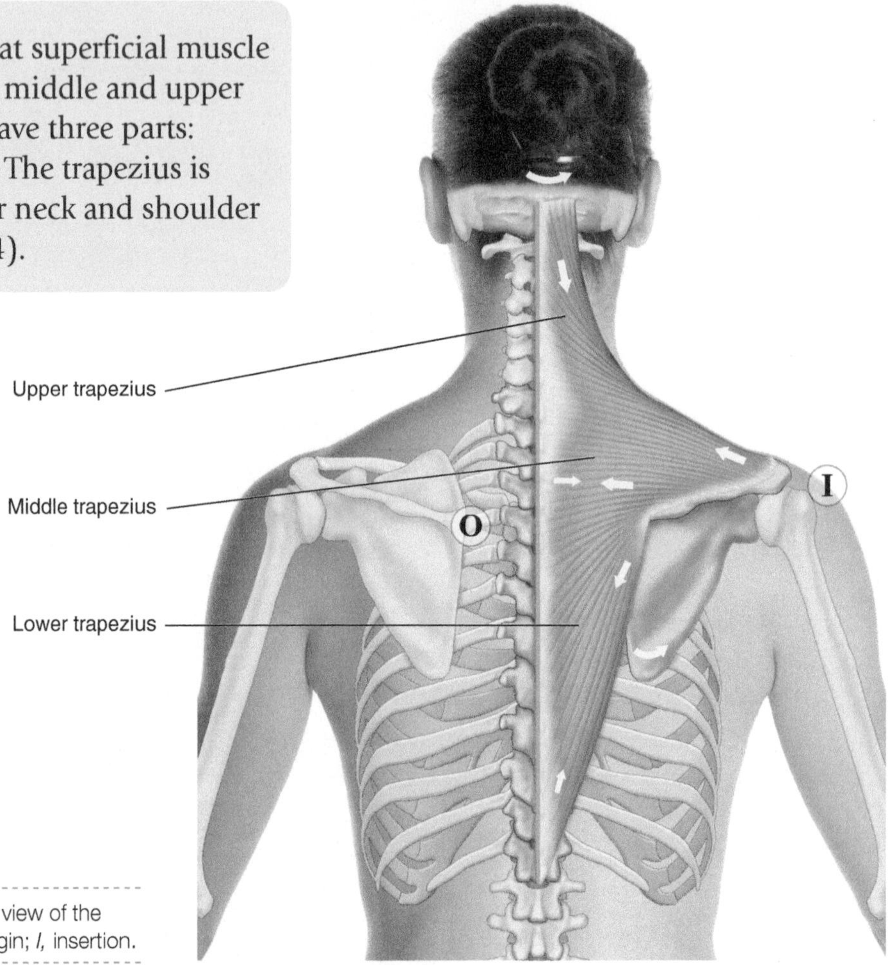

FIGURE 6-4 Posterior view of the right trapezius. *O*, Origin; *I*, insertion.

Upper trapezius

Middle trapezius

Lower trapezius

WHAT'S IN A NAME?

The name, *trapezius,* tells us that this muscle is shaped similar to a trapezoid (▱).

✳ **Derivation:**
   trapezius: Gr. a little table (or trapezoid shape)

ATTACHMENTS

Origin (Proximal/Medial Attachment)

■ External occipital protuberance, medial one third of the superior nuchal line of the occiput, nuchal ligament, and spinous processes of C7-T12

Insertion (Distal/Lateral Attachment)

■ Lateral one third of the clavicle, acromion process, and spine of the scapula

ACTIONS

The trapezius moves the scapula at the scapulocostal joint and moves the head and neck at the spinal joints.

Upper Fibers

■ Elevate the scapula.
■ Upwardly rotate the scapula.
■ Retract the scapula.
■ Extend the head and neck.
■ Laterally flex the head and neck.
■ Contralaterally rotate the head and neck.

Middle Fibers

■ Retract the scapula.

Lower Fibers

■ Depress the scapula.
■ Upwardly rotate the scapula.

STABILIZATION

1. Stabilizes the shoulder girdle.

2. Stabilizes the head, neck, and trunk.

   Stabilization Function Note: The upper trapezius is extremely important for stabilizing the shoulder girdle when the arm is abducted and/or flexed at the glenohumeral joint.

INNERVATION

- Spinal accessory nerve (cranial nerve [CN] XI)

PALPATION

1. Ask the client to lie prone with the arm resting on the table at the side of the body.

2. To palpate the lower and middle trapezius, place the palpating finger pads just lateral to the lower and middle thoracic spine. Then ask the client to abduct the arm to 90 degrees with the elbow joint extended; and slightly retract the scapula by pinching the shoulder blade toward the spine. Adding gentle resistance to the client's arm abduction with your support hand is usually helpful. Palpate perpendicular to the fibers between the spine and scapula (Figure 6-5, *A*).

3. To palpate the upper trapezius, ask the client to extend the head slightly. Look for the engagement of the upper trapezius and palpate it in the neck up to its occipital attachment (Figure 6-5, *B*).

4. Note that the upper trapezius is quite narrow; it only attaches to the medial one third of the superior nuchal line of the occiput. The semispinalis capitis muscle, the largest muscle in the neck, is deep to the upper trapezius.

TREATMENT CONSIDERATIONS

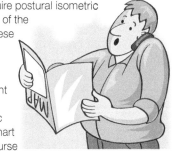

- Many positions require postural isometric contraction overuse of the upper trapezius. These positions include holding the head inclined anteriorly when working in front of the body using a hand-held electronic device such as a smart phone, carrying a purse or bag on the shoulder (regardless of the weight), crimping a telephone between the ear and the shoulder, holding the arm outward in an abducted position, or carrying a heavy weight in the hand.

- Weakness of the trapezius can contribute to the condition of rounded/slumped shoulders.

- Because the greater occipital nerve pierces through the upper trapezius, when the upper trapezius is tight, it can compress this nerve, which causes a tension headache. This condition is also known as *greater occipital neuralgia*.

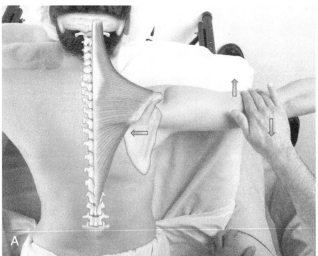
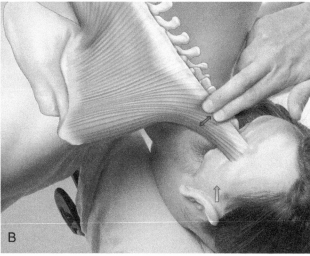

FIGURE 6-5 *A,* To engage the entire right trapezius, the client abducts the arm at the glenohumeral joint (resistance can be added as shown) and slightly retracts the scapula at the scapulocostal joint. ***B,*** Palpation of the upper trapezius is shown. Asking the client to extend the head and neck slightly at the spinal joints facilitates palpation of the upper trapezius. For all three parts of the trapezius, palpate by strumming perpendicular to the fiber direction as shown.

SHOULDER GIRDLE AND ARM
Rhomboid Major; Rhomboid Minor

Pronunciation · **ROM-boyd MAY-jor** • **ROM-boyd MY-nor**

The rhomboid muscles are located in the interscapular region between the spine and the scapula, deep to the trapezius and superficial to the erector spinae and transversospinalis musculature (Figure 6-6).

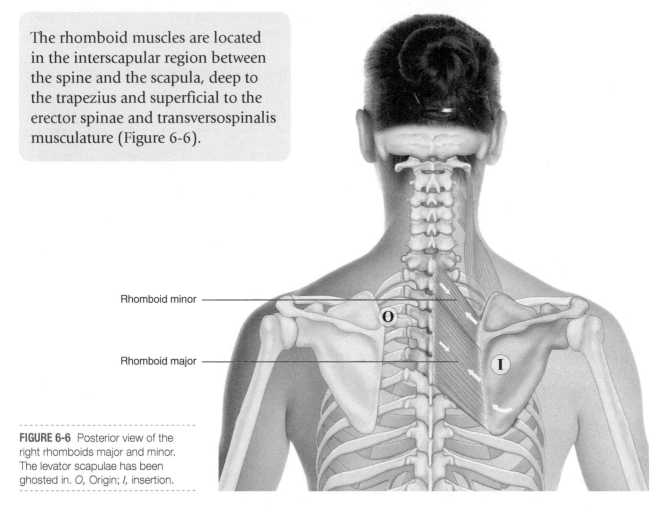

Rhomboid minor

Rhomboid major

FIGURE 6-6 Posterior view of the right rhomboids major and minor. The levator scapulae has been ghosted in. *O,* Origin; *I,* insertion.

WHAT'S IN A NAME?

The name, *rhomboids,* tells us that these muscles have the geometric shape of a rhombus (a parallelogram or diamond shape). Major and minor tell us that the rhomboid major is larger than the rhomboid minor.

✳ **Derivation:**
rhomb: Gr. rhombos (geometric shape)
oid: Gr. shape, resemblance
major: L. larger
minor: L. smaller

ATTACHMENTS

Origin (Proximal/Medial Attachment)
- Minor: spinous processes of C7-T1
- Major: spinous processes of T2-T5

Insertion (Distal/Lateral Attachment)
- Minor: medial border of the scapula at the root of the spine of the scapula
- Major: medial border of the scapula between the root of the spine and the inferior angle of the scapula

ACTIONS

The rhomboids move the scapula at the scapulocostal joint. Upper fibers:

- Retract the scapula.
- Elevate the scapula.
- Downwardly rotate the scapula.

STABILIZATION

1. Stabilize the shoulder girdle.
2. Stabilize the C7-T5 vertebrae.

INNERVATION

- Dorsal scapular nerve

PALPATION

1. Ask the client to lie prone or sit with the hand resting in the small of the back.
2. Ask the client to lift the hand away from the small of the back.
3. First look for the lower border of the rhomboids to become visible; then palpate the rhomboids between the spine and scapula (Figure 6-7).

TREATMENT CONSIDERATIONS

- *Rounded/slumped shoulders* is a common postural condition in which the scapulas are protracted (abducted) and depressed and the arms are medially rotated. Considering the rhomboids' actions of both retraction and elevation of the scapula, when they are weak, they can contribute to this common condition because they are unable to oppose efficiently the tight protractors and depressors of the scapula (pectoralis muscles).

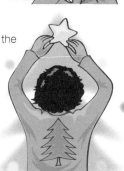

- The rhomboids often blend into the serratus anterior on the anterior side of the scapula; they are both part of the spiral line myofascial meridian.

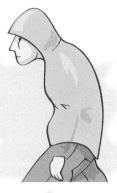

- A good way to remember the direction of fibers of the rhomboids is to think of them as the "Christmas Tree Muscles."

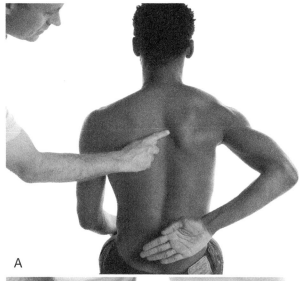

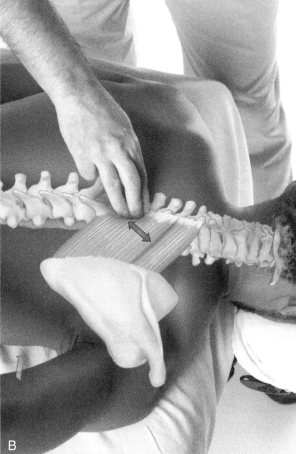

FIGURE 6-7 *A,* The inferior border of the rhomboids is often visible. *B,* Palpate perpendicular to the fiber direction of the rhomboids.

SHOULDER GIRDLE AND ARM
Levator Scapulae

Pronunciation **le-VAY-tor SKAP-you-lee**

The levator scapulae is a muscle of the shoulder girdle and neck. At its scapular attachment, it is located deep to the trapezius; at its spinal attachment, it is located deep to the sternocleidomastoid; its mid belly is superficial in the posterior triangle of the neck (Figure 6-8).

Levator scapulae

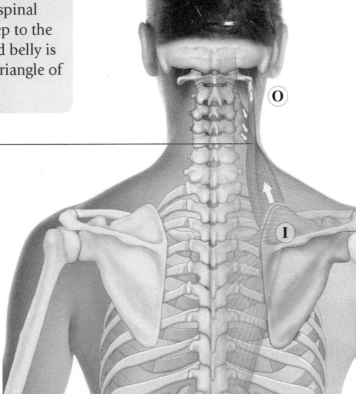

FIGURE 6-8 Posterior view of the right levator scapulae. The trapezius has been ghosted in. *O*, Origin; *I*, insertion.

WHAT'S IN A NAME?

The name, *levator scapulae*, tells us that this muscle elevates the scapula.

* **Derivation:**
  levator: L. lifter
  scapulae: L. of the scapula

ATTACHMENTS

Origin (Proximal/Superior Attachment)
■ Transverse processes of C1-C4

Insertion (Distal/Inferior Attachment)
■ Medial border of the scapula, between the superior angle and the root of the spine of the scapula

ACTIONS

The levator scapulae moves the scapula at the scapulocostal joint and moves the neck at the spinal joints.

■ Elevates the scapula.
■ Downwardly rotates the scapula.
■ Extends the neck.
■ Laterally flexes the neck.
■ Ipsilaterally rotates the neck

STABILIZATION

1. Stabilizes the shoulder girdle.
2. Stabilizes the upper cervical spinal joints.

INNERVATION

- Dorsal scapular nerve

PALPATION

1. Ask the client to lie prone or sit with the hand resting in the small of the back (Figure 6-9, *A*). Place palpating finger pads immediately superior to the superior angle of the scapula.

2. Ask the client to perform a gentle, very short range of motion of elevation of the scapula and feel for the levator scapulae deep to the trapezius (Figure 6-9, *B*).

3. Continue palpating superiorly until you are off the trapezius and in the posterior triangle of the neck. Now you can ask the client to elevate the scapula more forcefully (Figure 6-9, *C*).

4. Follow superiorly and anteriorly toward the transverse processes of C1-C4.

   Note: The transverse process of C1 is immediately inferior to the ear.

TREATMENT CONSIDERATIONS

- Many positions require postural isometric contraction overuse of the levator scapulae. These positions include holding the head inclined anteriorly when working in front of the body using a hand-held electronic device such as a "smart phone," carrying a purse or bag on the shoulder (regardless of the weight), crimping a telephone between the ear and shoulder, or carrying a heavy weight in the hand.

- The levator scapulae often becomes tight and visible in middle and older age as it contracts to maintain the posture of the upper neck and head.

- At approximately the midpoint of the levator scapulae, a twist in the fibers creates an increased density that may be mistaken for a trigger point.

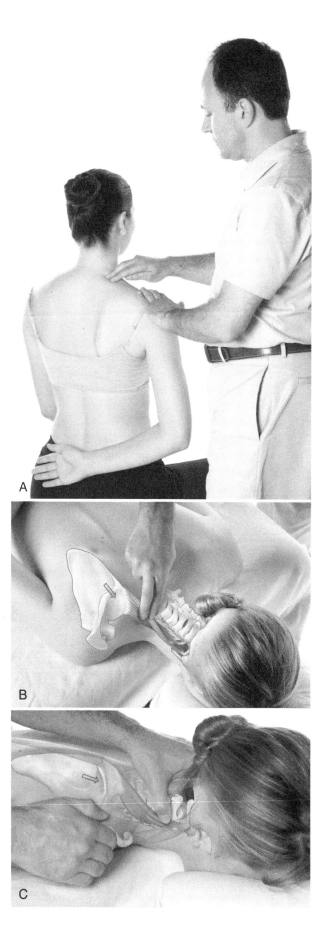

FIGURE 6-9 *A,* The levator scapulae can be easily palpated with the client seated. ***B,*** Palpation near the superior angle of the scapula is shown (where the levator scapulae is deep to the trapezius). ***C,*** Palpation is shown where the levator scapulae is superficial in the posterior triangle of the neck.

6

SHOULDER GIRDLE AND ARM
Serratus Anterior

Pronunciation **ser-A-tus an-TEE-ri-or**

The serratus anterior is a broad muscle that is located between the scapula and rib cage wall (along with the subscapularis). It hugs the rib cage wall and is superficial on the lateral rib cage wall, below the axilla (armpit) (Figure 6-10). When well developed, its slips of tissue look similar to ribs.

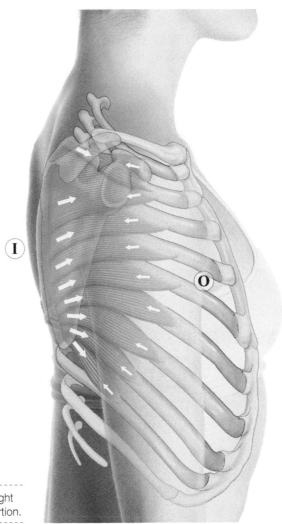

FIGURE 6-10 Lateral view of the right serratus anterior. *O,* Origin; *I,* insertion.

WHAT'S IN A NAME?

The name, *serratus anterior,* tells us that this muscle has a serrated appearance and is anterior (to the serratus posterior superior and serratus posterior inferior)

＊ **Derivation:**
  serratus: L. notching
  anterior: L. in front

ATTACHMENTS

Origin (Proximal/Anterior Attachment)
- Ribs one through nine

Insertion (Distal/Posterior Attachment)
- Anterior surface of the entire medial border of the scapula

ACTIONS

The serratus anterior moves the scapula at the scapulo-costal joint:

- Protracts the scapula.
- Upwardly rotates the scapula.

STABILIZATION

1. Stabilizes the shoulder girdle.
2. Stabilizes the rib cage.

> Stabilization Function Note: The serratus anterior stabilizes the scapula to prevent winging (lateral tilt) of the scapula.

INNERVATION

- Long thoracic nerve

PALPATION

1. The client is supine with the arm straight up in the air pointed toward the ceiling; place the finger pads against the lateral rib cage wall, directly inferior to the axilla (armpit).

2. Resist the client from reaching the hand toward the ceiling (Figure 6-11, *A*).

3. Palpate the serratus anterior where it is superficial on the rib cage (Figure 6-11, *B*); then palpate the rest of the muscle, reaching deep to the pectoralis major and the scapula.

TREATMENT CONSIDERATIONS

- When weak, the serratus anterior can contribute to winging (lateral tilt) of the scapula.

- The serratus anterior usually blends into the rhomboids on the anterior side of the scapula.

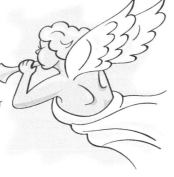

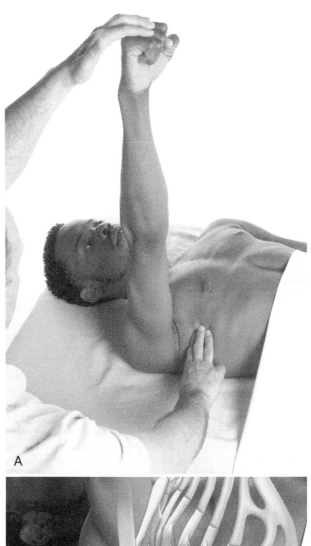

A

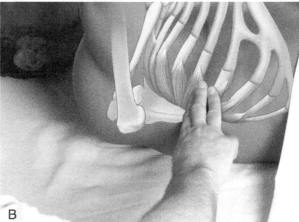

B

FIGURE 6-11 *A,* Starting position for supine palpation of the right serratus anterior. *B,* Palpation of the right serratus anterior against the lateral rib cage wall.

SHOULDER GIRDLE AND ARM: Pectoralis Group
Pectoralis Major; Pectoralis Minor

Pronunciation   **PEK-to-ra-lis MAY-jor • PEK-to-ra-lis MY-nor**

The pectoralis major and minor muscles are located in the pectoral (chest) region. The pectoralis major is considered to have two heads, a clavicular head and a sternocostal head; it is superficial, attaches to the arm, and creates the anterior axillary fold of tissue that borders the axilla (the armpit) anteriorly. The pectoralis minor is deep to the pectoralis major and attaches to the scapula (Figure 6-12).

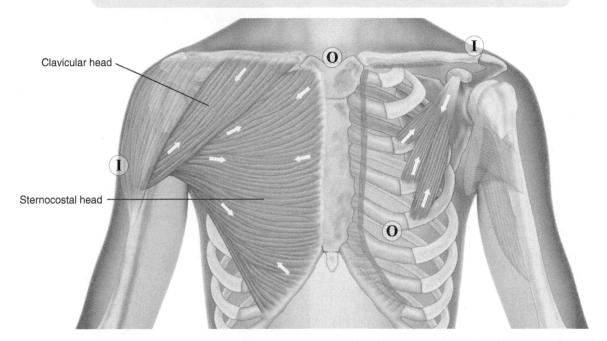

FIGURE 6-12 Anterior view of the right pectoralis major and left pectoralis minor. The deltoid has been ghosted in on the right side. The coracobrachialis and cut pectoralis major have been ghosted in on the left side. *O,* Origin; *I,* insertion.

WHAT'S IN A NAME?

The name, *pectoralis,* tells us that these muscles are located in the pectoral (chest) region. Major and minor tell us that the pectoralis major is larger than the pectoralis minor.

❋ **Derivation:**
pectoralis: L. refers to the chest
major: L. larger
minor: L. smaller

ATTACHMENTS

Pectoralis Major

Origin (Proximal/Medial Attachment)
■ Medial clavicle, sternum, and the costal cartilages of ribs one through seven

Insertion (Distal/Lateral Attachment)
■ Lateral lip of the bicipital groove of the humerus

Pectoralis Minor

Origin (Proximal/Anterior Attachment)
■ Ribs three through five

Insertion (Distal/Posterior Attachment)
■ Coracoid process of the scapula

ACTIONS

Pectoralis Major

The pectoralis major moves the arm at the glenohumeral joint and moves the scapula at the scapulocostal joint.

- Adducts the arm (entire muscle).
- Medially rotates the arm (entire muscle).
- Flexes the arm (clavicular fibers).
- Extends the arm (sternocostal fibers).
- Protracts the scapula.

PECTORALIS MAJOR STABILIZATION

1. Stabilizes the glenohumeral joint.
2. Stabilizes the shoulder girdle.

Pectoralis Minor

The pectoralis minor moves the scapula at the scapulocostal joint and moves the ribs at the sternocostal and costospinal joints.

- Protracts the scapula.
- Depresses the scapula.
- Downwardly rotates the scapula.
- Elevates ribs three through five.

PECTORALIS MINOR STABILIZATION

1. Stabilizes the shoulder girdle.
2. Stabilizes ribs three through five.

INNERVATION

- Medial and lateral pectoral nerves

   Note: The medial and lateral pectoral nerves innervate both the pectoralis major and minor.

PALPATION

Pectoralis Major

1. Client is supine with the arm resting at the side.
2. To palpate the sternocostal head, place palpating finger pads over the lower aspect of the anterior axillary fold of tissue. Ask the client to adduct the arm against resistance and feel for the contraction of the sternocostal head; palpate toward its proximal (medial) attachment (Figure 6-13, *A*).

3. To palpate the clavicular head, place palpating finger pads just inferior to the medial clavicle. Ask the client to move the arm obliquely between flexion and adduction against resistance and feel for the contraction of the clavicular head; palpate toward the distal attachment (Figure 6-13, *B*)

Pectoralis Minor

1. Client is supine with the hand under the body in the small of the back or seated with the hand in the small of the back. Place palpating finger pads just inferior to the coracoid process of the scapula.
2. Ask the client to press the hand and forearm down against the table if supine or move the hand posteriorly away from the small of the back if seated; feel for the contraction of the pectoralis minor through the pectoralis major (Figure 6-14, *A-B*).
3. Palpate to the rib attachments, strumming perpendicular to the fibers.

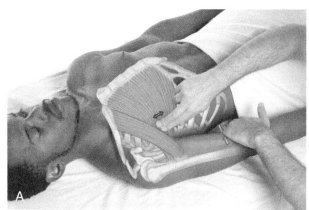

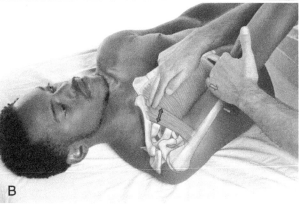

FIGURE 6-13 Palpation of the right pectoralis major. *A,* Palpation of the sternocostal head is demonstrated as the client performs adduction against resistance. *B,* Palpation of the clavicular head is demonstrated as the client performs an oblique plane motion of flexion and adduction against resistance.

Turn page to more.

6

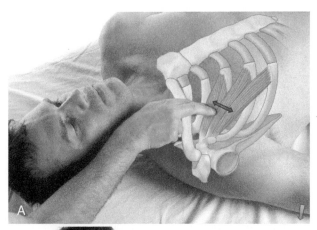

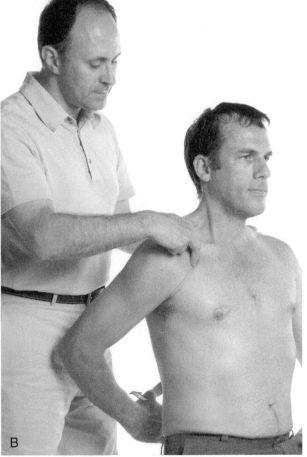

TREATMENT CONSIDERATIONS

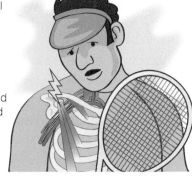

- If the pectoralis muscles are tight, they pull the shoulder girdle into protraction, causing the postural condition known as *rounded/slumped shoulders*.

- The brachial plexus of nerves and the subclavian artery and vein are sandwiched between the pectoralis minor and the rib cage. Therefore this region is a common entrapment site for these nerves and blood vessels. If the pectoralis minor is tight, then these vessels and nerves may be compressed and the condition is called *pectoralis minor syndrome*—one of the three types of *thoracic outlet syndrome*.

- A tight pectoralis minor, by rounding the shoulders, can also contribute to the clavicle dropping toward the first rib, causing compression of the brachial plexus of nerves and subclavian artery and vein. This occurrence is called *costoclavicular syndrome*—one of the three types of *thoracic outlet syndrome*.

FIGURE 6-14 *A,* Palpation of the right pectoralis minor is perpendicular to the fibers as the client presses the hand and forearm down against the table. ***B,*** Having the client seated is the easiest position for palpating the pectoralis minor, because the client can comfortably place the hand in the small of the back and move it posteriorly when asked to do so.

Detour to Subclavius

Pronunciation **sub-KLAY-vee-us**

The subclavius is a small muscle located between the clavicle and first rib, deep to the pectoralis major (Figure 6-15).

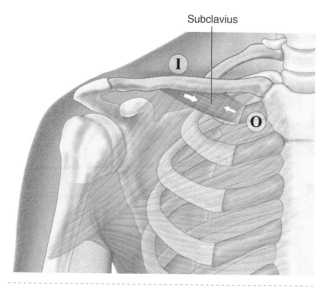

FIGURE 6-15 Anterior view of the right subclavius. The pectoralis major has been ghosted in. *O*, Origin; *I*, insertion.

WHAT'S IN A NAME?

The name, *subclavius,* tells us that this muscle is under (inferior to) the clavicle.

✳ **Derivation**
   sub: L. under
   clavius: L. key

ATTACHMENTS

Origin (Proximal/Inferior Attachment)
■ First rib

Insertion (Distal/Superior Attachment)
■ Clavicle

ACTIONS

The subclavius moves the clavicle at the sternoclavicular joint and moves the first rib at the sternocostal and costospinal joints.

■ Depresses the clavicle.

■ Elevates the first rib.

STABILIZATION

Stabilizes the clavicle and first rib.

INNERVATION

■ Nerve from the brachial plexus

PALPATION

1. Client is supine with the arm adducted and resting on the chest.

2. Curl the palpating fingers around the clavicle so that the finger pads are on the inferior surface of the clavicle; feel for the subclavius (Figure 6-16).

3. To palpate while engaged, ask the client to depress the shoulder girdle; feel for the contraction of the subclavius.

TREATMENT CONSIDERATION

■ If the subclavius is tight, it can pull the clavicle and first rib toward each other, causing compression of the brachial plexus of nerves and the subclavian artery and vein. This condition is called *costoclavicular syndrome*—one of the three types of *thoracic outlet syndrome.*

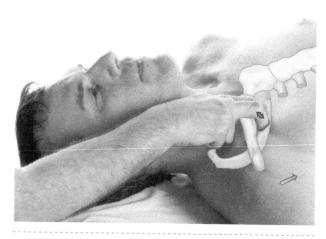

FIGURE 6-16 Palpation of the right subclavius is visualized as the client depresses the shoulder girdle.

SHOULDER GIRDLE AND ARM
Latissimus Dorsi (Lat); Teres Major

Pronunciation   **la-TIS-i-mus DOOR-si • TE-reez MAY-jor**

The latissimus dorsi commonly known as the *lat*, is a broad flat superficial muscle of the back that attaches to the arm. The teres major, often referred to as the *lat's helper*, is a thick round muscle that runs parallel to the lat. Together, they form the posterior axillary fold of tissue that borders the axilla (armpit) posteriorly (Figure 6-17). In the armpit, the teres major is deep to the lat.

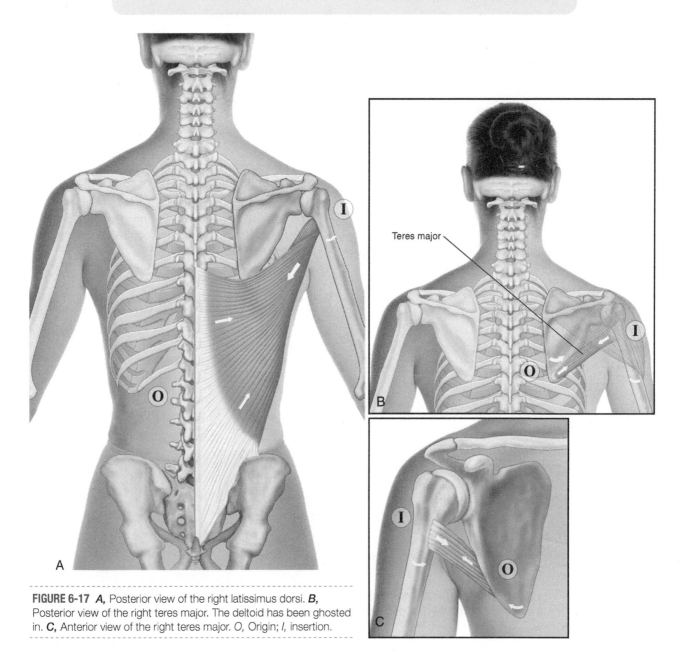

FIGURE 6-17 A, Posterior view of the right latissimus dorsi. **B,** Posterior view of the right teres major. The deltoid has been ghosted in. **C,** Anterior view of the right teres major. *O*, Origin; *I,* insertion.

WHAT'S IN A NAME?

The name, *latissimus dorsi*, tells us that this muscle is a wide muscle of the back. The name, *teres major*, tells us that this muscle is round and larger than the teres minor.

❊ **Derivation**
latissimus: L. wide
dorsi: L. of the back
teres: L. round
major: L. larger

ATTACHMENTS

Latissimus Dorsi

Origin (Proximal Attachment)

- Inferior angle of the scapula, spinous processes of T7-L5, posterior sacrum, and the posterior iliac crest

Insertion (Distal Attachment)

- Medial lip of the bicipital groove of the humerus

Teres Major

Origin (Proximal Attachment)

- Inferior angle and inferior lateral border of the scapula

Insertion (Distal Attachment)

- Medial lip of the bicipital groove of the humerus

ACTIONS

Latissimus Dorsi and Teres Major

The latissimus dorsi and teres major move the arm at the glenohumeral joint.

- Extend the arm.
- Adduct the arm.
- Medially rotate the arm

STABILIZATION

1. Both muscles stabilize the glenohumeral joint and scapula.

2. The latissimus dorsi also stabilizes the spinal joints and pelvis.

INNERVATION

- Thoracodorsal nerve (latissimus dorsi)
- Lower subscapular nerve (teres major)

PALPATION

Latissimus Dorsi

1. The client is prone with the arm relaxed at the side. Place the palpating fingers pads on the posterior axillary fold of tissue.

2. Ask the client to extend the arm; feel for the contraction of the latissimus dorsi (Figure 6-18, *A*).

3. Palpate to its proximal attachment on the pelvis; and palpate to its distal tendon attachment in the axilla on the humerus (Figure 6-18, *B*).

   Note: The latissimus dorsi can also be palpated with the client standing with the arm resting on your shoulder. When the client presses down against your shoulder toward extension and adduction, the latissimus dorsi can be felt to contract and palpated from attachment to attachment (Figure 6-18, *C-D*).

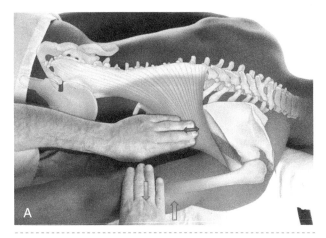

FIGURE 6-18 *A,* Palpation of the right latissimus dorsi is demonstrated as the client extends the arm against resistance. Palpation of the latissimus dorsi in the posterior axillary fold is noted.

Continued

Turn page to 👁 more.

6

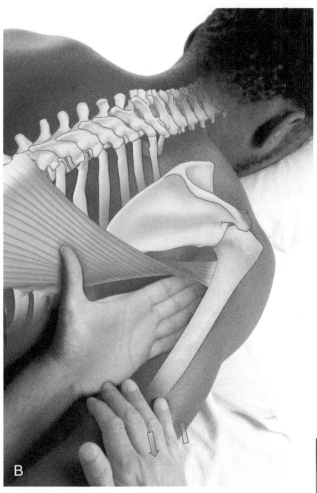

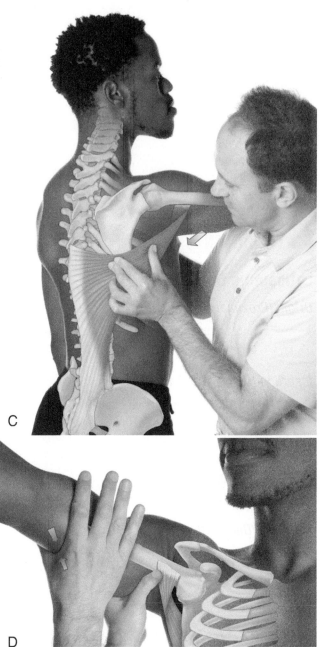

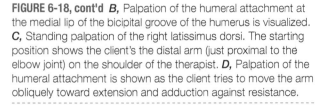

FIGURE 6-18, cont'd B, Palpation of the humeral attachment at the medial lip of the bicipital groove of the humerus is visualized. **C,** Standing palpation of the right latissimus dorsi. The starting position shows the client's the distal arm (just proximal to the elbow joint) on the shoulder of the therapist. **D,** Palpation of the humeral attachment is shown as the client tries to move the arm obliquely toward extension and adduction against resistance.

Teres Major

1. The client is prone with the arm resting on the table and the forearm hanging off the table and located between the therapist's knees; place the palpating finger pads just lateral to the lower aspect of the lateral border of the scapula.

2. Ask the client to rotate the arm medially at the glenohumeral joint against the resistance of your knee; feel for the contraction of the teres major (Figure 6-19).

3. Continue palpating the teres major distally toward the humerus.

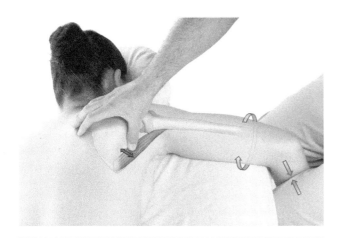

FIGURE 6-19 Palpation of the right teres major is demonstrated as the client medially rotates the arm against resistance.

▮ TREATMENT CONSIDERATIONS

■ Swimming the freestyle stroke (the crawl) involves extension, adduction, and medial rotation of the arm; all three are actions of the latissimus dorsi and teres major. Therefore swimmers heavily use these muscles. In fact, the latissimus dorsi is often called the *swimmer's muscle*.

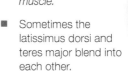
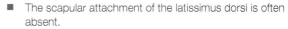
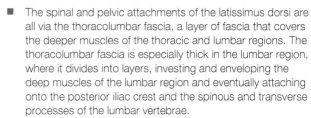

■ Sometimes the latissimus dorsi and teres major blend into each other.

■ The scapular attachment of the latissimus dorsi is often absent.

■ The spinal and pelvic attachments of the latissimus dorsi are all via the thoracolumbar fascia, a layer of fascia that covers the deeper muscles of the thoracic and lumbar regions. The thoracolumbar fascia is especially thick in the lumbar region, where it divides into layers, investing and enveloping the deep muscles of the lumbar region and eventually attaching onto the posterior iliac crest and the spinous and transverse processes of the lumbar vertebrae.

6

SHOULDER GIRDLE AND ARM: Rotator Cuff Group
Supraspinatus; Infraspinatus; Teres Minor; Subscapularis

Pronunciation   SOO-pra-spy-NAY-tus • IN-fra-spy-NAY-tus • TE-reez MY-nor •
sub-skap-u-LA-ris

The rotator cuff group is composed of four muscles that attach from the scapula proximally to the tubercles of the humerus distally; they conjoin to form a cuff on the humerus, hence the name. These muscles are the <u>S</u>upraspinatus, <u>I</u>nfraspinatus, and <u>T</u>eres minor posteriorly and the <u>S</u>ubscapularis more anteriorly; they are commonly referred to as the **SITS** muscles (Figure 6-20). The rotator cuff muscles are important as stabilizers of the glenohumeral joint.

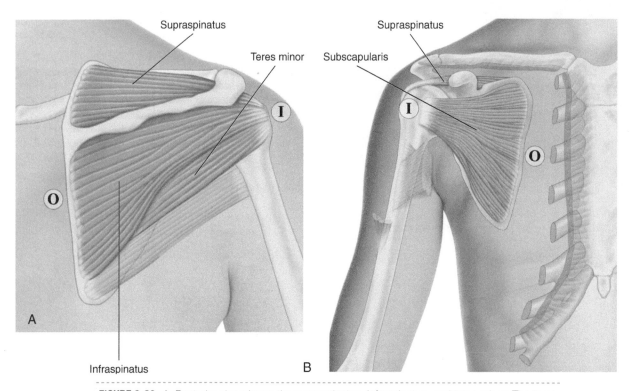

FIGURE 6-20 **A,** Posterior view shows the supraspinatus, infraspinatus, and teres minor. The teres major has been ghosted in. **B,** Anterior view shows the supraspinatus and subscapularis. The cut deltoid and pectoralis major have been ghosted in. *O,* Origin; *I,* insertion.

WHAT'S IN A NAME?

The name, *supraspinatus*, tells us that this muscle attaches into the supraspinous fossa of the scapula.

The name, *infraspinatus*, tells us that this muscle attaches into the infraspinous fossa of the scapula.

The name, *teres minor,* tells us that this muscle is round and smaller than the teres major.

The name, *subscapularis*, tells us that this muscle attaches into the subscapular fossa of the scapula.

✳ **Derivation**
supraspinatus: L. above the spine (of the scapula)
infraspinatus: L. below the spine (of the scapula)
teres: L. round
minor: L. smaller
subscapularis: L. refers to the subscapular fossa

ATTACHMENTS

Supraspinatus

The belly of the supraspinatus is located deep to the trapezius and acromion process of the scapula; its distal tendon is located deep to the deltoid.

Origin (Proximal Attachment)
- Supraspinous fossa of the scapula

Insertion (Distal Attachment)
- Greater tubercle of the humerus

Infraspinatus

The infraspinatus is a flat muscle located on the posterior scapula. Most of the infraspinatus is deep to the deltoid.

Origin (Proximal Attachment)
- Infraspinous fossa of the scapula

Insertion (Distal Attachment)
- Greater tubercle of the humerus

Teres Minor

The teres minor is a small round muscle that runs parallel with the infraspinatus. It is located between the infraspinatus and teres major. Most of the teres minor is deep to the deltoid.

Origin (Proximal Attachment)
- Superior lateral border of the scapula

Insertion (Distal Attachment)
- Greater tubercle of the humerus

Subscapularis

The subscapularis is located between the scapula and rib cage wall, along with the serratus anterior. Whereas the serratus anterior hugs the rib cage wall, the subscapularis hugs along the scapula and humerus.

Origin (Proximal Attachment)
- Subscapular fossa of the scapula

Insertion (Distal Attachment)
- Lesser tubercle of the humerus

ACTIONS

All four rotator cuff muscles move the arm at the glenohumeral joint.

Supraspinatus
- Abducts the arm.
- Flexes the arm.

Infraspinatus and Teres Minor
- Laterally rotate the arm.

Subscapularis
- Medially rotates the arm.

STABILIZATION

All four muscles stabilize the glenohumeral joint.

> Isometric Stabilization Function Note: The rotator cuff muscles are extremely important as stabilizers of the humeral head at the glenohumeral joint.

INNERVATION

- Suprascapular nerve (supraspinatus and infraspinatus)
- Axillary nerve (teres minor)
- Upper and lower subscapular nerves (subscapularis)

PALPATION

Supraspinatus

1. The client is prone with the arm resting on the table at the side; place the palpating finger pads just superior to the spine of the scapula in the supraspinous fossa.
2. Ask the client to perform a very short range of motion of abduction of the arm (approximately 10 to 20 degrees); feel for the contraction of the supraspinatus. Gentle resistance can be added (Figure 6-21, *A*).
3. The distal tendon can be palpated deep to the deltoid. Locate the acromion process of the scapula and drop off it just distally and laterally onto the distal tendon of the supraspinatus. Strum horizontally across it.

> Note: The supraspinatus can be easily palpated with the client seated. Ask the client to perform a short range of motion that is obliquely between abduction and flexion; feel for the contraction of the supraspinatus (Figure 6-21, *B*).

Turn page to 👁 more.

6

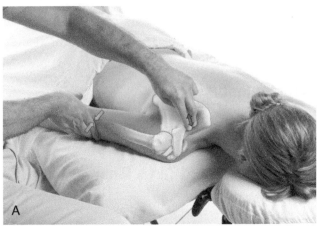

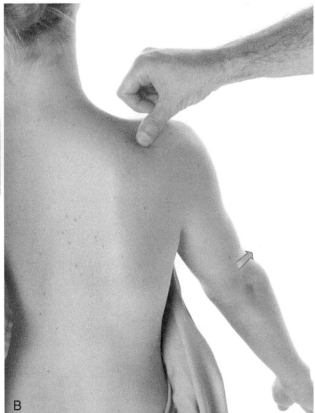

FIGURE 6-21 Palpation of the right supraspinatus. *A,* Palpation of the belly is shown superior to the spine of the scapula. *B,* The supraspinatus can also be easily palpated with the client seated. To engage the supraspinatus, the client performs either a very short range of motion (approximately 10 to 20 degrees) of abduction of the arm at the glenohumeral joint with the hand in the small of the back (to reciprocally inhibit the upper trapezius) or a short range of motion (approximately 10 to 20 degrees) of the arm halfway between abduction and flexion at the glenohumeral joint as seen here.

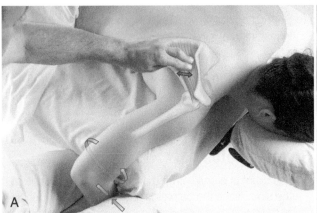

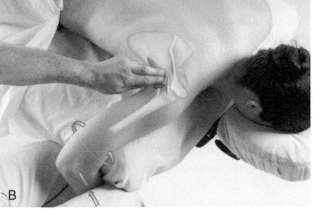

FIGURE 6-22 Palpation of the right infraspinatus and teres minor is demonstrated as the client laterally rotates the arm against resistance of the therapist's knee. *A,* Palpation of the infraspinatus is shown. *B,* Palpation of the teres minor is shown.

Infraspinatus and Teres Minor

1. The client is prone with the arm resting on the table and the forearm hanging off the table and between your knees.

2. Ask the client to rotate the arm laterally against the resistance of your knee; feel for the contraction of the muscles (Figure 6-22, *A-B*).

3. Palpate the infraspinatus from just below the spine of the scapula to the greater tubercle of the humerus.

Palpate the teres minor from the superior lateral border of the scapula to the greater tubercle of the humerus.

Note: To discern the teres minor from the teres major located inferiorly to it, the teres minor will engage with lateral rotation of the arm and the teres major will engage with medial rotation of the arm.

Subscapularis

1. The client is supine with the arm resting on the trunk and the other side hand gently holding the elbow of the side being palpated.

2. Reach under the client's body with one hand to grip the medial border of the scapula and gently passively protract the scapula. Place the finger pads of the palpating hand against the anterior surface of the scapula (Figure 6-23, *A*).

3. Ask the client to take in a deep breath; as the client exhales, slowly but firmly press your finger pads in against the anterior surface of the client's scapula. To verify that you are on the subscapularis, ask the client to rotate the arm medially, which will cause the arm to lift slightly (Figure 6-23, *B*).

4. Palpate as much of the subscapularis as possible by gently but firmly pressing in deeper toward the medial border of the scapula.

TREATMENT CONSIDERATIONS

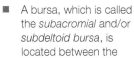

- The distal tendon of the supraspinatus is the most commonly injured tendon of the rotator cuff group because it is often pinched between the acromion process of the scapula and the greater tubercle of the humerus.

- A bursa, which is called the *subacromial* and/or *subdeltoid bursa*, is located between the supraspinatus and the acromion process and deltoid. This bursa is the commonly injured bursa of the shoulder joint.

- A bursa is usually located between the infraspinatus and the glenohumeral joint capsule.

- A bursa is usually located between the subscapularis and the scapula.

- The distal tendons of all four rotator cuff muscles adhere to the capsule of the glenohumeral joint, which is deep to them.

- A thick layer of fascia usually overlies the infraspinatus muscle (see Figure 6-1).

6

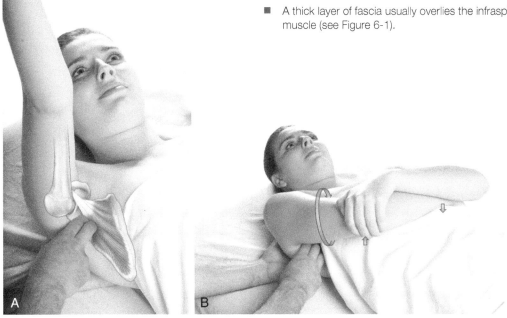

FIGURE 6-23 Palpation of the right subscapularis. **A,** Palpation of the belly is shown. Note: The client's arm is up so that the belly of the muscle is visualized. **B,** The arm may be down and resting on the chest as visualized, which shows the client medially rotating the arm to engage the subscapularis.

SHOULDER GIRDLE AND ARM
Deltoid

Pronunciation **DEL-toid**

The deltoid is a thick triangular muscle that is located over the glenohumeral joint. It is usually divided into three parts: anterior, middle, and posterior. The entire deltoid is superficial (Figure 6-24).

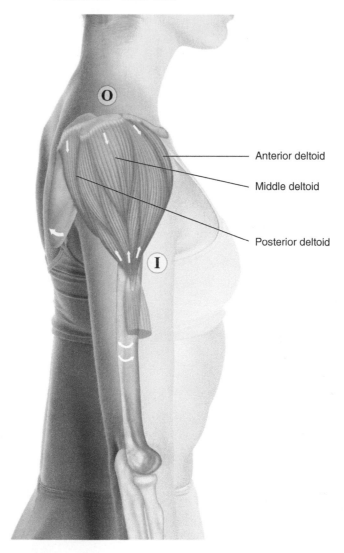

Anterior deltoid

Middle deltoid

Posterior deltoid

FIGURE 6-24 Lateral view of the right deltoid. The proximal end of the brachialis has been ghosted in. *O*, Origin; *I*, insertion.

WHAT'S IN A NAME?

The name, *deltoid*, tells us that this muscle has a triangular shape similar to the Greek letter delta (Δ).

＊ **Derivation**
delta: Gr. letter delta (Δ)
oid: Gr. resemblance

ATTACHMENTS

Origin (Proximal Attachment)
- Lateral clavicle, acromion process, and spine of the scapula

Insertion (Distal Attachment)
- Deltoid tuberosity of the humerus

ACTIONS

The deltoid moves the arm at the glenohumeral joint and moves the scapula at the glenohumeral and scapulocostal joints.

- Entire muscle:
  - Abducts the arm.
  - Downwardly rotates the scapula.
- Anterior fibers also:
  - Flex the arm.
  - Medially rotate the arm.
  - Horizontally flex the arm.
- Posterior fibers also:
  - Extend the arm.
  - Laterally rotate the arm.
  - Horizontally extend the arm.

STABILIZATION

1. Stabilizes the glenohumeral joint.
2. Stabilizes the shoulder girdle.

INNERVATION

- Axillary nerve

PALPATION

1. The client is seated, and you are standing behind the client.
2. To palpate the entire deltoid, place the palpating finger pads just distal to the acromion process of the scapula. Resist the client from abducting the arm; feel for the contraction of the deltoid (Figure 6-25, *A*).
3. To isolate the anterior deltoid, place the palpating finger pads just inferior to the lateral clavicle, resist the client from horizontally flexing the arm; feel for the contraction of the anterior fibers (Figure 6-25, *B*).

4. To isolate the posterior deltoid, place the palpating finger pads just inferior to the spine of the scapula, resist the client from horizontally extending the arm; feel for the contraction of the posterior fibers (Figure 6-25, *C*).

   Note: Resistance is added to the distal arm, not the forearm.

TREATMENT CONSIDERATIONS

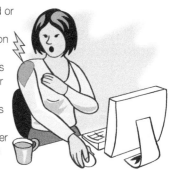

- The deltoid is often used or overused, stabilizing the arm in a position of flexion or abduction when performing such activities as working at a keyboard or using a smart phone in front of the body. For this reason, finding trigger points and taut and tender bands within the muscle is extremely common.
- Tendinitis at the distal attachment of the deltoid occurs often.

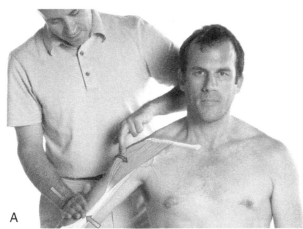

A

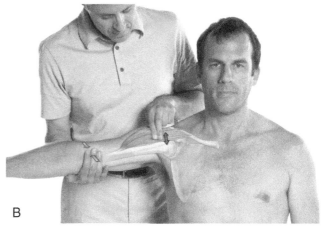

B

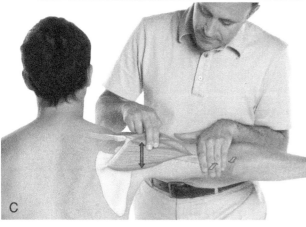

C

FIGURE 6-25 Palpation of the right deltoid. *A,* Palpation of the middle deltoid as the client abducts the arm against resistance. *B,* Palpation of the anterior deltoid as the client horizontally flexes the arm against resistance. *C,* Palpation of the posterior deltoid as the client horizontally extends the arm against resistance.

SHOULDER GIRDLE AND ARM
Coracobrachialis

Pronunciation   **KOR-a-ko-BRA-key-AL-is**

The coracobrachialis is a slender muscle that is located in the axillary (armpit) region. In anatomic position, it is deep to the pectoralis major and anterior deltoid (Figure 6-26). Abducting and laterally rotating the arm exposes this muscle from the anterior perspective.

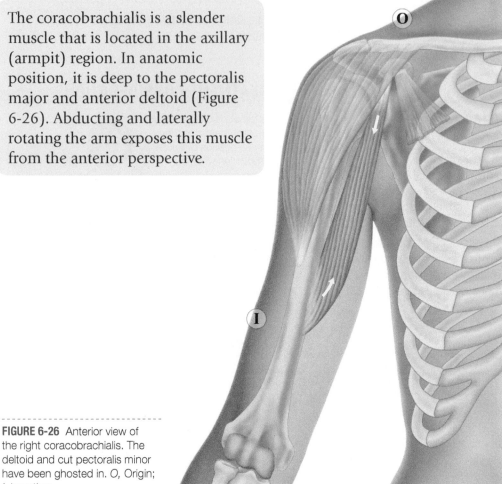

FIGURE 6-26 Anterior view of the right coracobrachialis. The deltoid and cut pectoralis minor have been ghosted in. *O,* Origin; *I,* insertion.

WHAT'S IN A NAME?

The name, *coracobrachialis*, tells us that this muscle attaches to the coracoid process and the brachium (the arm/humerus).

✳ **Derivation**
coraco: Gr. refers to the coracoid process of the scapula
brachialis: L. refers to the arm

ATTACHMENTS

Origin (Proximal Attachment)
- Coracoid process of the scapula

Insertion (Distal Attachment)
- Medial shaft of the humerus

ACTIONS

The coracobrachialis moves the arm at the glenohumeral joint.
- Flexes the arm.
- Adducts the arm.

STABILIZATION

1. Stabilizes the glenohumeral joint.
2. Stabilizes the shoulder girdle.

INNERVATION

- Musculocutaneous nerve

PALPATION STEPS

1. The client is seated with the arm abducted 90 degrees and laterally rotated, and the forearm is flexed approximately 90 degrees.

2. Place the palpating finger pads on the medial aspect of the proximal half of the client's arm.

3. Resist the client's horizontal flexion of the arm; feel for the contraction of the coracobrachialis (Figure 6-27).

   Note: Resistance is added to the distal arm, not the forearm.

TREATMENT CONSIDERATIONS

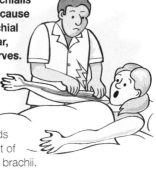

- **Palpation of the coracobrachialis must be done prudently because of the presence of the brachial artery and the median, ulnar, and musculocutaneous nerves.**

- The musculocutaneous nerve pierces through the coracobrachialis.

- The proximal attachment of the coracobrachialis blends with the proximal attachment of the short head of the biceps brachii.

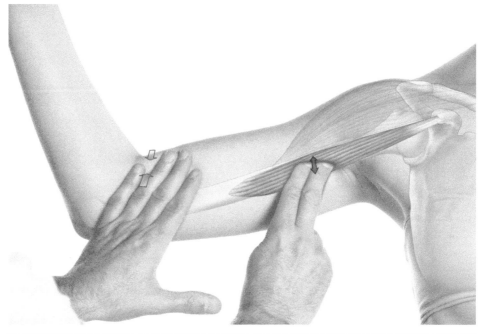

FIGURE 6-27 Palpation of the right coracobrachialis as the client horizontally flexes the arm at the glenohumeral joint against resistance. The deltoid has been ghosted in.

SHOULDER GIRDLE AND ARM
Biceps Brachii

Pronunciation   **BY-seps BRAY-key-eye**

The biceps brachii is a two-headed muscle that overlies the anterior arm. Both of its heads cross the elbow and glenohumeral joints. It is superficial except proximally, where it is deep to the deltoid (Figure 6-28).

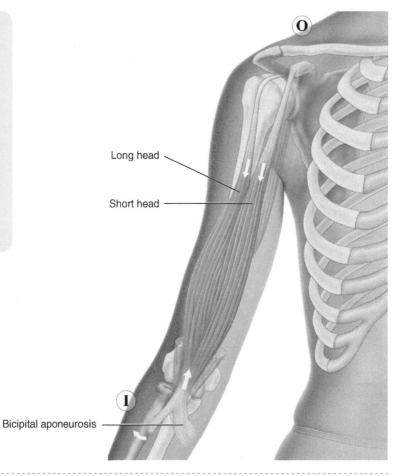

Long head

Short head

Bicipital aponeurosis

FIGURE 6-28 Anterior view of the right biceps brachii. The coracobrachialis and cut distal end of the brachialis have been ghosted in. *O,* Origin; *I,* insertion.

WHAT'S IN A NAME?

The name, *biceps brachii*, tells us that this muscle has two heads and lies over the brachium (the arm).

✳ **Derivation**
   biceps: L. two heads
   brachii: L. of the arm

ATTACHMENTS

Origin (Proximal Attachment)

- Long head: Supraglenoid tubercle of the scapula
- Short head: Coracoid process of the scapula

Insertion (Distal Attachment)

- Radial tuberosity and fascia at the medial elbow

ACTIONS

The biceps brachii moves the forearm at the elbow and the radioulnar joints and moves the arm at the glenohumeral joint.

- Flexes the forearm (elbow joint).
- Supinates the forearm (radioulnar joints).
- Flexes the arm.

STABILIZATION

1. Stabilizes the elbow, radioulnar, and glenohumeral joints.
2. Stabilizes the shoulder girdle.

INNERVATION

- Musculocutaneous nerve

PALPATION STEPS

1. The client is seated with the arm relaxed and the forearm fully supinated and resting on the client's thigh (not shown). Place palpating finger pads on the middle of the anterior arm.

2. With mild-to-moderate force, resist the client from flexing the forearm; feel for the contraction of the biceps brachii (Figure 6-29).

3. Strumming perpendicular to the fibers, first palpate to the distal tendon on the radius and then palpate toward the proximal attachments as far as possible.

   Note: Resistance is added to the distal forearm, not the hand.

TREATMENT CONSIDERATIONS

- Tendinitis of the long head of the biceps brachii occurs fairly often.

- The proximal attachment of the short head of the biceps brachii blends with the proximal attachment of the coracobrachialis at the coracoid process of the scapula.

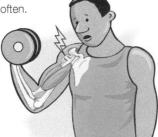

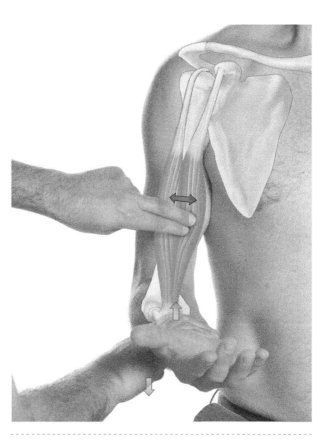

FIGURE 6-29 Palpation of the right biceps brachii is shown as the client flexes the forearm at the elbow joint against resistance.

6

6

SHOULDER GIRDLE AND ARM
Brachialis

Pronunciation   **BRAY-key-AL-is**

The brachialis is a thick muscle of the arm. From the anterior perspective, it is located deep to the biceps brachii; however, much of the brachialis is superficial from the lateral perspective (Figure 6-30).

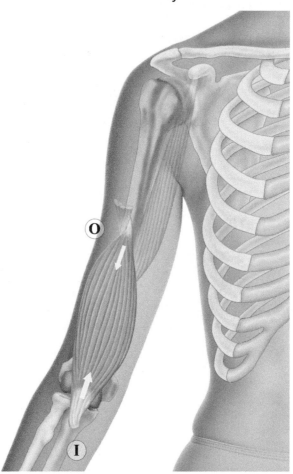

FIGURE 6-30 Anterior view of the right brachialis. The coracobrachialis and distal cut end of the deltoid have been ghosted in. *O,* Origin; *I,* insertion.

WHAT'S IN A NAME?

The name, *brachialis*, tells us that this muscle attaches to the brachium (the arm).

❋ **Derivation**
brachialis: L. refers to the arm

ATTACHMENTS

Origin (Proximal Attachment)
- Distal one half of the anterior shaft of the humerus

Insertion (Distal Attachment)
- Ulnar tuberosity

ACTIONS

The brachialis moves the forearm at the elbow joint.
- Flexes the forearm.

STABILIZATION

Stabilizes the elbow joint.

INNERVATION

- Musculocutaneous nerve

PALPATION STEPS

1. The client is seated with the arm relaxed, and the forearm is fully pronated and resting on the client's thigh (not shown). Place the palpating finger pads on the lateral side of the distal arm (slightly toward the anterior side, immediately posterior to the biceps brachii).

2. With gentle force, resist the client from flexing the forearm with the forearm fully pronated; feel for the contraction of the brachialis (Figure 6-31).

3. Strumming perpendicular to the fibers, palpate the lateral side of the brachialis to its proximal attachment and then to its distal attachment. Follow the same procedure to palpate the brachialis through the relaxed biceps brachii.

Note: Resistance is gentle and added to the distal forearm, not to the hand.

TREATMENT CONSIDERATIONS

- The brachialis is a strong and fairly large muscle, which accounts for much of the contour of the biceps brachii being so visible. "Behind every great biceps brachii is a great brachialis." ☺

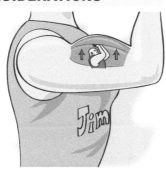

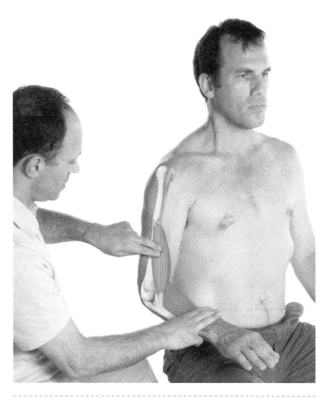

FIGURE 6-31 Palpation of the right brachialis as the client is gently resisted from flexing the forearm at the elbow joint, with the forearm in a fully pronated position.

6

SHOULDER GIRDLE AND ARM
Triceps Brachii

Pronunciation **TRY-seps BRAY-key-eye**

> The triceps brachii is a large three-headed muscle of the posterior arm. All three of its heads cross the elbow joint; only the long head crosses the glenohumeral joint. It is superficial except proximally where it is deep to the posterior deltoid (Figure 6-32).

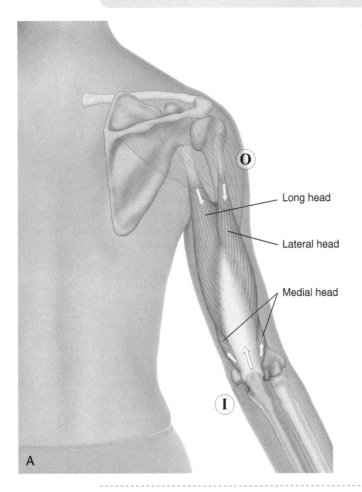

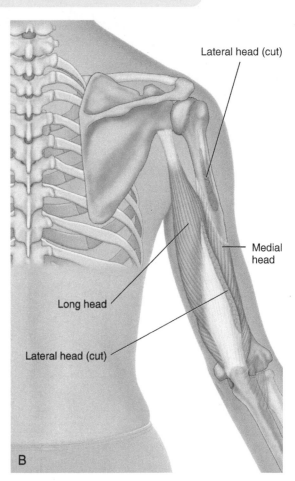

FIGURE 6-32 Posterior views of the right triceps brachii. **A,** Superficial view. The deltoid has been ghosted in. **B,** The lateral head has been cut to show the medial head. The anconeus has been ghosted in. *O,* Origin; *I,* insertion.

WHAT'S IN A NAME?

The name, *triceps brachii*, tells us that this muscle has three heads and attaches to the brachium (the arm/humerus).

✷ **Derivation**
 triceps: L. three heads
 brachii: L. of the arm

ATTACHMENTS

Origin (Proximal Attachment)
- Long head: Infraglenoid tubercle of the scapula
- Lateral head: Posterior shaft of the humerus
- Medial (deep) head: Posterior shaft of the humerus

Insertion (Distal Attachment)
- Olecranon process of the ulna

ACTIONS

The triceps brachii moves the forearm at the elbow joint and moves the arm at the glenohumeral joint.

- Extends the forearm.
- Extends the arm (long head).

STABILIZATION

1. Stabilizes the elbow and glenohumeral joints.
2. Stabilizes the shoulder girdle.

INNERVATION

- Radial nerve

PALPATION

1. The client is seated with the arm relaxed and hanging vertically, and the forearm resting on the client or therapist's thigh. Place the palpating finger pads on the posterior surface of the arm.
2. Ask the client to extend the forearm by pressing the forearm against the thigh; feel for the contraction of the triceps brachii (Figure 6-33).
3. Strumming perpendicular to the fibers, first palpate to the distal attachment and then palpate as far proximally as possible.
4. The triceps brachii can also be easily palpated with the client prone with the arm resting on the table and the forearm hanging off the side of the table.

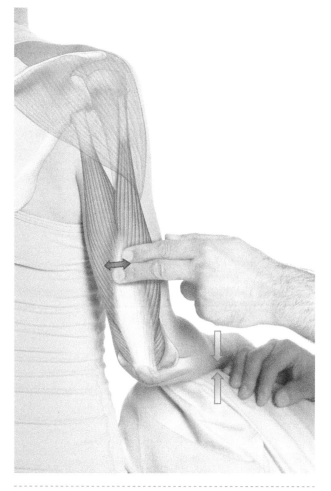

FIGURE 6-33 Palpation of the belly of the right triceps brachii is demonstrated as the client extends the forearm against resistance.

TREATMENT CONSIDERATIONS

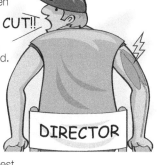

- The radial nerve runs between the medial and lateral heads of the triceps brachii. Because of its location here, the radial nerve is often injured.

- The medial head of the triceps brachii is the most active of the three heads, which means that it is engaged most often by the nervous system; however, the lateral head is the strongest.

SHOULDER GIRDLE AND ARM
Anconeus

Pronunciation   **an-KO-nee-us**

The anconeus is a small muscle located at the posterior elbow (Figure 6-34).

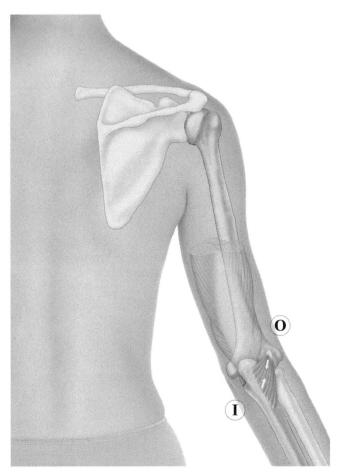

FIGURE 6-34 Posterior view of the right anconeus. The triceps brachii has been cut and ghosted in. *O*, Origin; *I*, insertion.

WHAT'S IN A NAME?

The name, *anconeus*, tells us that this muscle is involved with the elbow.

＊ **Derivation**
anconeus: Gr. elbow

ATTACHMENTS

Origin (Proximal Attachment)
■ Lateral epicondyle of the humerus

Insertion (Distal Attachment)
■ Posterior proximal ulna

ACTIONS

The anconeus moves the forearm at the elbow joint.

■ Extends the forearm.

STABILIZATION

Stabilizes the ulna and elbow joint.

> Stabilization Function Note: Some sources state that the major function of the anconeus is to stabilize the ulna when the forearm is pronating.

INNERVATION

■ Radial nerve

PALPATION

1. With the client seated, locate the point halfway between the olecranon process of the ulna and the lateral epicondyle of the humerus, and then place your palpating finger pads approximately ½ inch distal to that point.

2. Ask the client to extend the forearm at the elbow joint against resistance; feel for the contraction of the anconeus (Figure 6-35).

3. Palpate the entirety of the anconeus.

▌ TREATMENT CONSIDERATIONS

■ Because the anconeus attaches to the lateral epicondyle of the humerus, it can be involved in tennis elbow, which is also known as lateral epicondylitis or lateral epicondylosis.

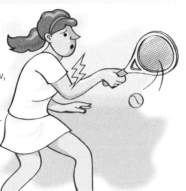

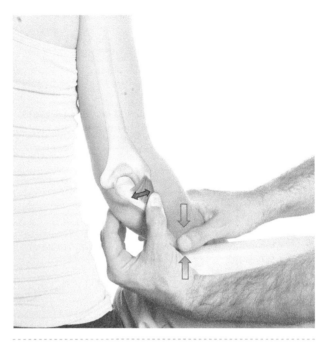

FIGURE 6-35 Palpation of the right anconeus is visualized as the client extends the forearm against resistance.

REVIEW QUESTIONS

Circle or fill in the correct answer for each of the following questions. More study resources, including audio pronunciations of muscle names, are provided on the Evolve website at http://evolve.elsevier.com/Muscolino/knowthebody.

1. **Which of the following muscles can both elevate and depress the scapula at the scapulocostal joint?**
   a. Rhomboids
   b. Trapezius
   c. Levator scapulae
   d. Subscapularis

2. **What muscle attaches from the distal one half of the anterior shaft of the humerus to the ulnar tuberosity?**
   a. Biceps brachii
   b. Coracobrachialis
   c. Brachialis
   d. Triceps brachii

3. **Which one of the following muscles can supinate the forearm at the radioulnar joints?**
   a. Brachialis
   b. Coracobrachialis
   c. Biceps brachii
   d. Anconeus

4. **What muscles attach to the lateral clavicle, acromion process, and spine of the scapula?**
   a. Deltoid and coracobrachialis
   b. Trapezius and serratus anterior
   c. Serratus anterior and latissimus dorsi
   d. Trapezius and deltoid

5. **Which of the following is an action of the pectoralis minor?**
   a. Retraction of the scapula at the scapulocostal joint
   b. Flexion of the arm at the glenohumeral joint
   c. Abduction of the arm at the glenohumeral joint
   d. Protraction of the scapula at the scapulocostal joint

6. **Which of the following is a glenohumeral joint action of the subscapularis?**
   a. Lateral rotation
   b. Medial rotation
   c. Flexion
   d. Adduction

7. **Which of the following muscles is antagonistic to the supraspinatus?**
   a. Pectoralis major
   b. Teres minor
   c. Brachialis
   d. Rhomboids

8. **Name the four muscles of the rotator cuff group.**

   _____

   _____

   _____

   _____

9. **What muscle attaches from the scapula to ribs one through nine?**

   _____

10. **What muscle can both flex and extend the arm at the glenohumeral joint?**

   _____

CASE STUDY 1

A client arrives for a massage therapy session with mild pain in the anterior left arm. The client is a 42-year-old man in good shape with no pathologic history or prior injury to the arm. The pain is mild and located directly distal to the glenohumeral (GH) joint in the anterior deltoid muscle. On a pain scale of 0 to 10, the intensity is approximately 3 when at rest and approximately 6 with exertion.

Verbal history reveals that the client was involved in a motor vehicle accident (MVA) 6 months earlier. The client was the driver; he hit a vehicle in front of him that was stopped at a red light. The client was wearing a seat belt at the time of the accident and had his left hand on the steering wheel. Damage to the vehicle was minor; the air bag did not deploy. The client saw his personal physician who ordered a magnetic resonance image (MRI) of the arm; the MRI report was negative for osseous damage. His physician also ordered a minor analgesic medication to be taken as needed for the soft-tissue pain. No physical therapy was prescribed. The client's pain was more intense immediately after the accident, but it decreased to the present level within approximately 3 months; it has remained at this level since then.

A physical examination revealed that active range of motion (ROM) of the GH joint into flexion is limited to 120 degrees. Active and passive ROM of the GH joint into extension is limited to 30 degrees. Manual resistance to GH joint flexion reveals reduced muscle strength and pain starting at approximately 45 degrees with total loss of strength at 120 degrees. Pain reaches an intensity of 6 at 120 degrees. Palpatory assessment revealed tightness and adhesions in the anterior deltoid, pectoralis major and minor, biceps brachii, and coracobrachialis muscles.

QUESTIONS

1. **Why did the MVA cause arm pain?**

   _____

   _____

   _____

   _____

   _____

   _____

   _____

2. **What treatment would be most beneficial for this client?**

   _____

   _____

   _____

   _____

   _____

   _____

   _____

   _____

   _____

   _____

6

CASE STUDY 2

A female client, age 34 years, well toned, and an active offshore competitive swimmer, complains of pain and decreased range of motion of her right shoulder. Her condition began approximately 1 week earlier. The client describes an inability to raise her arm fully to the side of her body and reports that she is experiencing a pain intensity that varies from 2 to 5 on a scale of 0 to 10. She points to the right anterior glenohumeral joint region as the site of maximal pain. The pain and stiffness are most acute when she first starts working out and also in the mornings when she first wakes up. She states that the range of motion increases after her workout but not fully; and that the pain is reduced to a 2 after her workout. She has been applying heat after her workouts and taking ibuprofen for pain: 200 mg, two times a day, for the last 5 days with little noticeable benefit. The client states that she has not experienced any traumatic injuries, accidents, or other pathologic issues.

This client has been an active swimmer for 2 years; her training consists of local pool workouts with a Swim Masters coach 2 days each week and open-water swims with competitors 2 days per week. The Swim Masters coach has noticed a change in her right arm stroke during her last two workouts. He can see that she is not lifting her right arm completely out of the water but is, instead, dragging it across the top of the water. In open-water training the client notices that her right arm does not seem to manage wave impacts as effectively as her left arm. Two weeks earlier, she added three weight training sessions to her weekly regimen.

Palpation during physical examination produces a pain intensity of 5 to 7 in the shoulder joint from the superior angle of the scapula to the head of the humerus anteromedially. Moderate muscle spasm is present diffusely throughout the entire right shoulder region, but it is strongest in the upper trapezius, supraspinatus, and anterior deltoid muscles. The client is very vigilant and noticeably guards herself when she fears that pain will occur. Mild swelling is present in the tissues around the glenohumeral joint. Manual muscle testing against resistance for all glenohumeral joint ranges of motion causes a pain intensity of 5 to 8.

QUESTIONS

1. **What activities could have caused the recent change?**

   _____

   _____

   _____

   _____

   _____

   _____

2. **What treatment plan would you recommend?**

   _____

   _____

   _____

   _____

   _____

   _____

   _____

3. **What self-care would you recommend?**

   _____

   _____

   _____

   _____

   _____

   _____

Muscles of the Forearm and Hand

The muscles of this chapter are involved with motions of the forearm (radius and ulna) at the radioulnar joints, the hand at the wrist (radiocarpal) joint, and the fingers at the metacarpophalangeal (MCP) and/or the proximal interphalangeal (PIP) and distal interphalangeal (DIP) joints; the thumb also moves at the first carpometacarpal (CMC) (saddle) joint.

Forearm muscles are usually divided into an anterior flexor compartment and a posterior extensor compartment. The flexor compartment has three layers: superficial, intermediate, and deep. The extensor compartment has two layers: superficial and deep. A third group, called the radial group (also known as the *wad of three*), is sometimes designated. It consists of the brachioradialis of the anterior compartment and the extensors carpi radialis longus and brevis of the posterior compartment.

‗‗‗‗ Two other structures of importance in the forearm are the common flexor tendon and the common extensor tendon. The common flexor tendon attaches to the medial epicondyle of the humerus. Five muscles attach into the common flexor tendon: (1) flexor carpi radialis, (2) palmaris longus, (3) flexor carpi ulnaris, (4) pronator teres, and (5) flexor digitorum superficialis. The common extensor tendon attaches to the lateral epicondyle of the humerus. Four muscles attach into the common extensor tendon: (1) extensor carpi radialis brevis, (2) extensor digitorum, (3) extensor digiti minimi, and (4) extensor carpi ulnaris.

‗‗‗‗ Muscles that move the fingers are often divided into extrinsic and intrinsic hand/finger muscles. Intrinsic hand muscles are wholly located within the hand; in other words, they originate and insert within the hand. Intrinsic muscles on the palmar side of the hand can be divided into three groups: (1) thenar eminence, (2) hypothenar eminence, and (3) central compartment.

‗‗‗‗ Extrinsic finger muscles have their origin (proximal attachment) outside of the hand, in the forearm or arm. Because they also cross the wrist and/or elbow joints, they can also move those joints.

‗‗‗‗ A structure of importance in the hand is the dorsal digital expansion. The dorsal digital expansion is a fibrous expansion of the extensor digitorum and extensor pollicis longus muscles' distal tendons on the dorsal side of the fingers (digits).

‗‗‗‗ As a general rule, muscles that move the elbow joint have their origin (proximal attachment) on the arm (humerus) and their insertion (distal attachment) on the forearm (radius or ulna) or hand. Muscles that pronate or supinate the forearm usually have their origin (proximal attachment) on the radius and their insertion (distal attachment) on the ulna. Muscles that move the wrist joint usually have their origin (proximal attachment) on the arm or forearm and their insertion (distal attachment) on the hand. Finger muscles may be extrinsic or intrinsic as previously discussed.

‗‗‗‗ As a rule, flexor and pronator muscles attach to the medial epicondyle of the humerus via the common flexor tendon.

‗‗‗‗ As a rule, extensor and supinator muscles attach to the lateral epicondyle of the humerus via the common extensor tendon.

The companion CD at the back of this book allows you to examine the muscles of this body region, layer by layer, and individual muscle palpation technique videos are available in the Chapter 7 folder on Evolve.

OVERVIEW OF FUNCTION: MUSCLES OF THE ELBOW AND RADIOULNAR JOINTS

The following general rules regarding actions can be stated for the functional groups of the muscles of the elbow and radioulnar joints.

- If a muscle crosses the elbow joint anteriorly with a vertical direction to its fibers, it can flex the forearm at the elbow joint by moving the anterior surface of the forearm toward the anterior surface of the arm.
- If a muscle crosses the elbow joint posteriorly with a vertical direction to its fibers, it can extend the forearm at the elbow joint by moving the posterior surface of the forearm toward the posterior surface of the arm.
- Reverse actions at the elbow joint involve moving the arm toward the forearm at the elbow joint. This movement usually occurs when the hand (and therefore the forearm) is fixed by holding onto an immovable object.*
- If a muscle crosses the radioulnar joints anteriorly with a horizontal orientation to its fibers, it will pronate the forearm at the radioulnar joints by crossing the radius over the ulna.

- If a muscle crosses the radioulnar joints posteriorly with a horizontal direction to its fibers, it will supinate the forearm at the radioulnar joints by moving the radius to be parallel with the ulna.
- Reverse actions of these standard mover actions at the radioulnar joints involve moving the ulna toward the radius at the radioulnar joints. This movement usually occurs when the hand (and therefore the radius) is fixed by holding onto an immovable object.*

OVERVIEW OF FUNCTION: MUSCLES OF THE WRIST JOINT

The following general rules regarding actions can be stated for the functional groups of the muscles of the wrist joint:

- If a muscle crosses the wrist joint anteriorly with a vertical direction to its fibers, it can flex the hand at the wrist joint by moving the palmar (anterior) surface of the hand toward the anterior surface of the forearm.
- If a muscle crosses the wrist joint posteriorly with a vertical direction to its fibers, it can extend the hand at the wrist joint by moving the dorsal (posterior)

surface of the hand toward the posterior surface of the forearm.

■ If a muscle crosses the wrist joint on the radial side (laterally) with a vertical direction to its fibers, it can radially deviate (abduct) the hand at the wrist joint by moving the radial side of the hand toward the radial side of the forearm.

■ If a muscle crosses the wrist joint on the ulnar side (medially) with a vertical direction to its fibers, it can ulnar deviate (adduct) the hand at the wrist joint by moving the ulnar side of the hand toward the ulnar side of the forearm.

■ Reverse actions of these standard mover actions involve the forearm being moved toward the hand at the wrist joint. These reverse actions usually occur when the hand is fixed, such as when holding onto an immovable object.*

OVERVIEW OF FUNCTION: MUSCLES OF THE FINGERS

The following general rules regarding actions can be stated for the functional groups of finger muscles:

■ Fingers two through five can move at three joints: (1) MCP, (2) PIP, and (3) DIP joints. If a muscle crosses only the MCP joint, it can move the finger only at the MCP joint. If the muscle crosses the MCP and PIP joints, it can move the finger at both of these joints. If the muscle crosses the MCP, PIP, and DIP joints, it can move the finger at all three joints.

Note: The little finger can also move at the CMC joint.

■ The thumb (finger one) can move at three joints: the CMC, MCP, and interphalangeal (IP) joints. Similarly, a muscle can only move the thumb at a joint or joints that it crosses.

■ If a muscle crosses the MCP, PIP, or DIP joints of fingers two through five on the anterior side, it can flex the finger at the joint(s) crossed; if a muscle crosses the MCP, PIP, or DIP joints of fingers two through five on the posterior side, it can extend the finger at the joint(s) crossed.

■ If a muscle crosses the MCP joint of fingers two, four, or five on the side that faces the middle finger, it can adduct the finger at the MCP joint. If a muscle crosses the MCP joint of fingers two, three, or four on the side that is away from the middle finger side, it can abduct the finger at the MCP joint (the middle finger abducts in both directions—radial and ulnar).

■ Muscles that cross the CMC, MCP, and IP joints of the thumb on the medial side can flex the thumb at the joint(s) crossed. Muscles that cross the CMC, MCP, and IP joints of the thumb on the lateral side can extend the thumb at the joint(s) crossed.

■ Muscles that cross the CMC joint of the thumb on the anterior side can abduct the thumb at the CMC joint. Muscles that cross the CMC joint of the thumb on the posterior side can adduct the thumb at the CMC joint.

■ Reverse actions involve the proximal attachment moving toward the distal attachment. This movement occurs when the fingers are holding onto a fixed, immovable object.*

7

---

*A standard (typical) mover action is when the insertion (distal attachment) moves toward the origin (proximal attachment). A reverse mover action occurs when the origin moves toward the insertion.

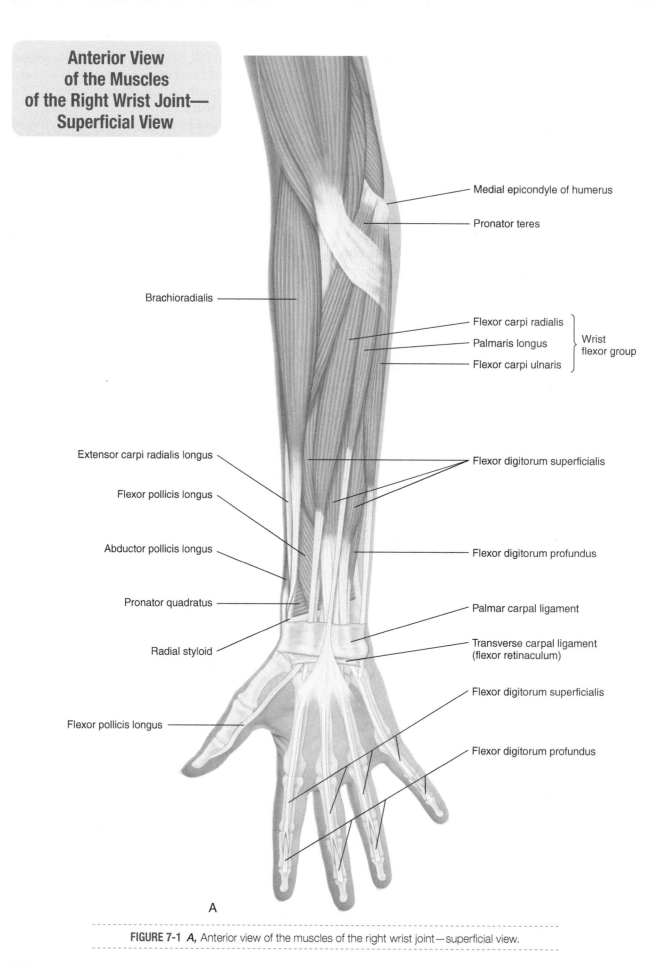

Anterior View of the Muscles of the Right Wrist Joint— Superficial View

Medial epicondyle of humerus

Pronator teres

Brachioradialis

Flexor carpi radialis

Palmaris longus

Flexor carpi ulnaris

Wrist flexor group

Extensor carpi radialis longus

Flexor pollicis longus

Abductor pollicis longus

Pronator quadratus

Radial styloid

Flexor pollicis longus

Flexor digitorum superficialis

Flexor digitorum profundus

Palmar carpal ligament

Transverse carpal ligament (flexor retinaculum)

Flexor digitorum superficialis

Flexor digitorum profundus

A

FIGURE 7-1 *A,* Anterior view of the muscles of the right wrist joint—superficial view.

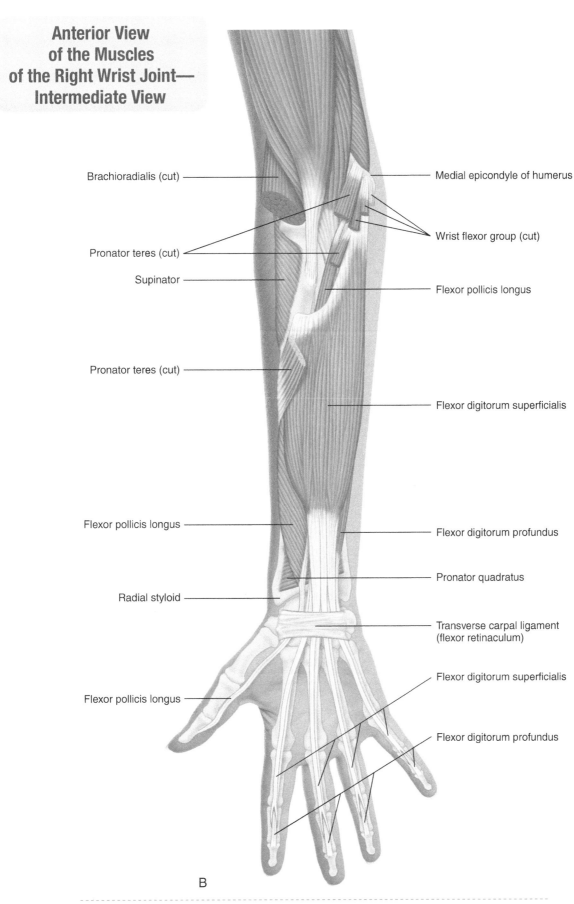

Anterior View of the Muscles of the Right Wrist Joint— Intermediate View

Brachioradialis (cut)

Pronator teres (cut)

Supinator

Pronator teres (cut)

Flexor pollicis longus

Radial styloid

Flexor pollicis longus

Medial epicondyle of humerus

Wrist flexor group (cut)

Flexor pollicis longus

Flexor digitorum superficialis

Flexor digitorum profundus

Pronator quadratus

Transverse carpal ligament (flexor retinaculum)

Flexor digitorum superficialis

Flexor digitorum profundus

B

FIGURE 7-1, cont'd B, Anterior view of the muscles of the right wrist joint—intermediate view.

Continued

7

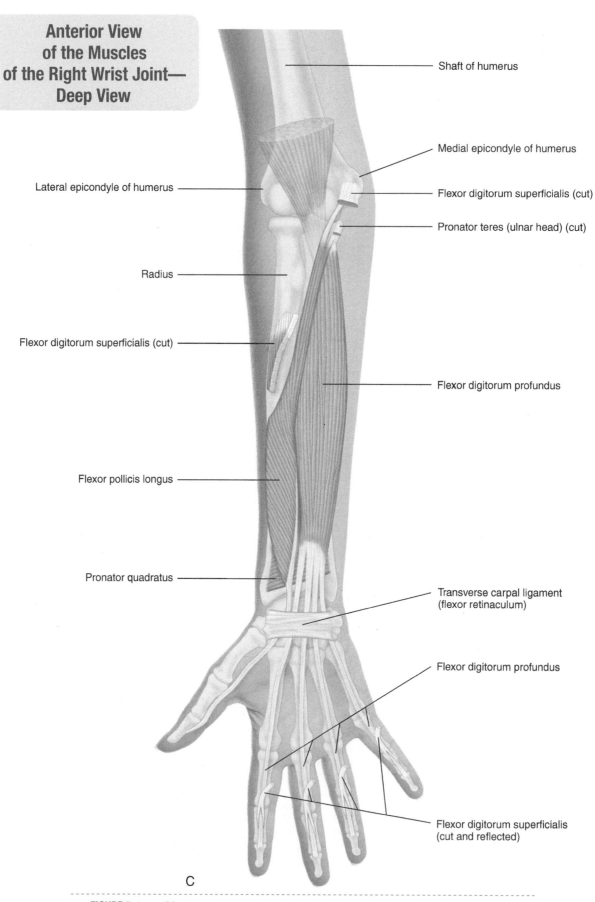

Anterior View of the Muscles of the Right Wrist Joint— Deep View

Shaft of humerus

Medial epicondyle of humerus

Lateral epicondyle of humerus

Flexor digitorum superficialis (cut)

Pronator teres (ulnar head) (cut)

Radius

Flexor digitorum superficialis (cut)

Flexor digitorum profundus

Flexor pollicis longus

Pronator quadratus

Transverse carpal ligament (flexor retinaculum)

Flexor digitorum profundus

Flexor digitorum superficialis (cut and reflected)

C

FIGURE 7-1, cont'd C, Anterior view of the muscles of the right wrist joint—deep view. The brachialis (cut) has been ghosted in.

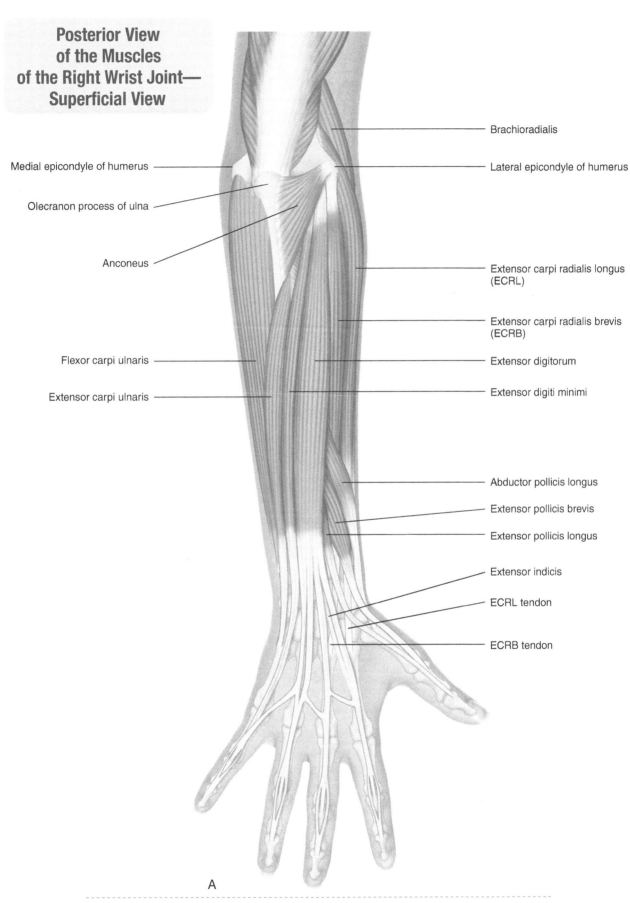

Posterior View of the Muscles of the Right Wrist Joint— Superficial View

Medial epicondyle of humerus

Olecranon process of ulna

Anconeus

Flexor carpi ulnaris

Extensor carpi ulnaris

Brachioradialis

Lateral epicondyle of humerus

Extensor carpi radialis longus (ECRL)

Extensor carpi radialis brevis (ECRB)

Extensor digitorum

Extensor digiti minimi

Abductor pollicis longus

Extensor pollicis brevis

Extensor pollicis longus

Extensor indicis

ECRL tendon

ECRB tendon

7

A

FIGURE 7-2 *A,* Posterior view of the muscles of the right wrist joint—superficial view.

Continued

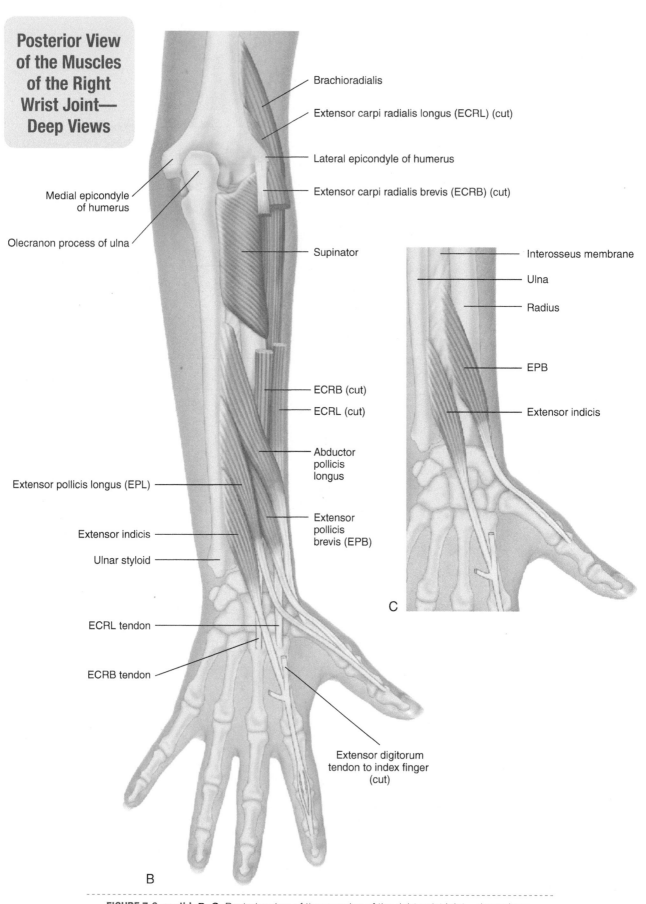

Posterior View of the Muscles of the Right Wrist Joint— Deep Views

Brachioradialis

Extensor carpi radialis longus (ECRL) (cut)

Lateral epicondyle of humerus

Extensor carpi radialis brevis (ECRB) (cut)

Medial epicondyle of humerus

Olecranon process of ulna

Supinator

Interosseus membrane

Ulna

Radius

EPB

Extensor indicis

ECRB (cut)

ECRL (cut)

Abductor pollicis longus

Extensor pollicis longus (EPL)

Extensor pollicis brevis (EPB)

Extensor indicis

Ulnar styloid

ECRL tendon

ECRB tendon

Extensor digitorum tendon to index finger (cut)

C

B

FIGURE 7-2, cont'd *B, C,* Posterior view of the muscles of the right wrist joint—deep views.

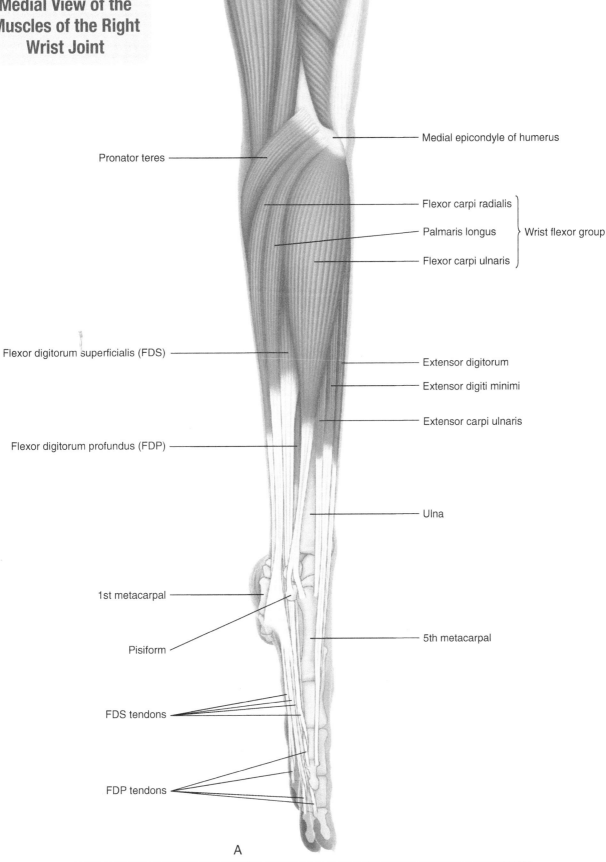

Medial View of the Muscles of the Right Wrist Joint

Pronator teres

Medial epicondyle of humerus

Flexor carpi radialis
Palmaris longus
Flexor carpi ulnaris
} Wrist flexor group

Flexor digitorum superficialis (FDS)

Extensor digitorum
Extensor digiti minimi
Extensor carpi ulnaris

Flexor digitorum profundus (FDP)

Ulna

1st metacarpal

Pisiform

5th metacarpal

FDS tendons

FDP tendons

A

FIGURE 7-3 *A,* Medial view of the muscles of the right wrist joint.

Continued

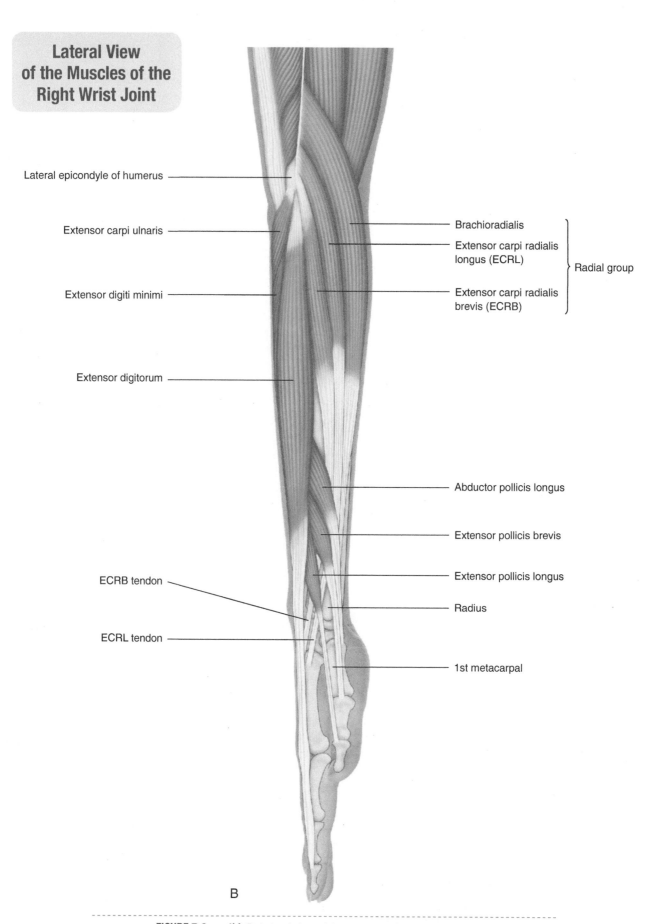

Lateral View of the Muscles of the Right Wrist Joint

Lateral epicondyle of humerus

Extensor carpi ulnaris

Extensor digiti minimi

Extensor digitorum

ECRB tendon

ECRL tendon

Brachioradialis

Extensor carpi radialis longus (ECRL)

Extensor carpi radialis brevis (ECRB)

Radial group

Abductor pollicis longus

Extensor pollicis brevis

Extensor pollicis longus

Radius

1st metacarpal

B

FIGURE 7-3, cont'd *B,* Lateral view of the muscles of the right wrist joint.

Cross Section of the Right Middle Forearm in the Transverse Plane

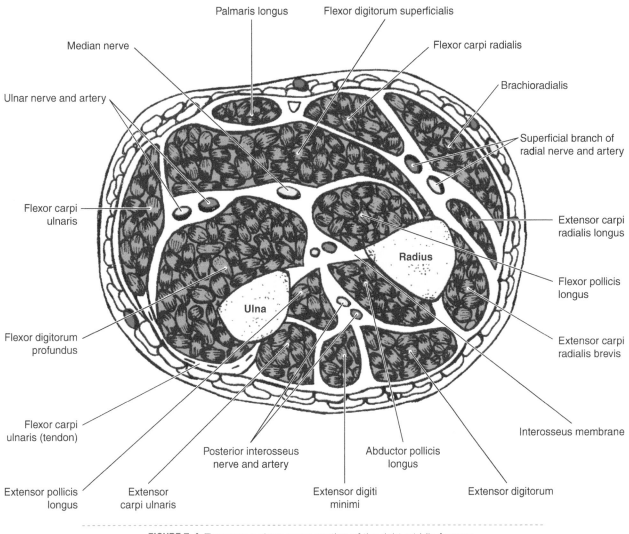

Palmaris longus

Flexor digitorum superficialis

Median nerve

Flexor carpi radialis

Ulnar nerve and artery

Brachioradialis

Superficial branch of radial nerve and artery

Flexor carpi ulnaris

Extensor carpi radialis longus

Radius

Flexor pollicis longus

Ulna

Extensor carpi radialis brevis

Flexor digitorum profundus

Flexor carpi ulnaris (tendon)

Interosseus membrane

Posterior interosseus nerve and artery

Abductor pollicis longus

Extensor pollicis longus

Extensor carpi ulnaris

Extensor digiti minimi

Extensor digitorum

FIGURE 7-4 Transverse plane cross section of the right middle forearm.

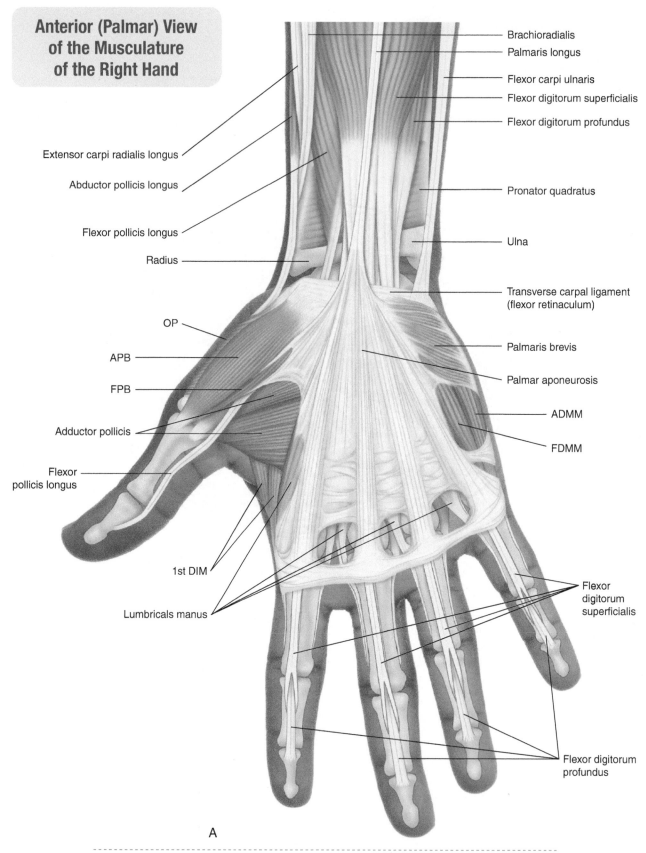

**Anterior (Palmar) View
of the Musculature
of the Right Hand**

Extensor carpi radialis longus

Abductor pollicis longus

Flexor pollicis longus

Radius

OP

APB

FPB

Adductor pollicis

Flexor
pollicis longus

1st DIM

Lumbricals manus

Brachioradialis

Palmaris longus

Flexor carpi ulnaris

Flexor digitorum superficialis

Flexor digitorum profundus

Pronator quadratus

Ulna

Transverse carpal ligament
(flexor retinaculum)

Palmaris brevis

Palmar aponeurosis

ADMM

FDMM

Flexor
digitorum
superficialis

Flexor digitorum
profundus

A

FIGURE 7-5 A, Superficial view of the hand with the palmar aponeurosis. *ADMM,* Abductor digiti
minimi manus; *APB,* abductor pollicis brevis; *DIM,* dorsal interosseus/interossei manus;
FDMM, flexor digiti minimi manus; *FPB,* flexor pollicis brevis; *OP,* opponens pollicis.

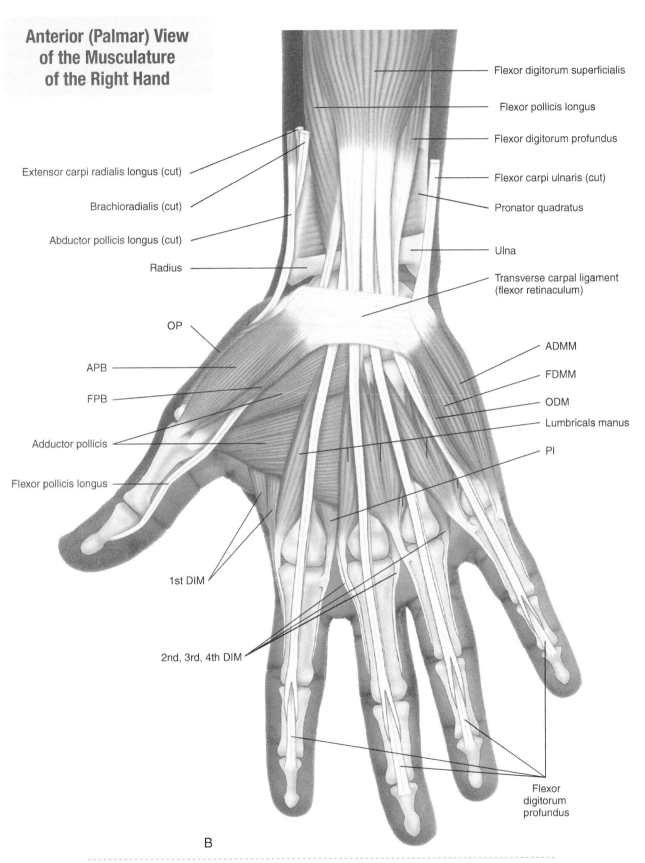

Anterior (Palmar) View of the Musculature of the Right Hand

Flexor digitorum superficialis

Flexor pollicis longus

Flexor digitorum profundus

Flexor carpi ulnaris (cut)

Pronator quadratus

Ulna

Transverse carpal ligament (flexor retinaculum)

ADMM

FDMM

ODM

Lumbricals manus

PI

Flexor digitorum profundus

Extensor carpi radialis longus (cut)

Brachioradialis (cut)

Abductor pollicis longus (cut)

Radius

OP

APB

FPB

Adductor pollicis

Flexor pollicis longus

1st DIM

2nd, 3rd, 4th DIM

B

FIGURE 7-5, cont'd B, Superficial view of the musculature of the hand with the palmar aponeurosis removed. *ADMM,* Abductor digiti minimi manus; *APB,* abductor pollicis brevis; *DIM,* dorsal interosseus/interossei manus; *FDMM,* flexor digiti minimi manus; *FPB,* flexor pollicis brevis; *ODM,* opponens digiti minimi; *OP,* opponens pollicis; *PI,* palmar interossei.

Continued

7

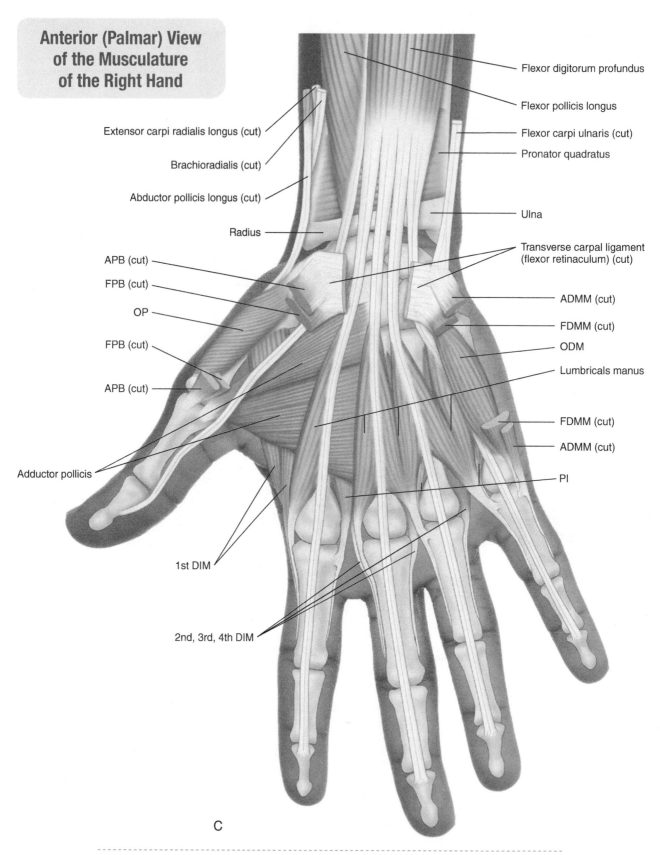

Anterior (Palmar) View of the Musculature of the Right Hand

Flexor digitorum profundus

Flexor pollicis longus

Flexor carpi ulnaris (cut)

Pronator quadratus

Extensor carpi radialis longus (cut)

Brachioradialis (cut)

Abductor pollicis longus (cut)

Radius

Ulna

Transverse carpal ligament (flexor retinaculum) (cut)

APB (cut)

FPB (cut)

OP

ADMM (cut)

FDMM (cut)

ODM

FPB (cut)

Lumbricals manus

APB (cut)

FDMM (cut)

ADMM (cut)

Adductor pollicis

PI

1st DIM

2nd, 3rd, 4th DIM

C

FIGURE 7-5, cont'd *C,* Intermediate view with the more superficial thenar and hypothenar muscles cut. *ADMM,* Abductor digiti minimi manus; *APB,* abductor pollicis brevis; *DIM,* dorsal interosseus/interossei manus; *FDMM,* flexor digiti minimi manus; *FPB,* flexor pollicis brevis; *ODM,* opponens digiti minimi; *OP,* opponens pollicis; *PI,* palmar interossei.

7

Anterior (Palmar) View
of the Musculature
of the Right Hand

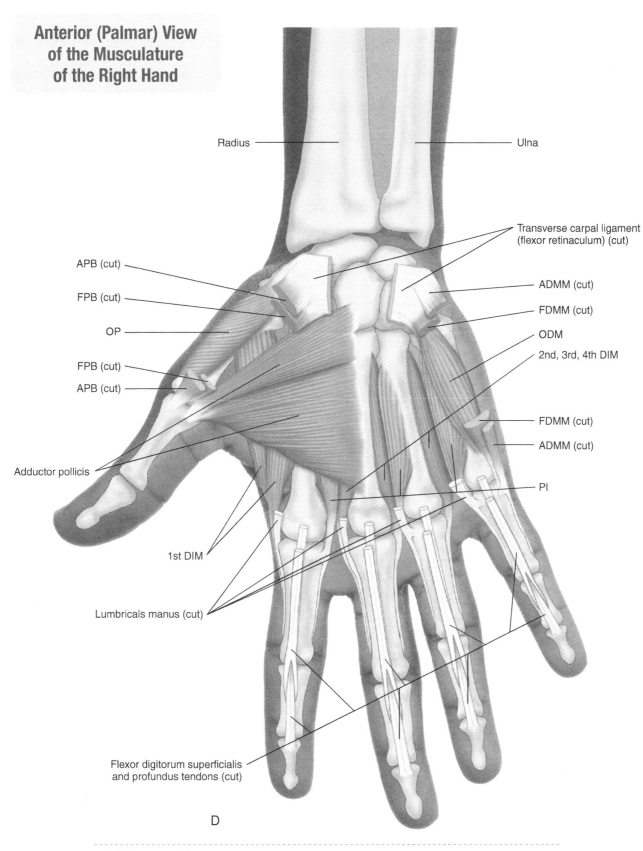

Radius

Ulna

APB (cut)

FPB (cut)

OP

FPB (cut)

APB (cut)

Adductor pollicis

Transverse carpal ligament
(flexor retinaculum) (cut)

ADMM (cut)

FDMM (cut)

ODM

2nd, 3rd, 4th DIM

FDMM (cut)

ADMM (cut)

PI

1st DIM

Lumbricals manus (cut)

Flexor digitorum superficialis
and profundus tendons (cut)

D

FIGURE 7-5, cont'd D, Deep view with the more superficial thenar and hypothenar muscles,
lumbricals manus, flexor digitorum muscles' tendons, and all forearm muscles cut and/or
removed. *ADMM,* Abductor digiti minimi manus; *APB,* abductor pollicis brevis; *DIM,* dorsal
interosseus/interossei manus; *FDMM,* flexor digiti minimi manus; *FPB,* flexor pollicis brevis;
ODM, opponens digiti minimi; *OP,* opponens pollicis; *PI,* palmar interossei.

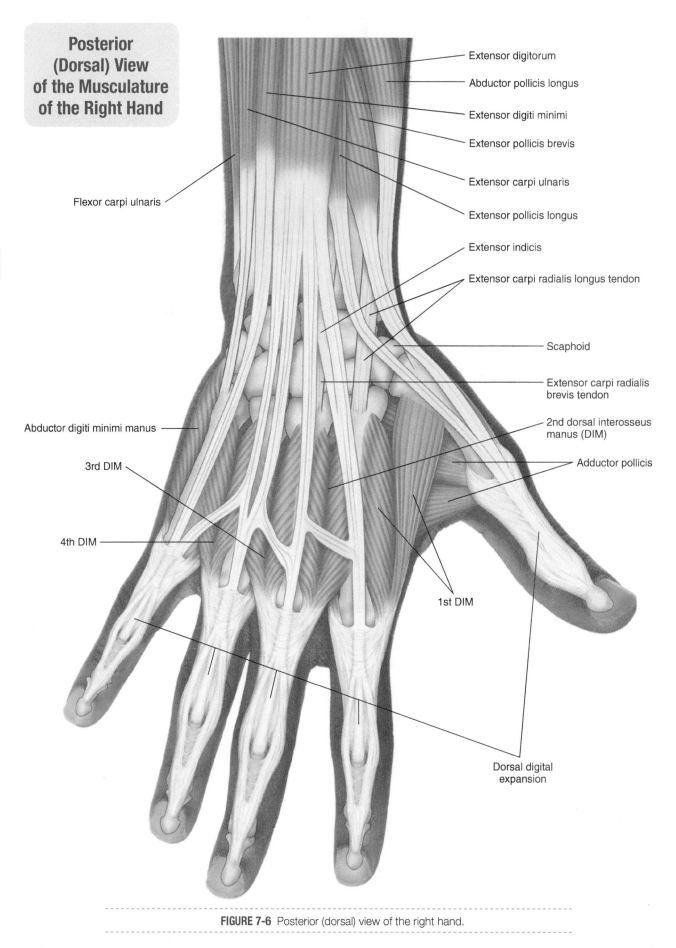

Posterior (Dorsal) View of the Musculature of the Right Hand

Extensor digitorum

Abductor pollicis longus

Extensor digiti minimi

Extensor pollicis brevis

Extensor carpi ulnaris

Extensor pollicis longus

Extensor indicis

Extensor carpi radialis longus tendon

Scaphoid

Extensor carpi radialis brevis tendon

2nd dorsal interosseus manus (DIM)

Adductor pollicis

Flexor carpi ulnaris

Abductor digiti minimi manus

3rd DIM

4th DIM

1st DIM

Dorsal digital expansion

FIGURE 7-6 Posterior (dorsal) view of the right hand.

Notes

FOREARM AND HAND: Wrist Flexor Group
Flexor Carpi Radialis; Palmaris Longus; Flexor Carpi Ulnaris

Pronunciation   FLEKS-or KAR-pie RAY-dee-A-lis • pall-MA-ris LONG-us •
FLEKS-or KAR-pie ul-NA-ris

The wrist flexor group is composed of three muscles that all originate (have their proximal attachment) on the medial epicondyle of the humerus via the common flexor tendon. They all cross the wrist joint anteriorly; therefore they can all flex the hand at the wrist joint, hence the name of the group. These muscles are the flexor carpi radialis, palmaris longus, and flexor carpi ulnaris. All three muscles of the wrist flexor group are superficial in the anterior forearm. At the wrist joint, the palmaris longus crosses dead center; the flexor carpi radialis crosses slightly to the radial (lateral) side; and the flexor carpi ulnaris crosses far to the ulnar (medial) side (Figure 7-7). In addition to the humeral attachment, the flexor carpi ulnaris also has an ulnar attachment. The humeral head is much thicker; the ulnar head is extremely thin.

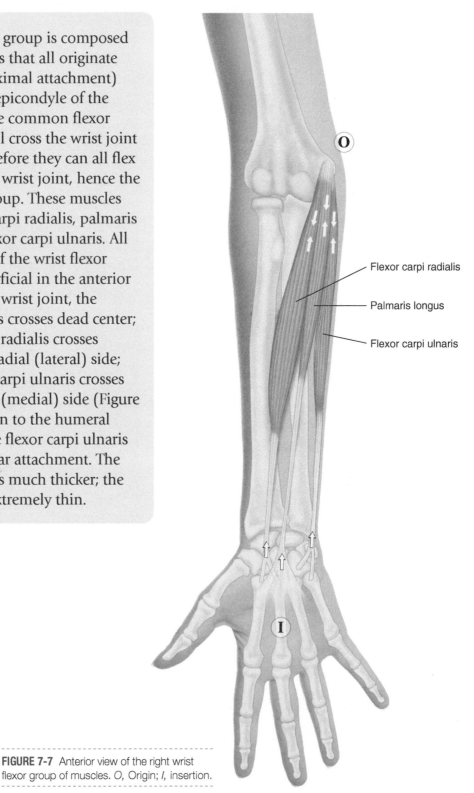

Flexor carpi radialis

Palmaris longus

Flexor carpi ulnaris

FIGURE 7-7 Anterior view of the right wrist flexor group of muscles. *O,* Origin; *I,* insertion.

WHAT'S IN A NAME?

The name, *flexor carpi radialis,* tells us that this muscle flexes *and* radially deviates (abducts); carpi tells us that these actions occur at the wrist joint.

The name, *flexor carpi ulnaris,* tells us that this muscle flexes *and* ulnar deviates (adducts) the wrist joint.

The name, *palmaris longus,* tells us that this muscle attaches into the palm of the hand and is long (longer than the palmaris brevis).

✳ **Derivation:**
flexor: L. muscle that flexes a body part
radialis: L. refers to the radial side (of the forearm)
ulnaris: L. refers to the ulnar side (of the forearm)
palmaris: L. refers to the palm
longus: L. longer
carpi: L. of the wrist

ATTACHMENTS

Flexor Carpi Radialis

The flexor carpi radialis is superficial in the anterior forearm and located between the pronator teres and the palmaris longus.

Origin (Proximal Attachment)

■ Medial epicondyle of the humerus via the common flexor tendon

Insertion (Distal Attachment)

■ Anterior hand on the radial side

Palmaris Longus

The palmaris longus is superficial in the anterior forearm and located between the flexor carpi radialis and the flexor carpi ulnaris.

Origin (Proximal Attachment)

■ Medial epicondyle of the humerus via the common flexor tendon

Insertion (Distal Attachment)

■ Palm of the hand

Flexor Carpi Ulnaris

The flexor carpi ulnaris is superficial in the anterior forearm and located medial to the palmaris longus.

Origin (Proximal Attachment)

■ Medial epicondyle of the humerus via the common flexor tendon, and the ulna

Insertion (Distal Attachment)

■ Anterior hand on the ulnar side

ACTIONS

■ All three muscles of the wrist flexor group flex the hand at the wrist joint.

■ The flexor carpi radialis also radially deviates the hand at the wrist joint.

■ The flexor carpi ulnaris also ulnar deviates the hand at the wrist joint.

STABILIZATION

As a group, the wrist flexor muscles stabilize the wrist, elbow, and radioulnar joints.

Stabilization Function Note: The flexor carpi ulnaris also stabilizes the pisiform bone of the carpal group when the abductor digiti minimi manus (intrinsic muscle of the hand) contracts, so that the abductor digiti minimi manus can efficiently abduct the little finger.

INNERVATION

■ Median and ulnar nerves

Note: The median nerve innervates the flexor carpi radialis and palmaris longus; the ulnar nerve innervates the flexor carpi ulnaris.

Turn page to 👁 more.

7

PALPATION

1. The client is seated with the arm relaxed. The forearm is flexed at the elbow joint and is fully supinated and resting on the client's thigh. Place your support/resistance hand on the client's hand, just proximal to the fingers.

2. Resist the client from flexing the hand at the wrist joint (be sure that you do not contact the fingers when offering resistance), and look for the distal tendons of all three wrist flexors to become visible. If they do not become visible, then they should be palpable by strumming perpendicularly across them. The flexor carpi ulnaris is usually the least visible.

3. Begin by palpating the flexor carpi radialis by strumming horizontally across it (Figure 7-8). Then palpate the palmaris longus and flexor carpi ulnaris in a similar manner.

4. Continue palpating each of these muscles proximally to the medial epicondyle by strumming across its fibers.

> Note: The flexor carpi radialis can be palpated with resisted radial deviation of the hand at the wrist joint; similarly, the flexor carpi ulnaris can be palpated with ulnar deviation. The palmaris longus can be palpated by asking the client to "cup the hand" (Figure 7-9).

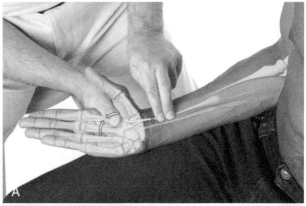

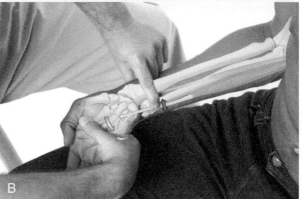

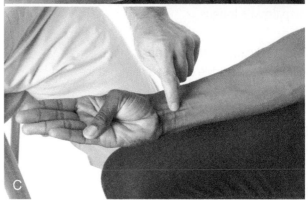

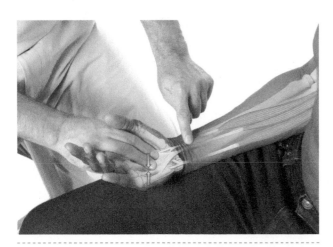

FIGURE 7-8 All three muscles of the right wrist flexor group are engaged with flexion of the hand against resistance. The distal tendons are often visible as shown. The tendon of the flexor carpi radialis is being palpated.

FIGURE 7-9 Palpation of the muscles of the right wrist flexor group. **A,** Palpation of the flexor carpi radialis as the client radially deviates the hand against resistance. The palmaris longus has been ghosted in. **B,** Palpation of the flexor carpi ulnaris as the client ulnar deviates the hand against resistance (the palmaris longus has been ghosted in). **C,** The palmaris longus is engaged when the client cups his hand.

TREATMENT CONSIDERATIONS

- Overuse of the wrist flexor group musculature can cause irritation and/or inflammation of the medial epicondyle and/or the common flexor tendon. This condition is known as *medial epicondylitis*, *medial epicondylosis*, or *golfer's elbow*.

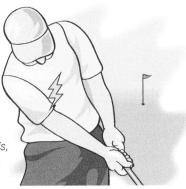

- In many individuals, the palmaris longus is bilaterally or unilaterally absent.

- The ulnar nerve passes between the two heads of the flexor carpi ulnaris. Compression of the ulnar nerve between the two heads of the flexor carpi ulnaris is called *cubital tunnel syndrome*.

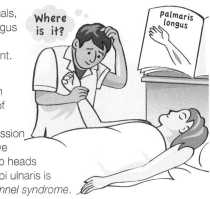

7

7

FOREARM AND HAND: Pronator Group
Pronator Teres; Pronator Quadratus

Pronunciation **pro-NAY-tor TE-reez** • **pro-NAY-tor kwod-RAY-tus**

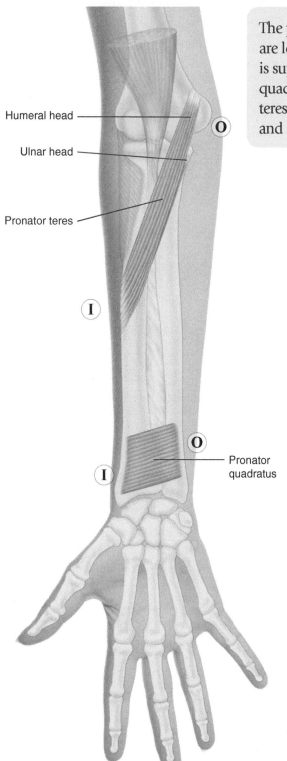

Humeral head

Ulnar head

Pronator teres

Pronator quadratus

The pronator teres and pronator quadratus muscles are located in the anterior forearm. The pronator teres is superficial in the proximal forearm; the pronator quadratus is very deep in the distal forearm. The pronator teres has two heads—a large, superficial humeral head and a small, deep ulnar head (Figure 7-10).

WHAT'S IN A NAME?

The name, *pronator*, tells us that these muscles pronate the forearm. *Teres* refers to being round in shape; *quadratus* refers to being square in shape.

❋ **Derivation:**
pronator: L. muscle that pronates a body part
teres: L. round
quadratus: L. squared

ATTACHMENTS

Pronator Teres

Origin (Proximal Attachment)
- Humeral head: Medial epicondyle of the humerus via the common flexor tendon
- Ulnar head: Coronoid process of the ulna

Insertion (Distal Attachment)
- Lateral radius

Pronator Quadratus

Origin (Proximal Attachment)
- Anterior distal ulna

Insertion (Distal Attachment)
- Anterior distal radius

ACTIONS

Pronator Teres
- Pronates the forearm at the radioulnar joints.
- Flexes the forearm at the elbow joint.

Pronator Quadratus
- Pronates the forearm at the radioulnar joints.

FIGURE 7-10 Anterior view. The supinator and brachialis (cut) have been ghosted in. *O,* Origin; *I,* insertion.

STABILIZATION

1. Both pronator muscles stabilize the radioulnar joints.
2. The pronator teres also stabilizes the elbow joint.

   Stabilization Function Note: The pronator quadratus is especially important for preventing the separation of the distal radius and ulna.

INNERVATION

- Median nerve

PALPATION

Pronator Teres

1. The client is seated with the arm relaxed and the forearm flexed at the elbow joint and in a position that is halfway between full pronation and full supination; the forearm is resting on the client's thigh. Place your palpating thumb or finger pads on the proximal anterior forearm, and gently but firmly grasp the client's distal forearm just proximal to the wrist joint with your support/resistance hand.
2. With moderate force, resist the client from pronating the forearm at the radioulnar joints and feel for the contraction of the pronator teres (Figure 7-11).
3. Strumming perpendicular to the fibers, palpate from attachment to attachment. Be sure to strum across the entire muscle belly.

Pronator Quadratus

1. The client is seated or supine with the forearm fully supinated. Place your palpating finger pads on the distal forearm, just proximal to the wrist.
2. Ask the client to pronate the forearm actively at the radioulnar joints, and feel for the contraction of the pronator quadratus. Resistance can be added if necessary (Figure 7-12).

   Note: The pronator quadratus is deep and can be difficult to palpate and discern. **Further, the median and ulnar nerves and radial and ulnar arteries are located in the anterior wrist; prudence must be exercised when palpating deeply here.**

TREATMENT CONSIDERATIONS

- The median nerve courses between the humeral head and the ulnar head of the pronator teres, making it a possible entrapment site. When the median nerve is entrapped here, it is termed *pronator teres syndrome* and may mimic symptoms of carpal tunnel syndrome or a pathologic cervical disc.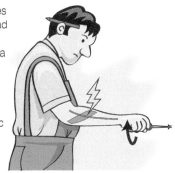

- Overuse of the pronator teres can cause irritation and/or inflammation of the medial epicondyle and/or the common flexor tendon. This condition is known as *medial epicondylitis, medial epicondylosis,* or *golfer's elbow.*

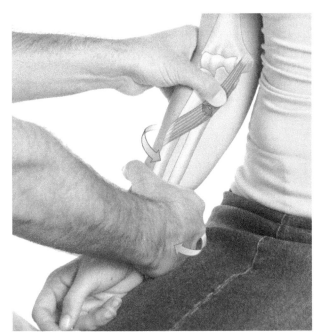

FIGURE 7-11 Palpation of the right pronator teres as the client pronates the forearm at the radioulnar joints against resistance.

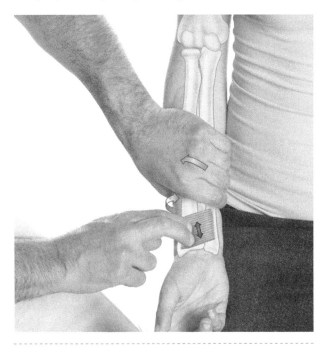

FIGURE 7-12 View of the right pronator quadratus being palpated as pronation of the forearm at the radioulnar joints is resisted.

FOREARM AND HAND
Brachioradialis

Pronunciation **BRAY-key-o-RAY-dee-AL-is**

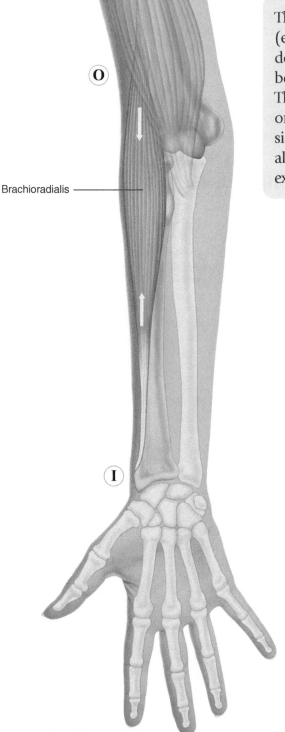

Brachioradialis

The brachioradialis is superficial for its entire course (except for a small part of its distal tendon that is deep to two small muscles of the thumb whose bellies are located deep in the posterior forearm). The brachioradialis is located in the anterior forearm on the radial (lateral) side. Because it is on the radial side, it is considered to be part of the "radial group," along with the extensor carpi radialis longus and extensor carpi radialis brevis (Figure 7-13).

WHAT'S IN A NAME?

The name, *brachioradialis,* tells us that this muscle attaches onto the brachium (the arm) and the radius.

✳ **Derivation:**
  brachio: L. refers to the arm
  radialis: L. refers to the radius

ATTACHMENTS

Origin (Proximal Attachment)
■ Lateral supracondylar ridge of the humerus

Insertion (Distal Attachment)
■ Styloid process of the radius

ACTIONS

The brachioradialis moves the forearm at the elbow and radioulnar joints.
■ Flexes the forearm at the elbow joint.
■ Supinates the forearm at the radioulnar joints.
■ Pronates the forearm at the radioulnar joints.

Action Note: If the forearm is fully pronated, the brachioradialis can supinate it to a position that is halfway between full pronation and full supination. If the forearm is fully supinated, the brachioradialis can pronate it to a position that is halfway between full pronation and full supination.

FIGURE 7-13 Anterior view of the right brachioradialis. The brachialis has been ghosted in. *O,* Origin; *I,* insertion.

STABILIZATION

Stabilizes the elbow and radioulnar joints.

INNERVATION

- Radial nerve

PALPATION

1. The client is seated with the arm relaxed and the forearm flexed at the elbow joint and in a position that is halfway between full pronation and full supination; the forearm is resting on the client's thigh. Place your support/resistance hand on the client's anterior distal forearm, just proximal to the wrist joint.

2. Ask the client to try to flex the forearm with moderate force against your resistance. First look for the contraction of the brachioradialis and then feel for its contraction at the proximal anterolateral forearm (Figure 7-14).

3. Strumming perpendicular to the fibers, palpate proximally to the lateral supracondylar ridge of the humerus and then distally to the styloid process of the radius.

Note: Contacting and adding resistance to the distal forearm, not the hand, is extremely important. If resistance is added to the hand, then the adjacent extensor carpi radialis longus will engage, making it difficult to discern the brachioradialis from this muscle.

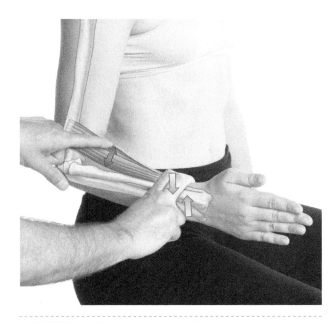

FIGURE 7-14 Palpation of the right brachioradialis with the forearm halfway between full supination and full pronation.

TREATMENT CONSIDERATIONS

- The brachioradialis is one of the three Bs of elbow joint flexion: (1) biceps brachii, (2) brachialis, and (3) brachioradialis. The biceps brachii flexes best when the forearm is fully supinated; the brachialis flexes best when the forearm is fully pronated; the brachioradialis flexes best when the forearm is halfway between fully supinated and fully pronated.

- The brachioradialis is sometimes nicknamed the *hitchhiker muscle* for the characteristic action of flexing the forearm in a position halfway between full pronation and full supination (with the thumb up) when hitchhiking. (Keep in mind that the brachioradialis has no action on the thumb itself.)

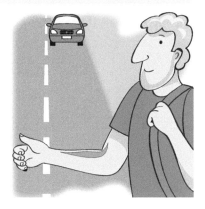

FOREARM AND HAND: Flexors Digitorum and Pollicis Group
Flexor Digitorum Superficialis: Flexor Digitorum Profundus; Flexor Pollicis Longus

Pronunciation **FLEKS-or dij-i-TOE-rum SOO-per-fish-ee-A-lis •
FLEKS-or dij-i-TOE-rum pro-FUN-dus • FLEKS-or POL-i-sis LONG-us**

The flexor digitorum superficialis, flexor digitorum profundus, and flexor pollicis longus are all long, extrinsic flexors of the fingers. Both flexor digitorum muscles flex fingers 2 through 5; and the flexor pollicis muscle flexes the thumb (finger 1). These muscles are considered to be long extrinsic finger muscles because they originate (have their proximal attachment) outside of the hand. The flexor digitorum superficialis is in the intermediate layer of anterior forearm muscles, directly deep to the muscles of the wrist flexor group. The flexor digitorum profundus and flexor pollicis longus are in the deep layer of the anterior forearm, deep to the flexor digitorum superficialis (Figure 7-15).

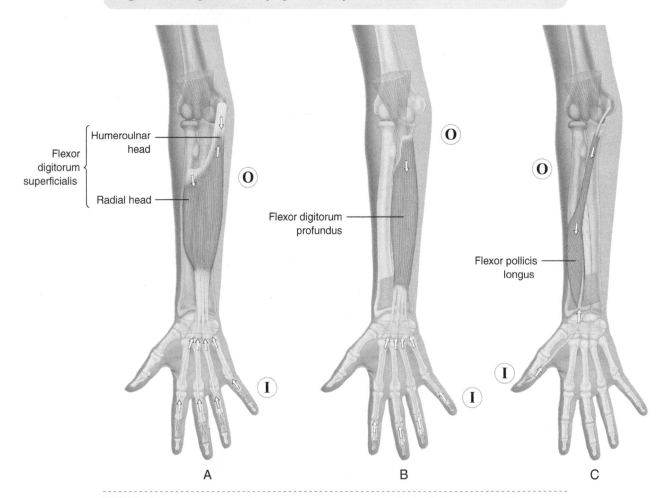

FIGURE 7-15 A, Anterior view of the right flexor digitorum superficialis. **B,** Anterior view of the right flexor digitorum profundus. **C,** Anterior view of the right flexor pollicis longus. The distal end of the brachialis has been ghosted in all three figures. The pronator quadratus has been ghosted in **B** and **C**. O, Origin; I, insertion.

WHAT'S IN A NAME?

The name, *flexor digitorum superficialis,* tells us that this muscle flexes the digits (i.e., fingers) and is superficial to the flexor digitorum profundus.

The name, *flexor digitorum profundus,* tells us that this muscle flexes the digits (i.e., fingers) and is deep to the flexor digitorum superficialis.

The name, *flexor pollicis longus,* tells us that this muscle flexes the thumb and is long (i.e., longer than the flexor pollicis brevis).

✳ **Derivation:**
flexor: L. muscle that flexes a body part
digitorum: L. refers to a digit (finger)
pollicis: L. thumb
superficialis: L. superficial (near the surface)
profundus: L. deep
longus: L. long

ATTACHMENTS

Flexor Digitorum Superficialis

Origin (Proximal Attachment)
- Medial epicondyle of the humerus via the common flexor tendon, and the anterior ulna and radius

Insertion (Distal Attachment)
- Anterior surfaces of fingers two through five

Flexor Digitorum Profundus

Origin (Proximal Attachment)
- Medial and anterior ulna

Insertion (Distal Attachment)
- Anterior surfaces of fingers two through five

Flexor Pollicis Longus

Origin (Proximal Attachment)
- Anterior surface of the radius, and the ulna and medial epicondyle of the humerus

Insertion (Distal Attachment)
- Thumb

ACTIONS

- The flexors digitorum superficialis and profundus flex fingers two through five at the MCP and IP joints (proximal and distal IP joints are the PIP and DIP joints).
- The flexor pollicis longus flexes the thumb at the CMC (saddle), MCP, and IP joints.
- Because these muscles also cross the wrist joint, they can move the hand at the wrist joint.

Flexor Digitorum Superficialis

- Flexes fingers two through five at the MCP and PIP joints.
- Flexes the hand at the wrist joint.

Flexor Digitorum Profundus

- Flexes fingers two through five at the MCP, PIP, and DIP joints.
- Flexes the hand at the wrist joint.

Flexor Pollicis Longus

- Flexes the thumb at the CMC, MCP, and IP joints.
- Flexes the hand at the wrist joint.

STABILIZATION

As a group, these muscles stabilize the CMC, MCP and IP joints of the fingers and thumb, as well as the wrist joint.

INNERVATION

- Median and ulnar nerves

  Note: The median nerve innervates all three muscles in this group. The ulnar nerve also innervates the flexor digitorum profundus.

7

Turn page to 👁 more.

█ PALPATION

Flexor Digitorum Superficialis and Flexor Digitorum Profundus

1. The client is seated with the arm relaxed; the forearm is flexed at the elbow joint and fully supinated and resting on the client's thigh.

2. For the flexor digitorum superficialis, place your palpating finger pads on the proximal medial forearm, slightly distal and anterior to the medial epicondyle of the humerus. Ask the client to flex the proximal phalanges of fingers two through five at the MCP joints.

   Note: If resistance is given, be sure to isolate your pressure against the proximal phalanges of the fingers (Figure 7-16, *A*).

3. Feel for the contraction of the flexor digitorum superficialis. Palpate the flexor digitorum superficialis by strumming perpendicular to the fibers from the proximal attachment at the medial epicondyle to the distal tendons at the anterior wrist.

4. For the flexor digitorum profundus, place your palpating finger pads on the proximal medial forearm, slightly distal and posterior to the medial epicondyle and against the shaft of the ulna. Ask the client to flex the middle and distal phalanges of fingers two through five at the proximal and distal IP joints and feel for the contraction of the flexor digitorum profundus (Figure 7-16, *B*).

5. Palpate the flexor digitorum profundus as far distally as possible by strumming perpendicular to the fibers.

Flexor Pollicis Longus

1. The client is seated with the arm relaxed, and the forearm is flexed at the elbow joint and fully supinated and resting on the client's thigh. Place your palpating finger pads just proximal to the wrist joint on the radial side.

2. Ask the client to flex the distal phalanx of the thumb at the IP joint. With gentle pressure, feel for the contraction of the flexor pollicis longus near the wrist (Figure 7-16, *C*).

3. Continue palpating the flexor pollicis longus as far proximal as possible as the client alternately contracts and relaxes it by flexing the thumb at the IP joint.

   Note: Because this muscle is so deep, trying to strum perpendicular to its fibers is usually not helpful.

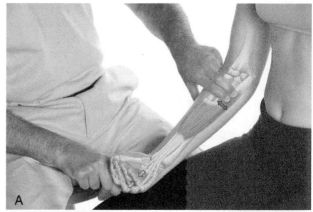

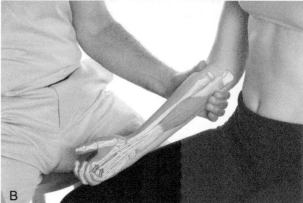

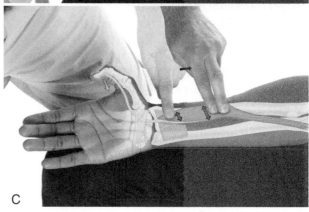

FIGURE 7-16 Palpation of the flexors digitorum and pollicis group. *A,* Palpation of the right flexor digitorum superficialis, starting distal and anterior to the medial epicondyle of the humerus. *B,* Palpation of the right flexor digitorum profundus, starting against the shaft of the ulna. Note the difference in the type of finger flexion that is performed by the client against resistance. *C,* Palpation of the belly of the right flexor pollicis longus as the thumb flexes at the interphalangeal (IP) joint. The pronator quadratus has been ghosted in.

TREATMENT CONSIDERATIONS

- The median nerve and the distal tendons of all three muscles in this group travel within synovial sheaths within the carpal tunnel. Overuse and irritation of these muscles can cause swelling, which can press on the median nerve, causing *carpal tunnel syndrome*.

- The flexor digitorum superficialis attaches to the common flexor tendon at the medial epicondyle of the humerus. Irritation or inflammation of the medial epicondyle and/or the common flexor tendon is known as *medial epicondylitis, medial epicondylosis,* or *golfer's elbow*.

- Overuse and irritation of the flexor pollicis longus is becoming more common as a result of the use of cell phones. This muscle is also often overused and injured in manual/massage therapists.

- The proximal attachments of the flexor pollicis longus are variable. The humeral and/or ulnar attachments are often missing.

VISIT DOCTOR. MY THUMBS HURT!

- **The radial artery is near the flexor pollicis longus, so if you feel a pulse, move off the artery.**

7

7

FOREARM AND HAND: Wrist Extensor Group
Extensor Carpi Radialis Longus; Extensor Carpi Radialis Brevis; Extensor Carpi Ulnaris

Pronunciation   **eks-TEN-sor KAR-pie RAY-dee-A-lis LONG-us •
eks-TEN-sor KAR-pie RAY-dee-A-lis BRE-vis • eks-TEN-sor KAR-pie ul-NA-ris**

The wrist extensor group is composed of three muscles that all originate (have their proximal attachment) either at the lateral epicondyle of the humerus via the common extensor tendon or nearby. They all cross the wrist joint posteriorly; therefore they can all extend the hand at the wrist joint, hence the name of the group. These muscles are the extensor carpi radialis longus, extensor carpi radialis brevis, and extensor carpi ulnaris. All three muscles of the wrist extensor group are superficial in the posterior forearm. At the wrist joint, both extensor carpi radialis muscles cross on the radial side, and the extensor carpi ulnaris crosses on the ulnar side (Figure 7-17). In addition to the humeral attachment, the extensor carpi ulnaris also has an ulnar attachment.

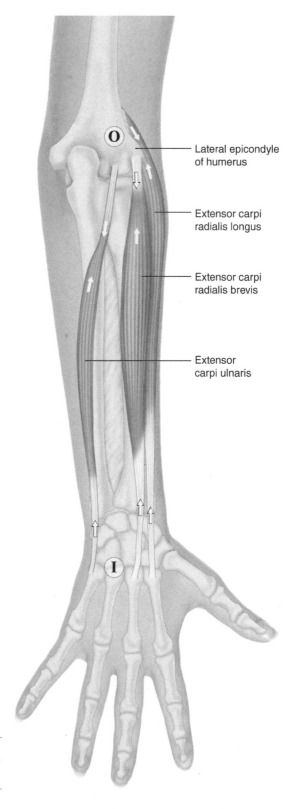

Lateral epicondyle of humerus

Extensor carpi radialis longus

Extensor carpi radialis brevis

Extensor carpi ulnaris

FIGURE 7-17 Posterior view of the right wrist extensor group of muscles. *O,* Origin; *I,* insertion.

WHAT'S IN A NAME?

The names, *extensor carpi radialis longus* and *extensor carpi radialis brevis,* tell us that these muscles extend and radially deviate (abduct). *Carpi* tells us that these actions occur at the wrist joint. *Longus* designates the muscle as being longer than the *brevis*.

The name, *extensor carpi ulnaris,* tells us that this muscle extends and ulnar deviates (adducts) the wrist joint.

✽ Derivation:
extensor: L. muscle that extends a body part
carpi: L. of the wrist
radialis: L. refers to the radial side (of the forearm)
ulnaris: L. refers to the ulnar side (of the forearm)
longus: L. longer
brevis: L. shorter

ATTACHMENTS

Extensor Carpi Radialis Longus

Origin (Proximal Attachment)
■ Lateral supracondylar ridge of the humerus

Insertion (Distal Attachment)
■ Posterior hand on the radial side

Extensor Carpi Radialis Brevis

Origin (Proximal Attachment)
■ Lateral epicondyle of the humerus via the common extensor tendon

Insertion (Distal Attachment)
■ Posterior hand on the radial side

Extensor Carpi Ulnaris

Origin (Proximal Attachment)
■ Lateral epicondyle of the humerus via the common extensor tendon, and the ulna

Insertion (Distal Attachment)
■ Posterior hand on the ulnar side

ACTIONS

The muscles of the wrist extensor group move the hand at the wrist joint.

Extensor Carpi Radialis Longus and Extensor Carpi Radialis Brevis

■ Extend the hand at the wrist joint.
■ Radially deviate the hand at the wrist joint.

Extensor Carpi Ulnaris

■ Extends the hand at the wrist joint.
■ Ulnar deviates the hand at the wrist joint.

STABILIZATION

Stabilizes the wrist and elbow joints.

INNERVATION

■ Radial nerve

PALPATION

Extensor Carpi Radialis Longus and Extensor Carpi Radialis Brevis

1. The client is seated with the arm relaxed and the forearm flexed at the elbow joint and in a position that is halfway between full pronation and full supination; the forearm is resting on the client's thigh.

2. The radial group is pinched with the palpating fingers and separated from the rest of the musculature of the forearm. Pinch the radial group of muscles between your thumb on one side and your index finger (or index and middle fingers) on the other side; gently pull them away from the forearm (Figure 7-18, *A*).

3. Move your palpating finger pads onto the extensors carpi radialis longus and brevis (posterior to the brachioradialis) and feel for their contraction as the client radially deviates the hand at the wrist joint (Figure 7-18, *B*). Resistance to radial deviation can be added with your support/resistance hand, if desired.

4. Continue palpating the extensor carpi radialis muscles toward their distal attachments by strumming perpendicularly across them.

7

Turn page to ◉ more.

7

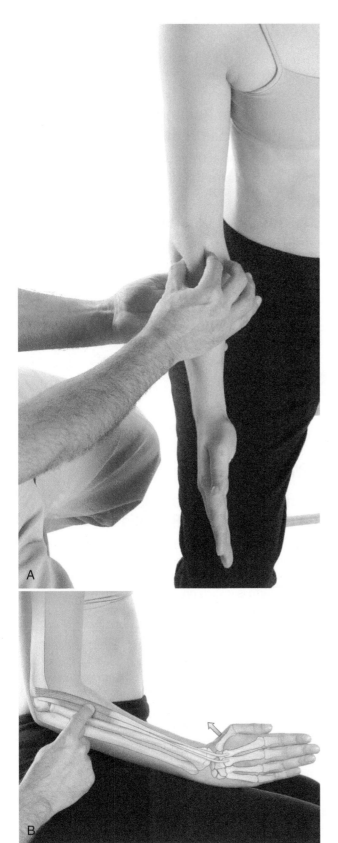

FIGURE 7-18 **A,** Right radial group of muscles is being pinched between the thumb and index finger of the therapist. **B,** Palpation of the extensors carpi radialis longus and brevis as the client radially deviates the hand at the wrist joint.

Extensor Carpi Ulnaris

1. The client is seated with the arm relaxed; the forearm is flexed at the elbow joint, fully pronated at the radioulnar joints, and resting on the client's thigh.

2. Place your palpating finger pads immediately posterior to the shaft of the ulna.

3. Ask the client to ulnar deviate the hand at the wrist joint and feel for the contraction of the extensor carpi ulnaris (Figure 7-19). If resistance is given, place your resistance hand on the ulnar side of the client's hand, proximal to the fingers.

4. Palpate proximally toward the lateral epicondyle and distally toward the fifth metacarpal by strumming perpendicular to the fibers as the client alternately contracts and relaxes the muscle.

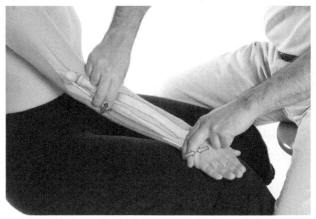

FIGURE 7-19 Palpation of the right extensor carpi ulnaris immediately posterior to the shaft of the ulna as the client ulnar deviates the hand at the wrist joint against resistance.

TREATMENT CONSIDERATIONS

■ Overuse of the wrist extensor group can cause irritation and/or inflammation of the lateral epicondyle and/or the common extensor tendon. This condition is known as *lateral epicondylitis, lateral epicondylosis,* or *tennis elbow*.

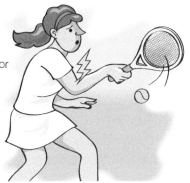

■ Stabilizing the wrist joint is an important action of the wrist extensor group, especially the extensor carpi radialis brevis. When the finger flexors contract to make a fist, wrist joint extensor muscles contract to prevent these finger flexor muscles from also flexing the hand at the wrist joint.

■ The attachment of the extensor carpi ulnaris onto the ulna blends with the ulnar attachment of the flexor carpi ulnaris and the flexor digitorum profundus.

7

7

FOREARM AND HAND
Extensor Digitorum; Extensor Digiti Minimi

Pronunciation   eks-TEN-sor dij-i-TOE-rum • eks-TEN-sor DIJ-i-tee MIN-i-mee

The extensor digitorum and extensor digiti minimi are superficial muscles in the posterior forearm and are located between the muscles of the wrist extensor group. They are considered to be long extrinsic finger muscles because they originate (have their proximal attachment) outside of the hand. They extend fingers two through five (Figure 7-20).

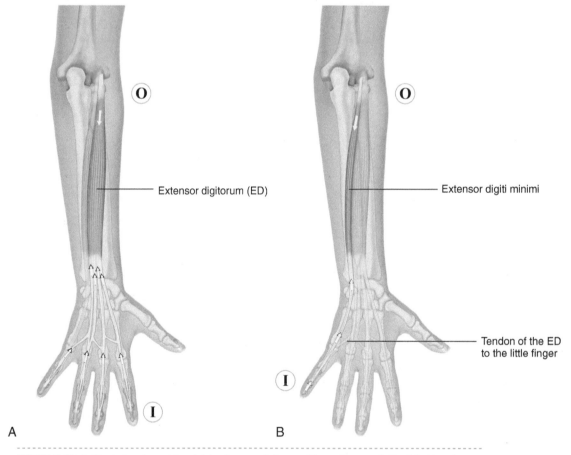

Extensor digitorum (ED)

Extensor digiti minimi

Tendon of the ED to the little finger

A   B

FIGURE 7-20 A, Posterior view of the right extensor digitorum. The extensor digiti minimi has been ghosted in. **B,** Posterior view of the right extensor digiti minimi. The extensor digitorum has been ghosted in. *O,* Origin; *I,* insertion.

WHAT'S IN A NAME?

The name, *extensor digitorum,* tells us that this muscle extends the digits (i.e., fingers).

The name, *extensor digiti minimi,* tells us that this muscle extends the little finger.

❊ **Derivation:**
    extensor: L. muscle that extends a body part
    digitorum: L. refers to a digit (finger)
    digiti: L. refers to a digit (finger)
    minimi: L. least

ATTACHMENTS

Extensor Digitorum

Origin (Proximal Attachment)

- Lateral epicondyle of the humerus via the common extensor tendon

Insertion (Distal Attachment)

- Posterior surfaces of fingers two through five

Extensor Digiti Minimi

Origin (Proximal Attachment)

- Lateral epicondyle of the humerus via the common extensor tendon

Insertion (Distal Attachment)

- Little finger (finger five)

ACTIONS

The extensor digitorum and extensor digiti minimi move the fingers at MCP joints and at the PIP and DIP joints; they also move the hand at the wrist joint.

Extensor Digitorum

- Extends fingers two through five at the MCP, PIP, and DIP joints.
- Extends the hand at the wrist joint.

Extensor Digiti Minimi

- Extends the little finger (finger five) at the MCP, PIP, and DIP joints.
- Extends the hand at the wrist joint.

STABILIZATION

1. Stabilizes the MCP, PIP, and DIP joints.
2. Stabilizes the wrist joint.
3. Stabilizes the fifth CMC joint.

INNERVATION

- Radial nerve

PALPATION

1. The client is seated with the arm relaxed; the forearm is flexed at the elbow joint, fully pronated at the radioulnar joints, and resting on the client's thigh. Place your palpating finger pads on the middle of the posterior proximal forearm.

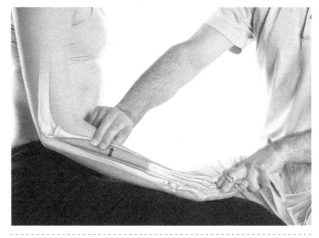

FIGURE 7-21 Palpation of the right extensor digitorum and extensor digiti minimi as the client extends fingers two through five against resistance.

2. Ask the client to extend fingers two through five fully at the MCP and IP joints (be sure that the client is not attempting to also extend the hand at the wrist joint), and feel for the contraction of the extensor digitorum and extensor digiti minimi (Figure 7-21).

   Note: Discerning the border of these two muscles is difficult.

3. If resistance is given, place your resistance hand on the posterior side of the fingers, not over the metacarpals of the hand.

4. Continue palpating toward the insertion and then the origin (distal and proximal attachments) by strumming perpendicular to the fibers of these two muscles.

   Note: The distal tendons of the finger extensors can often be seen on the posterior surface of the hand.

TREATMENT CONSIDERATIONS

- The distal attachment of the extensor digitorum spreads out to become a fibrous expansion that covers the posterior, medial, and lateral sides of the proximal phalanx. It then continues distally to attach onto the posterior sides of the middle and distal phalanges. This structure is called the *dorsal digital expansion*.

- Irritation and/or inflammation of the lateral epicondyle and/or the common extensor tendon is known as *lateral epicondylitis, lateral epicondylosis,* or *tennis elbow*.

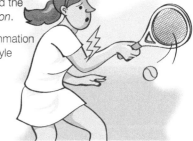

- The belly of the extensor digiti minimi often blends with the belly of the extensor digitorum.

FOREARM AND HAND
Supinator

Pronunciation   **SUE-pin-AY-tor**

The supinator is located proximally in the deep compartment of the posterior forearm (Figure 7-22).

WHAT'S IN A NAME?

The name, *supinator,* tells us that this muscle supinates the forearm.

❋ **Derivation:**
supinator: L. muscle that supinates a body part

ATTACHMENTS

Origin (Proximal Attachment)
- Lateral epicondyle of the humerus and the proximal ulna

Insertion (Distal Attachment)
- Proximal radius

ACTIONS

- Supinates the forearm at the radioulnar joints.

STABILIZATION

Stabilizes the radioulnar and elbow joints.

INNERVATION

- Radial nerve

PALPATION

1. The client is seated with the arm relaxed, and the forearm is flexed at the elbow joint in a position that is halfway between full pronation and full supination and is resting on the client's thigh. Place your resistance hand on the client's distal forearm, just proximal to the wrist joint.

2. With your palpating hand, pinch the radial group of muscles between your thumb on one side and your index and middle fingers on the other side, and gently pull them away from the forearm (see Figure 7-18, *A*). Now gently but firmly sink in (between the extensor carpi radialis brevis of the radial group and the extensor digitorum) with your thumb (if palpating with your right hand) toward the supinator attachment on the radius.

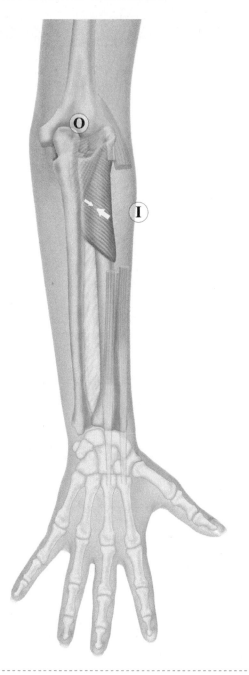

FIGURE 7-22 Posterior view of the right supinator. The anconeus, extensor carpi radialis longus (cut), and extensor carpi radialis brevis (cut) have been ghosted in. *O,* Origin; *I,* insertion.

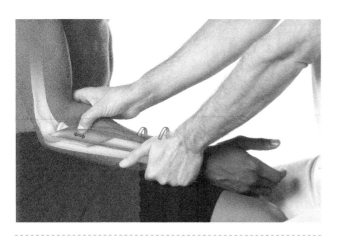

FIGURE 7-23 Palpation of the right supinator against the radius between the radial group of muscles and the extensor digitorum.

3. Ask the client to supinate the forearm against resistance, and feel for the contraction of the supinator (Figure 7-23).

4. Continue palpating the supinator (through the more superficial musculature) toward its proximal attachment, and feel for its contraction as the client alternately contracts and relaxes the supinator.

TREATMENT CONSIDERATIONS

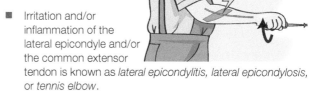

- Proximally, the supinator muscle has a superficial layer and a deep layer. A deep branch of the radial nerve runs between the two layers and may be entrapped there.

- Irritation and/or inflammation of the lateral epicondyle and/or the common extensor tendon is known as *lateral epicondylitis, lateral epicondylosis,* or *tennis elbow*.

- **The deep branch of the radial nerve runs through the supinator muscle. Be aware of this when pressing in deeply against the supinator.**

7

FOREARM AND HAND: Deep Distal Four Group
Abductor Pollicis Longus; Extensor Pollicis Brevis; Extensor Pollicis Longus; Extensor Indicis

Pronunciation ab-DUK-tor POL-i-sis LONG-us • eks-TEN-sor POL-i-sis BRE-vis • eks-TEN-sor POL-i-sis LONG-us • eks-TEN-sor IN-di-sis

The deep distal four group is a group of four muscles located distally in the deep compartment of the posterior forearm. Three of these muscles move the thumb; the fourth muscle moves the index finger (Figure 7-24).

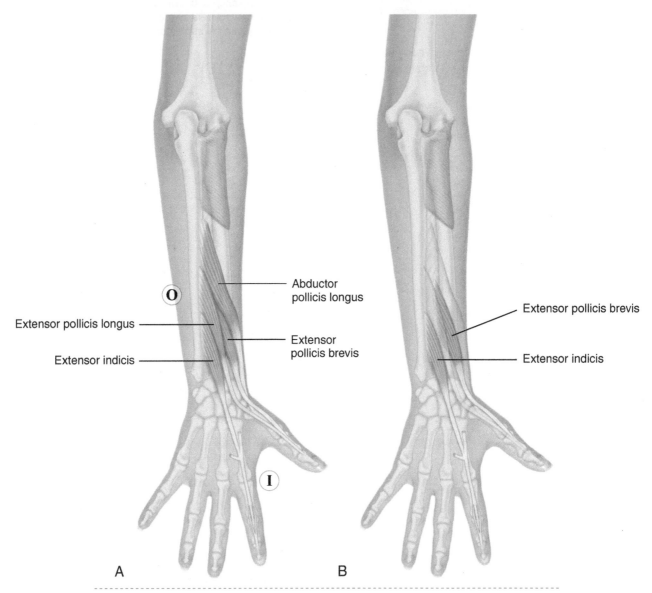

FIGURE 7-24 Posterior views of the muscles of the right deep distal four group. **A,** All four muscles are shown with the supinator ghosted in. **B,** The abductor pollicis longus and extensor pollicis longus have now been ghosted in. *O,* Origin; *I,* insertion.

The name, *abductor pollicis longus,* tells us that this muscle abducts the thumb and is long (longer than the abductor pollicis brevis).

The name, *extensor pollicis brevis,* tells us that this muscle extends the thumb and is shorter than the extensor pollicis longus.

The name, *extensor pollicis longus,* tells us that this muscle extends the thumb and is longer than the extensor pollicis brevis.

The name, *extensor indicis,* tells us that this muscle extends the index finger.

✳ **Derivation:**
abductor: L. muscle that abducts a body part
extensor: L. muscle that extends a body part
pollicis: L. thumb
indicis: L. index finger (finger two)
longus: L. longer
brevis: L. shorter

ATTACHMENTS

Abductor Pollicis Longus

Origin (Proximal Attachment)
- Posterior radius and ulna

Insertion (Distal Attachment)
- Thumb

Extensor Pollicis Brevis

Origin (Proximal Attachment)
- Posterior radius

Insertion (Distal Attachment)
- Thumb

Extensor Pollicis Longus

Origin (Proximal Attachment)
- Posterior ulna

Insertion (Distal Attachment)
- Thumb

Extensor Indicis

Origin (Proximal Attachment)
- Posterior ulna

Insertion (Distal Attachment)
- Index finger (finger two)

ACTIONS

The muscles of the deep distal four group move the thumb at the CMC (saddle), MCP, and IP joints, and the index finger at the MCP and proximal and distal IP (PIP and DIP) joints.

> Note: Abduction of the thumb is a sagittal plane motion in which the thumb is brought anteriorly away from the plane of the palm of the hand. Extension of the thumb is a frontal plane motion in which the thumb is moved away from the index finger.

Abductor Pollicis Longus
- Abducts the thumb at the CMC joint.
- Extends the thumb at the CMC joint.

Extensor Pollicis Brevis
- Extends the thumb at the CMC and MCP joints.
- Abducts the thumb at the CMC joint.

Extensor Pollicis Longus
- Extends the thumb at the CMC, MCP, and IP joints.

Extensor Indicis
- Extends the index finger at the MCP, PIP, and DIP joints.

STABILIZATION

1. Stabilizes the CMC (saddle), MCP, and IP joints of the thumb.
2. Stabilizes the MCP, PIP, and DIP joints of the index finger.

INNERVATION

- Radial nerve

7

Turn page to 👁 more.

▎ PALPATION

1. The client is seated with the arm relaxed; the forearm is flexed at the elbow joint, fully pronated at the radioulnar joints, and resting on the client's thigh.

2. Ask the client to actively extend the thumb (in the frontal plane) and look to see the distal tendons of this group that border the anatomic snuffbox.

3. Now begin palpating the distal tendons on the radial side of the posterior wrist.

   Note: The tendons of the abductor pollicis longus and extensor pollicis brevis are right next to one another and may appear to be one tendon; you can gently separate them with a fingernail.

4. Once located, palpate each of these muscles individually back to its proximal attachment by strumming perpendicular to the fibers as the client alternately contracts and relaxes each muscle by extending the thumb (Figure 7-25, *A*).

5. To palpate the extensor indicis, first locate its distal tendon on the posterior side of the hand by asking the client to extend the index finger at the MCP and IP joints (Figure 7-25, *B*).

6. Continue palpating the extensor indicis proximally by strumming perpendicular to its fibers as the client alternately contracts and relaxes the muscle.

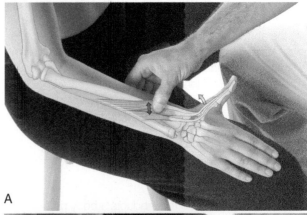

A

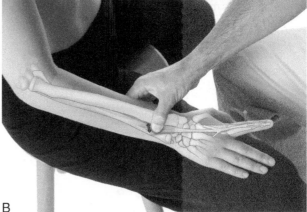

B

FIGURE 7-25 A, Palpation of the three thumb muscles of the right deep distal four group (abductor pollicis longus, and extensors pollicis brevis and longus) as the client fully extends the thumb. **B,** Palpation of the right extensor indicis of the deep distal four group as the client fully extends the index finger.

▎ TREATMENT CONSIDERATIONS

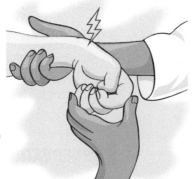

- The distal tendons of the three thumb muscles of the deep distal four group border the anatomic snuffbox. The abductor pollicis longus and extensor pollicis brevis create the lateral border (they are very close together and can be difficult to distinguish from each other); the extensor pollicis longus creates the medial border. The scaphoid bone is located within the anatomic snuffbox.

- The abductor pollicis longus and the extensor pollicis brevis share a common synovial sheath. With excessive movements of the thumb, the friction between the tendons of the abductor pollicis longus and/or the extensor pollicis brevis and the styloid process of the radius can cause atenosynovitis (inflammation of the synovial sheath). This condition is known as *de Quervain's disease*.

- The distal attachment of the extensor pollicis longus spreads out to become the fibrous dorsal digital expansion of the thumb.

Notes

FOREARM AND HAND: Thenar Eminence Group
Abductor Pollicis Brevis; Flexor Pollicis Brevis; Opponens Pollicis

Pronunciation   **ab-DUK-tor POL-i-sis BRE-vis •**
FLEKS-or POL-i-sis BRE-vis • op-PO-nens POL-i-sis

The thenar eminence group is composed of three muscles: (1) abductor pollicis brevis, (2) flexor pollicis brevis, and (3) opponens pollicis. These muscles are intrinsic hand muscles (wholly located within the hand) that attach onto and move the thumb. The abductor is the most superficial, the flexor is intermediate in depth, and the opponens is the deepest (Figure 7-26).

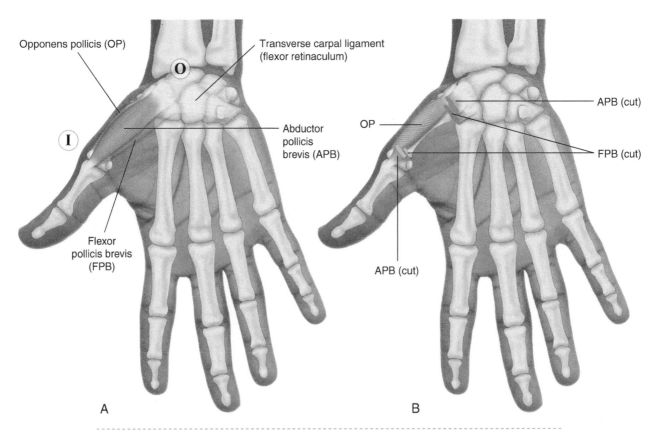

A

B

FIGURE 7-26 Anterior views of the right thenar group muscles. *A,* Superficial view. *B,* Deep view. The abductor pollicis brevis and flexor pollicis brevis have been cut. *O,* Origin; *I,* insertion.

The name, *abductor pollicis brevis,* tells us that this muscle abducts the thumb and is short (shorter than the abductor pollicis longus).

The name, *flexor pollicis brevis,* tells us that this muscle flexes the thumb and is short (shorter than the flexor pollicis longus).

The name, *opponens pollicis,* tells us that this muscle opposes the thumb.

✳ Derivation:
  abductor: L. muscle that abducts a body part
  flexor: L. muscle that flexes a body part
  opponens: L. opposing
  pollicis L. thumb
  brevis: L. shorter

ATTACHMENTS

Abductor Pollicis Brevis

Origin (Proximal Attachment)
  ▪ Flexor retinaculum and the scaphoid and trapezium

Insertion (Distal Attachment)
  ▪ Proximal phalanx of the thumb

Flexor Pollicis Brevis

Origin (Proximal Attachment)
  ▪ Flexor retinaculum and trapezium

Insertion (Distal Attachment)
  ▪ Proximal phalanx of the thumb

Opponens Pollicis

Origin (Proximal Attachment)
  ▪ Flexor retinaculum and trapezium

Insertion (Distal Attachment)
  ▪ First metacarpal (of the thumb)

ACTIONS

The thenar muscles move the thumb at the CMC (saddle) and MCP joints.

Note: Abduction of the thumb is a sagittal plane motion in which the thumb is brought anteriorly away from the plane of the palm of the hand. Flexion of the thumb is a frontal plane motion in which the thumb is brought toward the index finger. Opposition of the thumb occurs when the thumb pad meets the pad of another finger.

Abductor Pollicis Brevis
  ▪ Abducts the thumb at the CMC joint.

Flexor Pollicis Brevis
  ▪ Flexes the thumb at the CMC and MCP joints.

Opponens Pollicis
  ▪ Opposes the thumb at the CMC joint.

STABILIZATION

The thenar group stabilizes the CMC and MCP joints of the thumb.

INNERVATION

  ▪ Median nerve
  ▪ Ulnar nerve

  Note: The median nerve innervates all three thenar muscles; the ulnar nerve also innervates the flexor pollicis brevis and opponens pollicis.

PALPATION

1. The client is seated. Place your palpating finger pads on the lateral side of the thenar eminence of the client; place your resistance hand on the anterior surface of the proximal phalanx of the client's thumb.

2. For the abductor pollicis brevis, palpate the lateral side of the thenar eminence and feel for its contraction as you gently to moderately resist the client from abducting the thumb at the saddle joint.

3. Pinching the muscle between your thumb and index finger can be helpful (Figure 7-27, *A*).

4. Once felt, palpate the muscle to its proximal and distal attachments.

5. For the flexor pollicis brevis, palpate the most medial aspect of the thenar eminence and feel for its contraction as you moderately resist the client from flexing the thumb at the saddle joint (Figure 7-27, *B*).

Turn page to 👁 more.

7

7

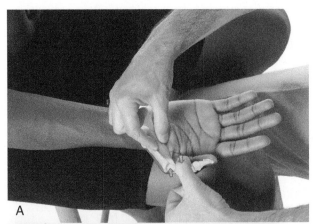

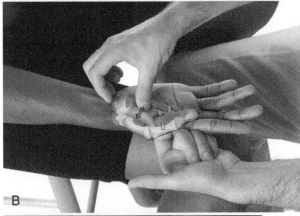

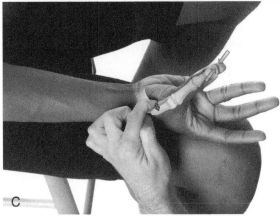

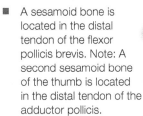

FIGURE 7-27 Palpation of the right thenar group. *A,* Palpation of the abductor pollicis brevis as the client abducts the thumb at the carpometacarpal (CMC) joint against resistance. *B,* Palpation of the flexor pollicis brevis as the client flexes the thumb at the CMC joint against resistance. *C,* Palpation of the opponens pollicis by curling around the metacarpal of the thumb as the client opposes the thumb at the CMC joint to the little finger.

6. Once felt, try to palpate it deep to the abductor pollicis brevis more laterally as the client alternately contracts the muscle against gentle resistance and relaxes it.

7. For the opponens pollicis, curl your palpating finger(s) around the shaft of the metacarpal of the thumb (Figure 7-27, *C*). Ask the client to oppose the thumb against the little finger, exerting gentle pressure against the pad of the little finger; feel for the contraction of the opponens pollicis.

8. Once felt against the metacarpal, attempt to palpate the rest of this muscle deep to the other thenar muscles.

Note: Discerning the opponens pollicis from the other thenar muscles can be very difficult. For this reason, palpating for tight spots in this muscle is usually more effective with the thenar musculature relaxed.

TREATMENT CONSIDERATIONS

■ With the tremendous increase of cell phone texting, the thumb muscles are being overused, which can lead to a repetitive-use syndrome that is called *texting thumb*. Manual therapists need to be especially aware of this condition, given that they already tend to use their thumbs so much when performing soft tissue manipulation.

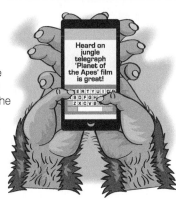

■ The overuse of our thumbs for texting will likely also increase the incidence of arthritic changes (degenerative joint disease) of the saddle joint of the thumb. This condition is known as *basilar arthritis*.

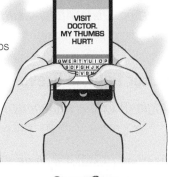

■ A sesamoid bone is located in the distal tendon of the flexor pollicis brevis. Note: A second sesamoid bone of the thumb is located in the distal tendon of the adductor pollicis.

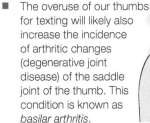

■ Apes can oppose their thumb, but it is so short that it is not very functional for grasping objects.

Notes

FOREARM AND HAND: Hypothenar Eminence Group
Abductor Digiti Minimi Manus; Flexor Digiti Minimi Manus; Opponens Digiti Minimi

Pronunciation   ab-DUK-tor DIJ-i-tee MIN-i-mee MAN-us •
FLEKS-or DIJ-i-tee MIN-i-mee MAN-us • op-PO-nens DIJ-i-tee MIN-i-mee

The hypothenar eminence group is composed of three muscles: (1) abductor digiti minimi manus, (2) flexor digiti minimi manus, and (3) opponens digiti minimi. Note the similarity to the thenar group—both groups have an abductor, flexor, and opponens. Hypothenar muscles are intrinsic hand muscles (wholly located within the hand) that attach onto and move the little finger. The abductor is the most superficial, the flexor is intermediate in depth, and the opponens is the deepest (Figure 7-28).

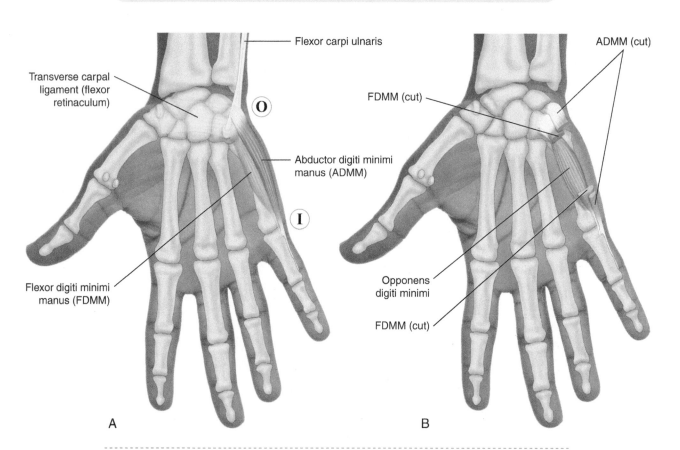

FIGURE 7-28 Anterior views of the right hypothenar group muscles. **A,** Superficial view. The flexor carpi ulnaris has been drawn in. **B,** Deep view. The abductor digiti minimi manus (ADMM) and flexor digiti minimi manus (FDMM) have been cut. *O,* Origin; *I,* insertion.

The name, *abductor digiti minimi manus,* tells us that this muscle abducts the little finger.

The name, *flexor digiti minimi manus,* tells us that this muscle flexes the little finger.

The name, *opponens digiti minimi,* tells us that this muscle opposes the little finger.

❋ **Derivation:**
abductor: L. muscle that abducts a body part
flexor: L. muscle that flexes a body part
opponens: L. opposing
digiti: L. refers to a digit (finger)
minimi: L. least
manus: L. refers to the hand

ATTACHMENTS

Abductor Digiti Minimi Manus

Origin (Proximal Attachment)
- Pisiform

Insertion (Distal Attachment)
- Proximal phalanx of the little finger (finger five)

Flexor Digiti Minimi Manus

Origin (Proximal Attachment)
- Flexor retinaculum and the hamate

Insertion (Distal Attachment)
- Proximal phalanx of the little finger (finger five)

Opponens Digiti Minimi

Origin (Proximal Attachment)
- Flexor retinaculum and the hamate

Insertion (Distal Attachment)
- Fifth metacarpal (of the little finger)

ACTIONS

The hypothenar muscles move the little finger at the CMC and MCP joints.

Abductor Digiti Minimi Manus
- Abducts the little finger at the MCP joint.

Flexor Digiti Minimi Manus
- Flexes the little finger at the MCP joint.

Opponens Digiti Minimi
- Opposes the little finger at the CMC joint.

STABILIZATION

Stabilizes the CMC and MCP joints of the little finger.

INNERVATION

- Ulnar nerve

PALPATION

1. The client is seated. Place your palpating finger pads on the medial side of the hypothenar eminence of the client. Place your resistance finger on the medial surface of the proximal phalanx of the client's little finger.

2. For the abductor digiti minimi manus, feel for its contraction at the medial side of the hypothenar eminence as you resist the client from abducting the little finger at the MCP joint (Figure 7-29, *A*).

3. Once felt, palpate distally to the medial side of the base of the proximal phalanx and proximally to the pisiform.

4. For the flexor digiti minimi manus, feel for its contraction on the lateral side of the hypothenar eminence as you resist the client from flexing the little finger at the MCP joint, while keeping the little finger extended at the IP joints (Figure 7-29, *B*).

   Note: Your resistance finger should be placed over the anterior surface of the proximal phalanx of the little finger.

5. Once felt, palpate distally to the anteromedial surface of the base of the proximal phalanx and proximally to the hook of the hamate.

6. For the opponens digiti minimi, feel for its contraction immediately distal to the hook of the hamate at the most lateral aspect of the hypothenar eminence as the client opposes the little finger against the thumb (Figure 7-29, *C*).

7. Once felt, palpate distally as far as possible deep to the other muscles of the hypothenar eminence.

8. Curling your palpating finger around to the anterior side of the shaft of the fifth metacarpal can usually palpate the metacarpal attachment of the opponens digiti minimi (Figure 7-29, *D*).

   Note: This palpation step is similar to how the opponens pollicis is palpated against the first metacarpal.

Turn page to 👁 more.

7

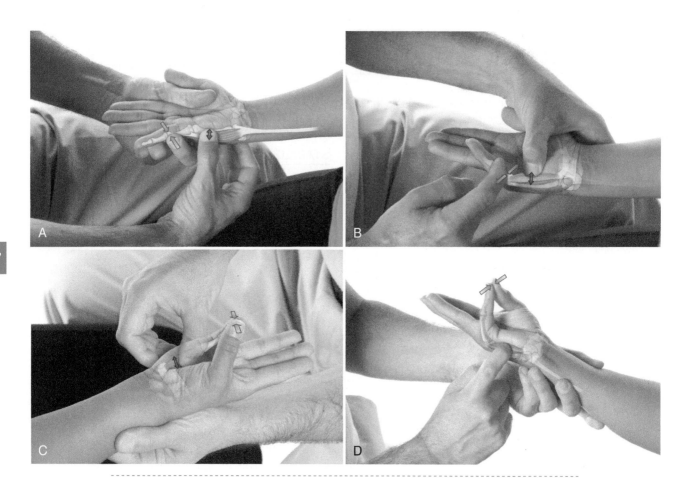

FIGURE 7-29 Palpation of the right hypothenar group. *A,* Palpation of the abductor digiti minimi manus at the medial side of the hypothenar eminence as the client abducts the little finger against resistance. *B,* Palpation of the flexor digiti minimi manus at the lateral side of the hypothenar eminence as the client flexes the proximal phalanx of the little finger against resistance. *C,* Palpation of the opponens digiti minimi at the far lateral side of the hypothenar eminence as the client opposes the little finger against resistance. *D,* Palpation of the opponens digiti minimi against the metacarpal of the little finger as the client opposes the little finger against resistance.

TREATMENT CONSIDERATIONS

■ The origin (proximal attachment) of the abductor digiti minimi manus is the pisiform. Whenever the abductor digiti minimi contracts, the flexor carpi ulnaris also contracts to fix (stabilize) the pisiform. This knowledge can be used to engage and palpate the flexor carpi ulnaris. Ask for the client to abduct the little finger actively; the distal tendon of the flexor carpi ulnaris at the distal wrist on the ulnar side can be felt to contract.

■ The flexor digiti minimi manus is often very small or entirely absent. When this occurs, the opponens digiti minimi will have relatively more superficial exposure.

■ We do not normally think of the little finger as having to work very hard; however, manual therapy can physically stress the hypothenar muscles of the little finger, especially if pinching (opposition) motions are performed often.

Notes

7

FOREARM AND HAND
Palmaris Brevis

Pronunciation **pall-MA-ris BRE-vis**

The palmaris brevis is technically not part of the hypothenar group because it does not attach onto and move the little finger. It is a very thin superficial muscle located within the fascia and dermis that overlie the hypothenar eminence. For this reason, it is being considered here (Figure 7-30).

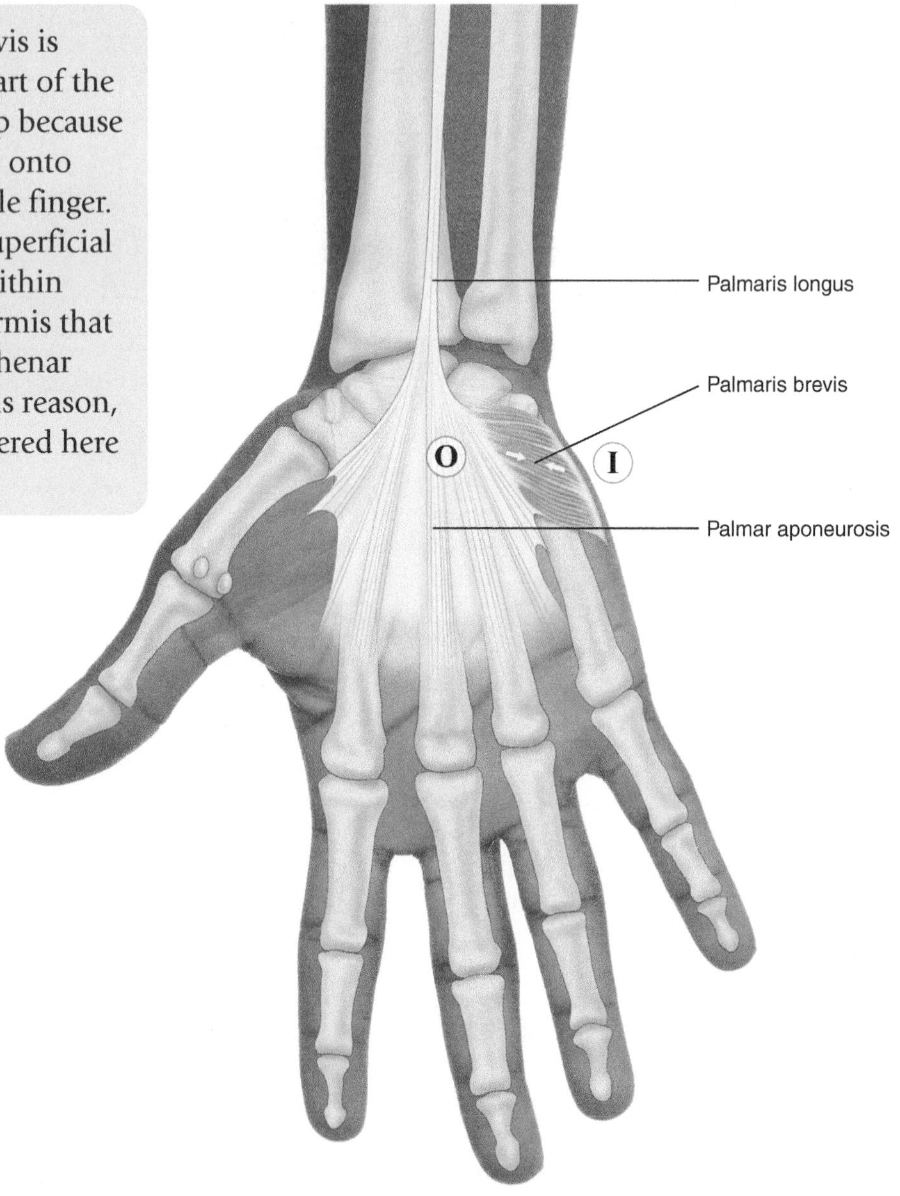

Palmaris longus

Palmaris brevis

O   I

Palmar aponeurosis

FIGURE 7-30 Anterior view of the right palmaris brevis. *O,* Origin; *I,* insertion.

WHAT'S IN A NAME?

The name, *palmaris brevis,* tells us that this muscle attaches into the palm of the hand and is short (shorter than the palmaris longus).

✳ **Derivation:**
   palmaris: L. refers to the palm
   brevis: L. shorter

ATTACHMENTS

Origin (Proximal Attachment)
■ Flexor retinaculum and the palmar aponeurosis

Insertion (Distal Attachment)
■ Dermis of the ulnar (medial) border of the hand

ACTIONS

- Wrinkles the skin of the palm.

STABILIZATION

The palmaris brevis has no joint stabilization function.

INNERVATION

- Ulnar nerve

PALPATION

1. The client is seated. Gently place your palpating finger pad(s) over the hypothenar eminence.

2. Ask the client to cup the palm of the hand; feel for this muscle's contraction (Figure 7-31). Be sure that the little finger is either not moved at all or moved as little as possible, or you will feel the contraction of the hypothenar muscles.

   Note: The palmaris brevis is extremely thin and difficult to discern from adjacent soft tissue.

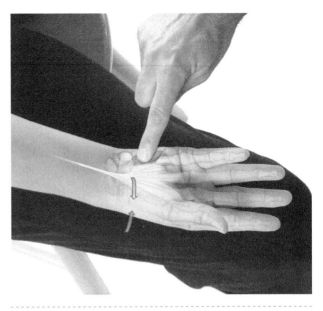

FIGURE 7-31 Palpation of the right palmaris brevis.

7

FOREARM AND HAND: Central Compartment Group
Adductor Pollicis; Lumbricals Manus; Palmar Interossei; Dorsal Interossei Manus

Pronunciation   ad-DUK-tor POL-i-sis • LUM-bri-kuls MAN-us •
PAL-mar IN-ter-OSS-ee-i • DOR-sul IN-ter-OSS-ee-i MAN-us

7

The central compartment is composed of intrinsic hand muscles that are located between the thenar and hypothenar eminences. The central compartment includes the adductor pollicis, four muscles of the lumbricals manus group, three muscles of the palmar interossei group, and four muscles of the dorsal interossei manus group (Figure 7-32). All of these muscles are found and palpated in the palm of the hand except for the dorsal interossei manus group, which is located on the dorsal side (the adductor pollicis is in the thumb web and can be palpated from both sides). The lumbricals manus, palmar interossei, and dorsal interossei manus are named by numbering them, beginning on the thumb (radial) side.

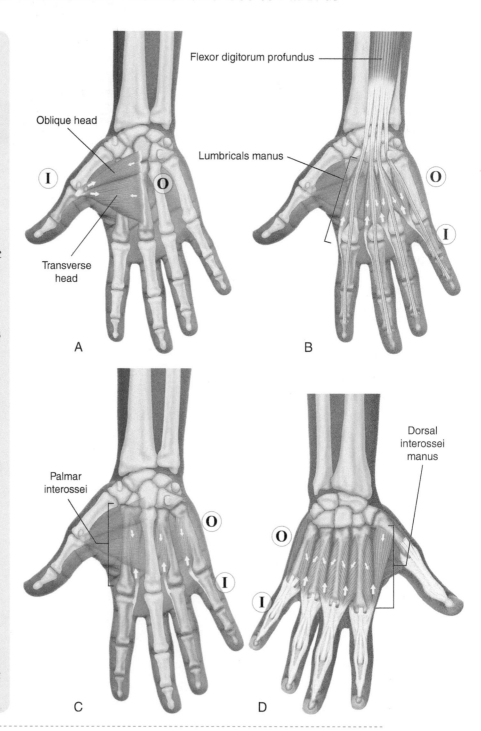

FIGURE 7-32 **A,** Anterior view of the right adductor pollicis. **B,** Anterior view of the right lumbricals manus. The flexor digitorum profundus muscle has been drawn in. **C,** Anterior view of the right palmar interossei. **D,** Posterior view of the right dorsal interossei manus. **B, C,** and **D** have the adductor pollicis ghosted in. *O,* Origin; *I,* insertion.

The name, *adductor pollicis,* tells us that this muscle adducts the thumb.

The name, *lumbricals manus,* tells us that these muscles are shaped like earthworms and are located in the hand.

The name, *palmar interossei,* tells us that these muscles are located between bones (metacarpals) on the palmar (anterior) side.

The name, *dorsal interossei manus,* tells us that these muscles are located between bones (metacarpals) on the dorsal (posterior) side and located in the hand.

❊ Derivation:
adductor: L. muscle that adducts a body part
pollicis: L. thumb
manus: L. refers to the hand
palmar: L. refers to the palm
dorsal: L. back
interossei: L. between bones
lumbricals: L. earthworms

- -

ATTACHMENTS

Adductor Pollicis

Origin (Proximal Attachment)
■ Third metacarpal and capitate

Insertion (Distal Attachment)
■ Proximal phalanx of the thumb

Lumbricals Manus

Origin (Proximal Attachment)
■ Distal tendons of the flexor digitorum profundus muscle

Insertion (Distal Attachment)
■ Distal tendons of the extensor digitorum muscle (the dorsal digital expansion)

Palmar Interossei

Origin (Proximal Attachment)
■ Metacarpals of fingers two, four, and five

Insertion (Distal Attachment)
■ Proximal phalanges of fingers two, four, and five on the "middle finger side"

Dorsal Interossei Manus

Origin (Proximal Attachment)
■ Metacarpals of fingers one through five

Insertion (Distal Attachment)
■ Proximal phalanges of fingers two, three, and four on the side that faces away from the center of the middle finger

ACTIONS

The central compartment muscles move the thumb at the CMC (saddle) joint, and move fingers two through five at the MCP joints.

Note: Abduction of fingers two through five is a motion during which the fingers move away from an imaginary line drawn through the middle finger when it is in anatomic position. The middle finger itself can abduct in both the radial and ulnar direction. Adduction of fingers two through five is a motion during which the fingers move toward the same imaginary reference line; the middle finger itself, by definition, cannot adduct.

Adduction of the thumb is a sagittal plane motion during which the thumb is brought posteriorly back toward the plane of the palm of the hand.

Adductor Pollicis
■ Adducts the thumb at the CMC joint.

Lumbricals Manus
■ Flexes fingers two through five at the MCP joints.

Palmar Interossei
■ Adducts fingers two, four, and five at the MCP joints.

Dorsal Interossei Manus
■ Abducts fingers two through four at the MCP joints.

STABILIZATION

1. The adductor pollicis stabilizes the thumb at the CMC and MCP joints of the thumb.
2. The other central compartment muscles stabilize the MCP joints of fingers two through five.
3. The first dorsal interosseus also stabilizes the CMC joint of the thumb.

7

Turn page to 👁 more.

INNERVATION

- Ulnar nerve
- Median nerve

The ulnar nerve innervates all central compartment muscles. The median nerve also innervates the lumbricals manus group. The median nerve innervates the first and second lumbricals; the ulnar nerve innervates the third and fourth lumbricals.

PALPATION

Adductor Pollicis

1. The client is seated. Place your palpating finger pad(s) on the anterior surface of the thumb web of the client's hand; place the fingers of the resistance hand on the posterior surface of the proximal phalanx of the client's thumb.

2. While palpating the anterior side of the thumb web of the hand, resist the client from adducting the thumb at the saddle joint; feel for the contraction of the adductor pollicis (Figure 7-33).

3. Once felt, palpate the entire adductor pollicis from the proximal phalanx of the thumb to the third metacarpal and capitate.

Lumbricals Manus

1. The client is seated. Palpating finger pad(s) are placed over the anterolateral surface of the shaft of each of the metacarpal bone of fingers two through five. If resistance is given, apply it to the anterior surface of the proximal phalanx of the finger of the same metacarpal bone.

2. To palpate the first lumbrical manus: Palpate over the anterolateral surface of the shaft of the second metacarpal, ask the client to flex the index finger at the MCP joint while keeping the IP joints completely extended, and feel for the contraction of the first lumbrical manus muscle (Figure 7-34, *A*). Once located, palpate from attachment to attachment.

3. To palpate the second lumbrical manus: Follow the same procedure as used for the first lumbrical manus muscle. Palpate over the anterolateral surface of the third metacarpal, and feel for its contraction as the client flexes the third finger at the MCP joint with the IP joints fully extended (Figure 7-34, *B*). Once located, palpate from attachment to attachment.

4. To palpate the third and fourth lumbricals manus: Follow the same protocol. For the third lumbrical manus, palpate between the third and fourth metacarpals. For the fourth lumbrical manus, palpate between the fourth and fifth metacarpals.

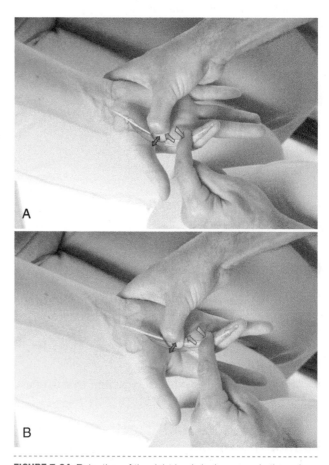

A

B

FIGURE 7-34 Palpation of the right lumbricals manus in the palm of the hand. **A,** Palpation of the first lumbrical manus on the lateral (radial) side of the metacarpal of the index finger. **B,** Palpation of the second lumbrical manus on the radial side of the metacarpal of the middle finger. The third and fourth lumbricals manus are palpated in a similar manner against the radial side of the metacarpals of the ring and little fingers, respectively.

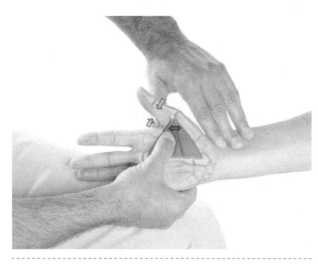

FIGURE 7-33 Palpation of the right adductor pollicis as the client adducts the thumb against resistance.

Palmar Interossei

1. The client is seated with a pencil or highlighter placed between the index and middle fingers. Palpating finger pad(s) are placed in the palm of the hand, between metacarpal bones.

2. To palpate the first palmar interosseus: Palpate in the palm against the second metacarpal between the second and third metacarpals. Ask the client to squeeze the highlighter between the index and middle fingers, and feel for the contraction of the first palmar interosseus muscle (Figure 7-35, *A*).

3. To palpate the second palmar interosseus: Follow the same procedure but palpate against the fourth metacarpal between the fourth and third metacarpals. Feel for the contraction of the second palmar interosseus as the client squeezes the highlighter between the ring and middle fingers (Figure 7-35, *B*).

4. To palpate the third palmar interosseus: Following the same procedure, palpate against the fifth metacarpal between the fifth and fourth metacarpals. Feel for the contraction of the third palmar interosseus as the client squeezes the highlighter between the little and ring fingers (Figure 7-35, *C*).

5. Once each palmar interosseus is located, follow it from attachment to attachment while the client alternately contracts and relaxes the muscle.

Dorsal Interossei Manus

1. The client is seated. Palpating finger pad(s) are placed on the dorsal side of the client's hand between the metacarpal bones. The contact for resistance will always be on the proximal phalanx.

2. To palpate the fourth dorsal interosseus manus: While palpating on the dorsal side of the hand between the fourth and fifth metacarpals, ask the client to abduct the ring finger against your resistance; feel for the contraction of the fourth dorsal interossei manus (DIM) (Figure 7-36, *A*).

3. To palpate the third dorsal interosseus manus: Following the same procedure, palpate between the third and fourth metacarpals while resisting ulnar abduction of the middle finger; feel for the contraction of the third DIM (Figure 7-36, *B*).

4. To palpate the second dorsal interosseus manus: Following the same procedure, palpate between the third and second metacarpals while resisting radial abduction of the middle finger; feel for the contraction of the second DIM (Figure 7-36, *C*).

5. To palpate the first dorsal interosseus manus: Palpate in the thumb web of the hand on the dorsal side, especially against the second metacarpal; feel for the contraction of the first DIM as the client abducts the index finger (Figure 7-36, *D*).

6. Once each dorsal interosseus manus is located, palpate from attachment to attachment as the client alternately contracts and relaxes the muscle.

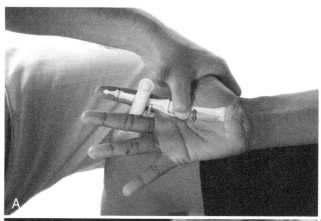

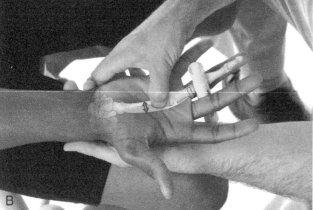

FIGURE 7-35 Palpation of the right palmar interossei (PI) in the palm of the hand. **A,** Palpation of the first PI as the client adducts the index finger against resistance (provided by a highlighter). **B,** Palpation of the second PI as the client adducts the ring finger against resistance. **C,** Palpation of the third PI as the client adducts the little finger against resistance.

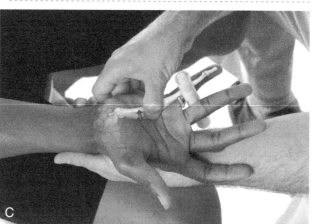

Turn page to 👁 more.

7

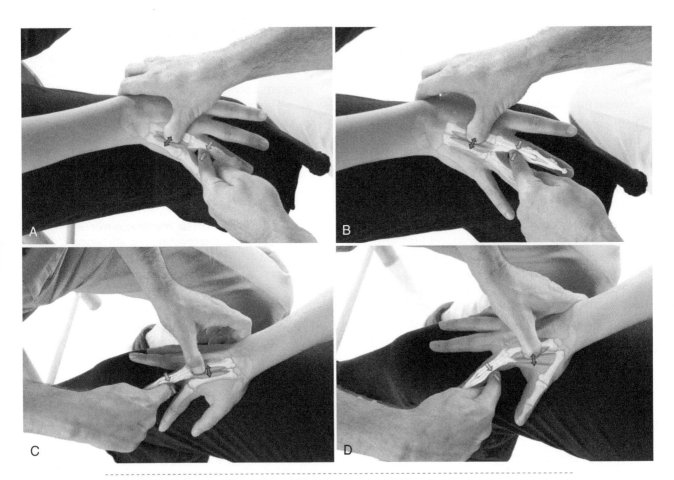

FIGURE 7-36 Palpation of the right dorsal interossei manus (DIM) on the dorsal surface of the hand. *A,* Palpation of the fourth DIM as the client abducts the ring finger against resistance. *B,* Palpation of the third DIM as the client ulnar abducts the middle finger against resistance. *C,* Palpation of the second DIM as the client radially abducts the middle finger against resistance. *D,* Palpation of the first DIM as the client abducts the index finger against resistance.

TREATMENT CONSIDERATIONS

- The oblique head of the adductor pollicis has a sesamoid bone located within it. Note: A second sesamoid bone of the thumb is located in the distal tendon of the flexor pollicis brevis.

- The majority of tissue of the thumb web of the hand is made up of the adductor pollicis and the first dorsal interosseus manus.

- The adductor pollicis contracts to create the pinching motion in which the thumb is brought toward the index finger in the sagittal plane (adduction at the saddle joint). Therapists who use this stroke technique often in their practice may find that their adductor pollicis becomes

fatigued and tight. Ironically, an ideal way to work a tight adductor pollicis in the thumb web is via a pinching stroke!

- The first dorsal interosseus manus muscle (the largest) is sometimes known as the abductor indicis.

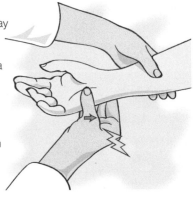

REVIEW QUESTIONS

Circle or fill in the correct answer for each of the following questions. More study resources, including audio pronunciations of muscle names, are provided on the Evolve website at http://evolve.elsevier.com/Muscolino/knowthebody.

1. What are the three muscles of the wrist flexor group?

   _____

   _____

   _____

2. What are the three muscles of the wrist extensor group?

   _____

   _____

   _____

3. What are the three muscles of the thenar group?

   _____

   _____

   _____

4. Which of the following muscles can flex and radially deviate the hand at the wrist joint?
   a. Palmaris longus
   b. Flexor carpi radialis
   c. Flexor carpi ulnaris
   d. Extensor carpi radialis longus

5. Which of the following muscles can flex the thumb at the IP joint?
   a. Pronator teres
   b. Flexor digitorum superficialis
   c. Flexor pollicis brevis
   d. Flexor pollicis longus

6. Which of the following muscles are intrinsic muscles of the hand?
   a. Flexor pollicis longus and flexor pollicis brevis
   b. Extensor pollicis brevis and adductor pollicis
   c. Abductor digiti minimi manus and palmar interossei
   d. Pronator teres and palmaris brevis

7. Which of the following muscles flexes and pronates the forearm?
   a. Flexor carpi ulnaris
   b. Pronator quadratus
   c. Biceps brachii
   d. Pronator teres

8. Which of the following muscles attaches to the medial epicondyle of the humerus via the common flexor tendon?
   a. Extensor carpi radialis longus
   b. Flexor carpi ulnaris
   c. Abductor pollicis longus
   d. Dorsal interossei manus

9. Which of the following muscles attach onto the thumb?
   a. Adductor pollicis and abductor pollicis brevis
   b. Flexor digitorum superficialis and flexor digitorum profundus
   c. Opponens pollicis and opponens digiti minimi
   d. Pronator teres and pronator quadratus

10. Which of the following muscles attach onto the styloid process of the radius?
    a. Brachioradialis
    b. Flexor digitorum superficialis
    c. Pronator teres
    d. Flexor carpi ulnaris

7

CASE STUDY 1

A client appears for his weekly massage appointment with complaints of pain in his left forearm. He is left-handed, 43 years of age, and in good shape. He has an active lifestyle; he likes to do carpentry jobs around the house and plays softball every week in a league.

Last weekend, he was working on a carpentry project at home with a manual screwdriver for many hours. That night, he felt soreness in his left anterior proximal forearm that radiated toward his elbow. The pain seemed to lessen over the next day or so. However, when he played softball Wednesday night, the pain returned. He felt sharp pain each time he threw the ball. As the game progressed, the intensity of the pain increased until it was constant and he could no longer play. He had to retire from the game. He immediately iced his forearm and took ibuprofen for pain relief. It is now Saturday; although his pain has lessened in intensity, it is still present. Visual examination shows that his proximal forearm is red and swollen.

QUESTIONS

1. **What activity of the client caused the injury, and what joint action and muscle was involved in the activity?**

   _____

   _____

   _____

   _____

   _____

   _____

2. **How would you assess this condition during the physical examination?**

   _____

   _____

   _____

   _____

   _____

   _____

   _____

   _____

   _____

3. **How would you treat this condition?**

   _____

   _____

   _____

   _____

   _____

   _____

   _____

   _____

   _____

   _____

CASE STUDY 2

A 34-year-old man comes to your office with pain and stiffness when he flexes and extends his left wrist joint. Using a pain scale of 0 to 10, the client feels pain at a 6 when he attempts to lift anything heavier than 25 pounds. The client is a mechanic and finds the pain is impeding his work. He has had this pain for 4 weeks. Two weeks earlier, he started to use over-the-counter pain medication for relief; it worked but only temporarily. After each workday, his left hand and forearm are significantly sore to the touch.

The client was asked if he had been involved in any form of accident or trauma or whether any change in his lifestyle had occurred. He responded negatively to both questions. As a follow-up question, the therapist asked, "Have you been doing any unexpected heavy or repetitive lifting?" The client responded that he was involved in moving large pieces of lumber that were both heavy and bulky a month ago.

On physical examination, the client has full and pain-free active and passive wrist joint range of motion into flexion, radial deviation, and ulnar deviation. However, active and passive extension is limited and he experiences pain in the anterior forearm with both. With manual resistance to motion, extension and ulnar deviation are negative for pain. Resisted radial deviation causes mild anterior forearm pain, and resisted flexion causes strong and immediate anterior forearm pain.

QUESTIONS

1. **What muscles would you expect to find tight and painful on palpation assessment?**

_____

_____

_____

_____

_____

_____

2. **Why did you choose those muscles?**

_____

_____

_____

_____

_____

_____

_____

_____

_____

3. **How would you treat this client?**

_____

_____

_____

_____

_____

_____

_____

_____

_____

_____

Muscles of the Spine and Rib Cage

The muscles of this chapter are primarily involved with movement of the trunk, neck, and head at the spinal joints. Some of these spinal muscles can also move the mandible at the temporomandibular joints (TMJs). In addition, muscles of the rib cage are presented in this chapter. These muscles move the ribs at the sternocostal and costospinal joints.

The following is an overview of the structure and function of the spinal joint muscles presented in this chapter.

The companion CD at the back of this book allows you to examine the muscles of this body region, layer by layer, and individual muscle palpation technique videos are available in the chapter 8 folder on the Evolve website.

OVERVIEW OF FUNCTION: MUSCLES OF THE SPINAL JOINTS

Muscles of the spinal joints may be categorized based on three factors: (1) the region of the spine, (2) their location, and (3) their depth. Regionally, they may be divided into three groups: (1) those that run the full length of the spine, (2) those that are primarily located only in the trunk, and (3) those that are primarily located only in the neck. Regarding location, they can be described as being anterior or posterior. Regarding their depth, they can be divided based on whether they are superficial or deep. Generally, the larger, more superficial muscles of the spine are important for creating motion; and the deeper, smaller muscles function to stabilize the spine.

The following general rules regarding actions can be stated for the functional groups of muscles of the spinal joints:

- If a muscle crosses the spinal joints anteriorly with a vertical direction to its fibers, it can flex the trunk, neck, and/or head at the spinal joints by moving the insertion (superior attachment) down toward the origin (inferior attachment) in front.
- If a muscle crosses the spinal joints posteriorly with a vertical direction to its fibers, it can extend the trunk, neck, and/or head at the spinal joints by moving the origin (superior attachment) down toward the insertion (inferior attachment) in back.
- If a muscle crosses the spinal joints laterally, it can perform same-side lateral flexion of the trunk, neck, and/or head at the spinal joints by moving the insertion (superior attachment) down toward the origin (inferior attachment) on that side of the body.
- Right and left rotators of the spine have a horizontal component to their fiber direction and wrap around the body part that they move.
- Reverse actions of these muscles involve the lower spine (origin; inferior attachment) being moved toward the upper spine (insertion; superior attachment) at the spinal joints. These reverse actions usually occur when the client is lying down so the lower attachment is free to move. If the muscle attaches onto the pelvis, the reverse action involves movement of the pelvis at the lumbosacral spinal joint as well.
- The reverse action of flexion of the upper spine relative to the lower spine is flexion of the lower spine relative to the upper spine, and posterior tilt of the pelvis if the muscle attaches to it.
- The reverse action of extension of the upper spine relative to the lower spine is extension of the lower spine relative to the upper spine, and anterior tilt of the pelvis if the muscle attaches to it.
- The reverse action of lateral flexion of the upper spine relative to the lower spine is lateral flexion of the lower spine relative to the upper spine, and elevation of the same side of the pelvis (and therefore depression of the opposite side of the pelvis) if the muscle attaches to it.

- The reverse action of ipsilateral rotation of the upper spine relative to the lower spine is contralateral rotation of the lower spine relative to the upper spine, and contralateral rotation of the pelvis if the muscle attaches to it.
- The reverse action of contralateral rotation of the upper spine relative to the lower spine is ipsilateral rotation of the lower spine relative to the upper spine, and ipsilateral rotation of the pelvis if the muscle attaches to it.

OVERVIEW OF MUSCLES THAT MOVE THE MANDIBLE*

Muscles that move the mandible at the TMJs attach to the mandible. The other attachment of these muscles is usually considered to be either superior or inferior to the mandible attachment.

The following general rules regarding actions can be stated for functional groups of muscles that move the mandible:

- If a muscle attaches to the mandible and its other attachment is inferior to the mandibular attachment, it can depress the mandible at the TMJs.
- Reverse actions of the suprahyoid muscles of the hyoid group occur when the mandible is fixed and the hyoid bone is moved superiorly toward the mandible.

OVERVIEW OF FUNCTION: MUSCLES OF THE RIB CAGE

Muscles that move the rib cage attach to the rib cage. The other attachment of these muscles is usually considered to be either superior or inferior to the rib attachment. These muscles may be located anteriorly, posteriorly, and/or laterally.

The following general rules regarding actions can be stated for the functional groups of muscles of the rib cage:

- If a muscle attaches to the rib cage and its other attachment is superior to the rib cage attachment, it can elevate the ribs to which it is attached at the sternocostal and costospinal joints.
- If a muscle attaches to the rib cage and its other attachment is inferior to the rib cage attachment, it can depress the ribs to which it is attached at the sternocostal and costospinal joints.
- As a rule, muscles that elevate ribs contract with inspiration and muscles that depress ribs contract with expiration.

The major muscles of mastication (that move the mandible) are discussed in Chapter 9, Muscles of the Head.

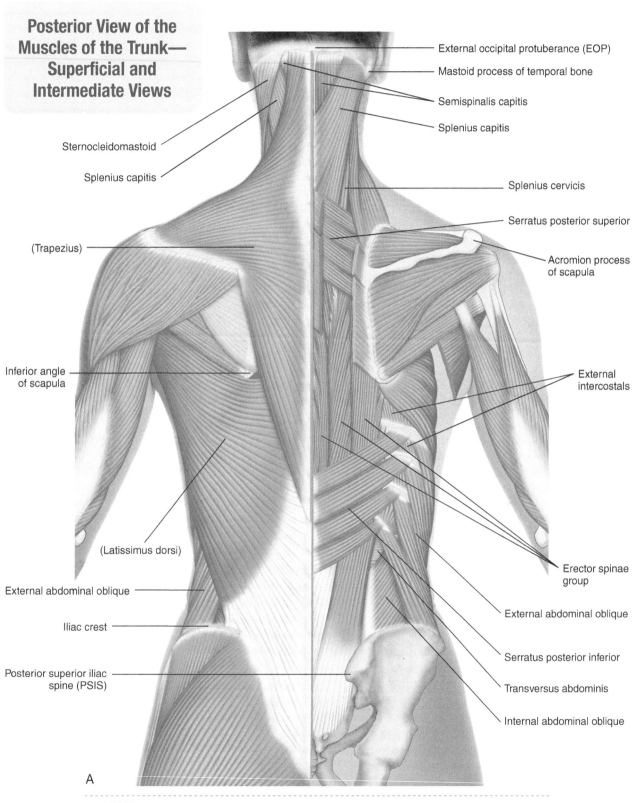

Posterior View of the Muscles of the Trunk— Superficial and Intermediate Views

External occipital protuberance (EOP)

Mastoid process of temporal bone

Semispinalis capitis

Splenius capitis

Sternocleidomastoid

Splenius capitis

Splenius cervicis

Serratus posterior superior

(Trapezius)

Acromion process of scapula

Inferior angle of scapula

External intercostals

(Latissimus dorsi)

Erector spinae group

External abdominal oblique

External abdominal oblique

Iliac crest

Serratus posterior inferior

Posterior superior iliac spine (PSIS)

Transversus abdominis

Internal abdominal oblique

A

FIGURE 8-1 A, Posterior view of the muscles of the trunk—superficial view on the left and an intermediate view on the right.

Continued

8

Posterior View of the Muscles of the Trunk—Deep Views

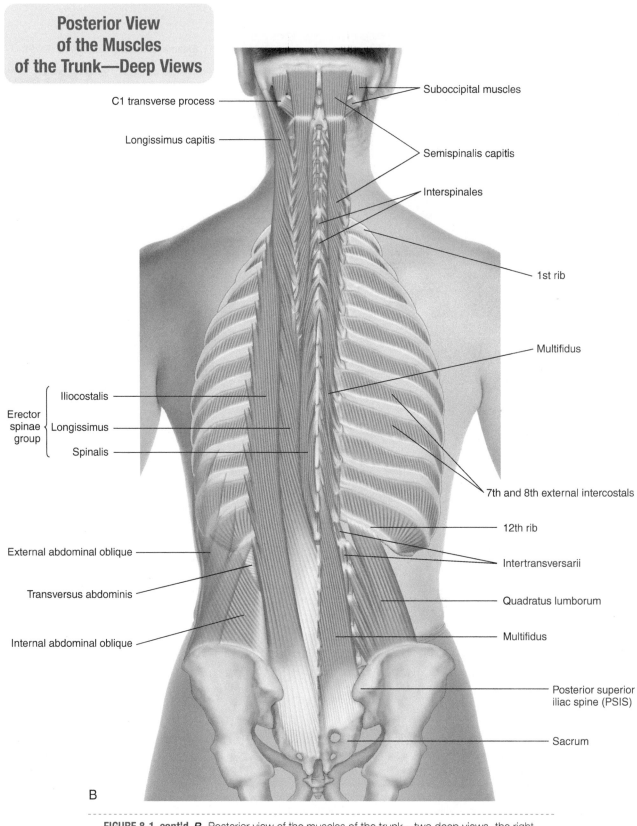

C1 transverse process

Longissimus capitis

Suboccipital muscles

Semispinalis capitis

Interspinales

1st rib

Multifidus

Erector spinae group
- Iliocostalis
- Longissimus
- Spinalis

7th and 8th external intercostals

12th rib

External abdominal oblique

Intertransversarii

Transversus abdominis

Quadratus lumborum

Internal abdominal oblique

Multifidus

Posterior superior iliac spine (PSIS)

Sacrum

B

FIGURE 8-1, cont'd B, Posterior view of the muscles of the trunk—two deep views, the right side deeper than the left. The external abdominal oblique has been ghosted in.

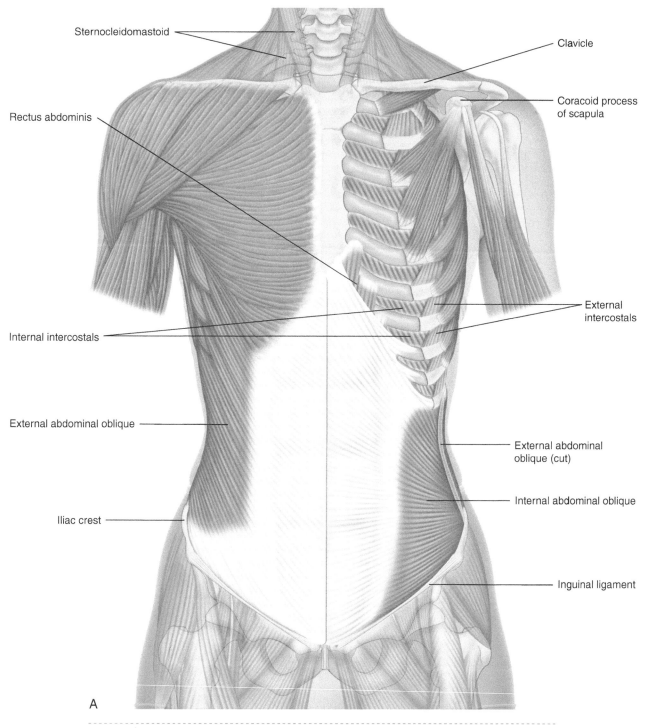

Sternocleidomastoid

Clavicle

Coracoid process of scapula

Rectus abdominis

External intercostals

Internal intercostals

External abdominal oblique

External abdominal oblique (cut)

Internal abdominal oblique

Iliac crest

Inguinal ligament

A

FIGURE 8-2 A, Anterior view of the muscles of the trunk—superficial view on the right and an intermediate view on the left. The muscles of the neck and thigh have been ghosted in.

Continued

8

**Anterior View
of the Muscles
of the Trunk—Deep Views**

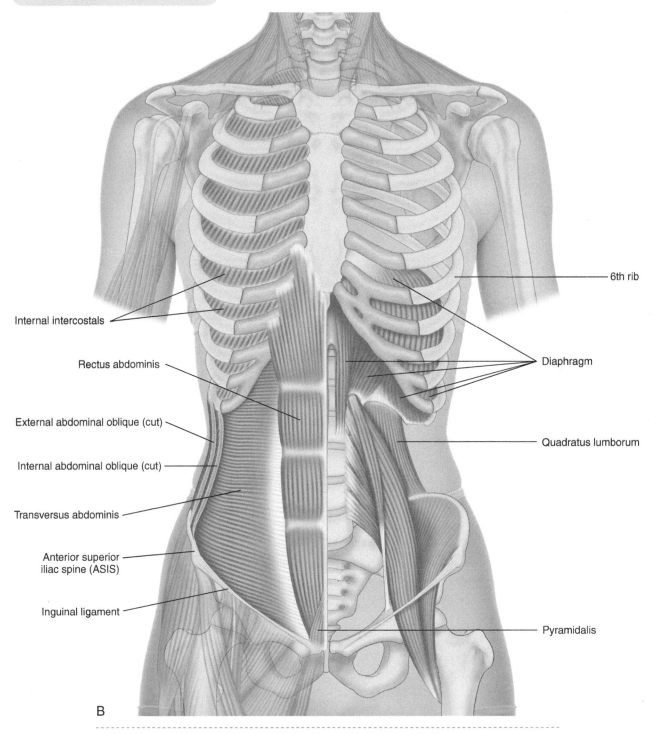

Internal intercostals

Rectus abdominis

External abdominal oblique (cut)

Internal abdominal oblique (cut)

Transversus abdominis

Anterior superior
iliac spine (ASIS)

Inguinal ligament

6th rib

Diaphragm

Quadratus lumborum

Pyramidalis

B

FIGURE 8-2, cont'd *B,* Anterior views of the muscles of the trunk—deep views with the posterior abdominal wall seen on the left. The muscles of the neck, arm, and thigh have been ghosted in.

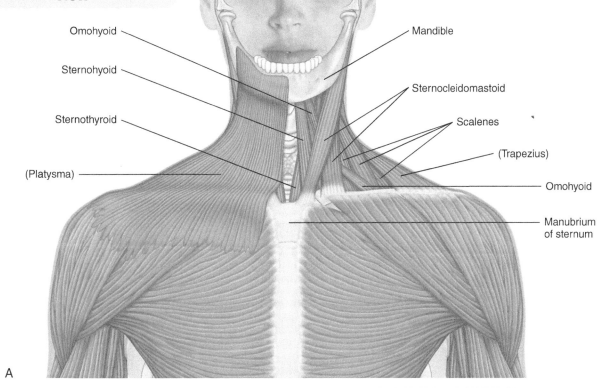

Omohyoid

Sternohyoid

Sternothyroid

(Platysma)

Mandible

Sternocleidomastoid

Scalenes

(Trapezius)

Omohyoid

Manubrium
of sternum

A

8

FIGURE 8-3 *A,* Anterior view of the neck and upper chest region—superficial view. The
platysma has been removed on the left side.

Continued

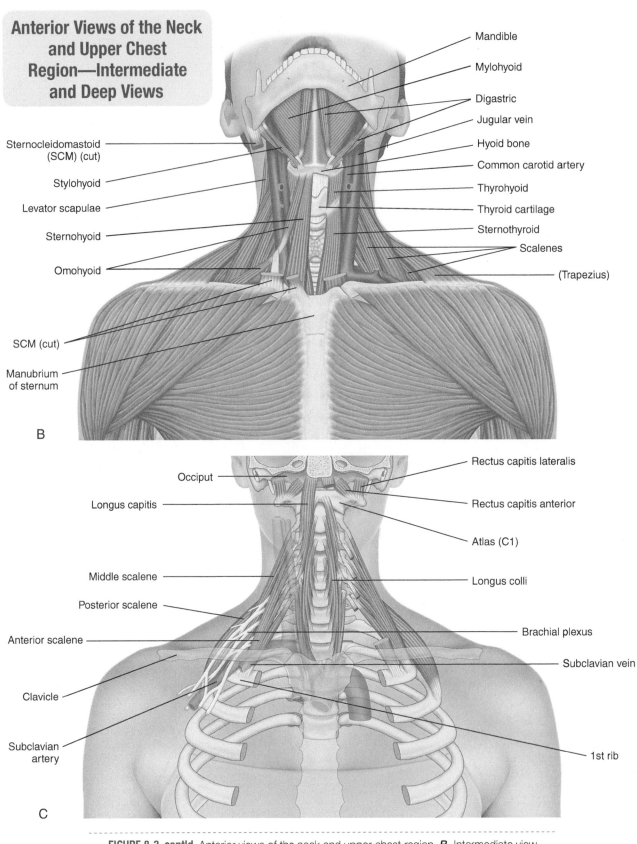

Mandible

Mylohyoid

Digastric

Jugular vein

Sternocleidomastoid (SCM) (cut)

Hyoid bone

Common carotid artery

Stylohyoid

Thyrohyoid

Levator scapulae

Thyroid cartilage

Sternohyoid

Sternothyroid

Scalenes

Omohyoid

(Trapezius)

SCM (cut)

Manubrium of sternum

B

Occiput

Rectus capitis lateralis

Longus capitis

Rectus capitis anterior

Atlas (C1)

Middle scalene

Longus colli

Posterior scalene

Anterior scalene

Brachial plexus

Subclavian vein

Clavicle

Subclavian artery

1st rib

C

FIGURE 8-3, cont'd Anterior views of the neck and upper chest region. **B,** Intermediate view with the head extended. The sternocleidomastoid (SCM) has been cut on the right side; the SCM and omohyoid have been removed and the sternohyoid has been cut on the left side. **C,** Deep view. The anterior scalene and longus capitis, as well as the brachial plexus of nerves and subclavian artery and vein, have been cut and/or removed on the left side. The clavicles and blood vessels have been ghosted in.

Right Lateral Views of the Muscles of the Trunk and Neck Region

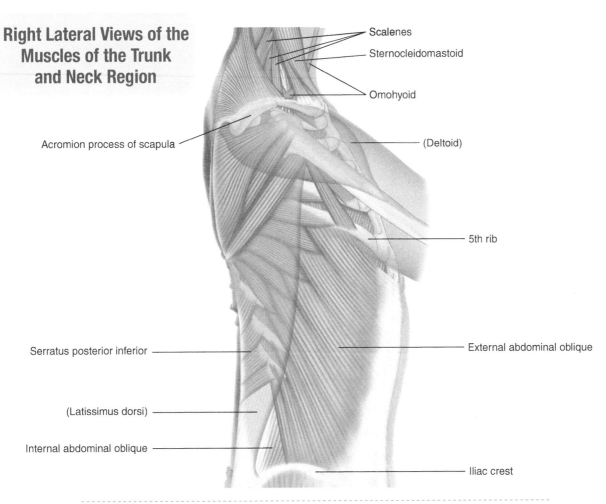

Scalenes

Sternocleidomastoid

Omohyoid

Acromion process of scapula

(Deltoid)

5th rib

Serratus posterior inferior

External abdominal oblique

(Latissimus dorsi)

Internal abdominal oblique

Iliac crest

FIGURE 8-4 Right lateral view of the muscles of the trunk. The latissimus dorsi and deltoid have been ghosted in.

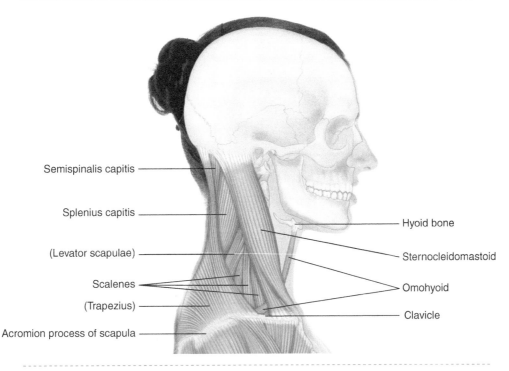

Semispinalis capitis

Splenius capitis

Hyoid bone

(Levator scapulae)

Sternocleidomastoid

Scalenes

Omohyoid

(Trapezius)

Clavicle

Acromion process of scapula

FIGURE 8-5 Right lateral view of the muscles of the neck region.

SPINE AND RIB CAGE: Erector Spinae Group
Iliocostalis; Longissimus; Spinalis

Pronunciation   **IL-ee-o-kos-TA-lis • lon-JIS-i-mus • spy-NA-lis**

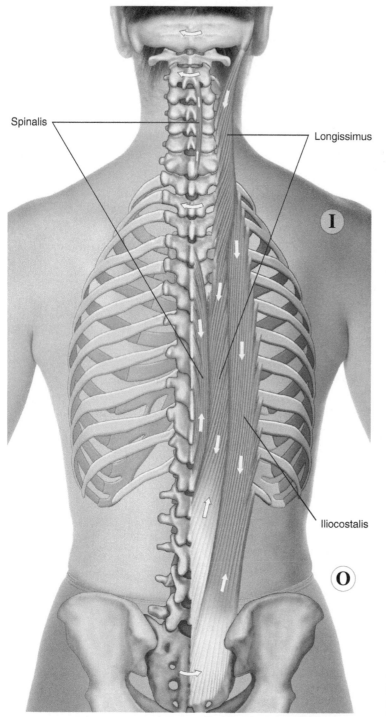

Spinalis

Longissimus

Iliocostalis

I

O

The erector spinae group is a large muscle group that runs parallel to the spine from the pelvis to the head. It is composed of three subgroups. From lateral to medial, they are the iliocostalis, longissimus, and spinalis (Figure 8-6). The erector spinae is most massive in the lumbar and thoracic regions. In the lumbar region, it is deep to the latissimus dorsi; in the thoracic region, it is deep to the trapezius and rhomboids. Very little erector spinae is present in the neck. Other than a small amount of spinalis, its presence in the neck is the longissimus capitis that is located more laterally and goes up to the mastoid process of the temporal bone. It is deep to the trapezius, splenius capitis, and splenius cervicis.

Note: The erector spinae group is also known as the *sacrospinalis group*. The term *paraspinal* musculature is also used to describe the erector spinae and the transversospinalis groups together.

FIGURE 8-6 Posterior view of the right erector spinae group. *O*, Origin; *I*, insertion.

WHAT'S IN A NAME?

The name, *erector spinae,* tells us that this muscle makes the spine erect. (Considering that the spine usually bends forward into flexion, to make it erect would be to perform extension of the spine.)

✳ **Derivation:**
erector: L. to erect
spinae: L. thorn (refers to the spine)

ATTACHMENTS

Origin (Proximal Attachment)

- Pelvis

Insertion (Distal Attachment)

- Spine, rib cage, and mastoid process of the temporal bone

ACTIONS

- Extends the trunk, neck, and head at the spinal joints.
- Anteriorly tilts the pelvis at the lumbosacral joint and extends the lower spine relative to the upper spine.
- Laterally flexes the trunk, neck, and head at the spinal joints.

STABILIZATION

1. Stabilizes the spinal joints.
2. Stabilizes the ribs at the sternocostal and costospinal joints.
3. Stabilizes the sacroiliac joint.

INNERVATION

- Spinal nerves

PALPATION

1. The client is prone. Place your palpating finger pads just lateral to the lumbar spine.
2. Ask the client to extend the trunk; feel for the contraction of the erector spinae musculature in the lumbar region (Figure 8-7). Palpate the erector spinae by strumming perpendicularly; palpate inferiorly to its origin on the pelvis.
3. Now ask the client to extend the trunk, neck, and head; continue palpating it superiorly as far as possible toward its mastoid process attachment.

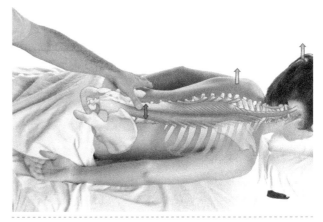

FIGURE 8-7 Palpation of the right erector spinae group as the client extends the head, neck, and trunk.

TREATMENT CONSIDERATIONS

- Each of the three subgroups of the erector spinae can be further subdivided into three subgroups: (1) iliocostalis lumborum, thoracis, and cervicis; (2) the longissimus thoracis, cervicis, and capitis; and (3) the spinalis thoracis, cervicis, and capitis. Note: The spinalis capitis often blends with and is therefore considered part of the semispinalis capitis of the transversospinalis group.

- Inferiorly, the erector spinae blends into the thick thoracolumbar fascia.

- The erector spinae is the principal musculature that works when we bend forward. It contracts eccentrically to guide our descent when we bend forward; it contracts isometrically when we hold a bent-forward posture; and it contracts concentrically when we stand back up.

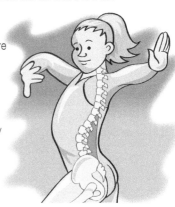

- Tight erector spinae musculature pulls the pelvis into anterior tilt, which then increases the lordotic curve of the lumbar spine.

SPINE AND RIB CAGE: Transversospinalis Group
Semispinalis; Multifidus; Rotatores

Pronunciation   SEM-ee-spy-NA-lis • mul-TIF-id-us • ro-ta-TO-reez

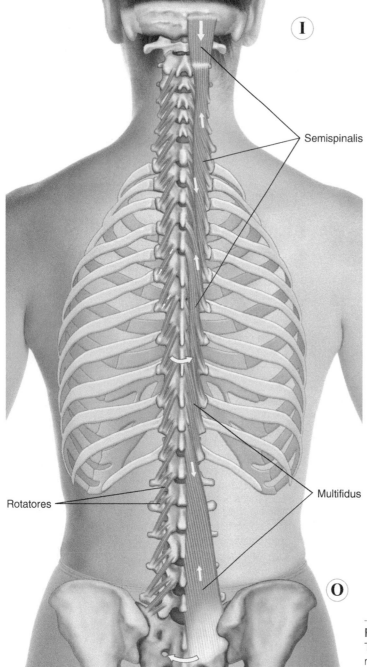

The transversospinalis group musculature is deep and makes up the mass of musculature that fills the laminar groove of the spine between the transverse and spinous processes. The transversospinalis muscle group can be divided into three subgroups: from superficial to deep, they are the semispinalis, the multifidus, and the rotatores (Figure 8-8). The rotatores attach superiorly to the vertebrae one to two levels above the inferior attachment; the multifidus attaches superiorly to vertebrae three to four levels above the inferior attachment; the semispinalis attaches superiorly to vertebrae five or more levels above the inferior attachment. The multifidus is the largest muscle of the low back; the semispinalis is the largest muscle of the neck. Of the three subgroups of the transversospinalis, only the multifidus attaches onto the pelvis, and only the semispinalis attaches onto the head. The term *paraspinal* musculature is used to describe the erector spinae and the transversospinalis groups together.

FIGURE 8-8 Posterior view of the transversospinalis group. The semispinalis and multifidus are seen on the right; the rotatores are seen on the left. *O*, Origin; *I*, insertion.

WHAT'S IN A NAME?

■ The name, *transversospinalis*, tells us that this muscle group attaches from the transverse processes (inferiorly) to the spinous processes (superiorly).

✳ **Derivation:**
transverso: L. refers to transverse processes
spinalis: L. refers to spinous processes

ATTACHMENTS

Origin (Proximal Attachment)

- Pelvis and transverse processes of spine

Insertion (Distal Attachment)

- Spinous processes of spine, and the head

ACTIONS

- Extends the trunk, neck, and head at the spinal joints.
- Anteriorly tilts the pelvis at the lumbosacral joint and extends the lower spine relative to the upper spine.
- Laterally flexes the trunk, neck, and head at the spinal joints.
- Contralaterally rotates the trunk and neck at the spinal joints.

STABILIZATION

1. Stabilizes the spinal joints.
2. Stabilizes the sacroiliac joint.

INNERVATION

- Spinal nerves

PALPATION

1. The client is prone. Place your palpating finger pads just lateral to the spinous processes of the lumbar spine within the laminar groove.
2. Ask the client to extend and rotate the trunk slightly to the opposite side of the body (contralaterally rotate) at the spinal joints. Feel for the contraction of the transversospinalis musculature of the lumbar spine (Figure 8-9).
3. Repeat this procedure superiorly up the spine.
4. To palpate the semispinalis group in the cervical region, have the client prone with the hand in the small of the back. Place your palpating fingers over the laminar groove of the cervical spine and ask the client to extend the head and neck slightly at the spinal joints. Feeling for the contraction of the semispinalis deep to the upper trapezius (Figure 8-10).

5. Once located, follow the semispinalis up to the attachment on the head by strumming perpendicular to the direction of fibers.

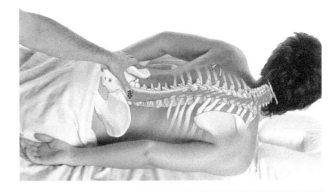

FIGURE 8-9 Palpation of the right lumbar multifidus as the client extends and contralaterally rotates (left) the trunk.

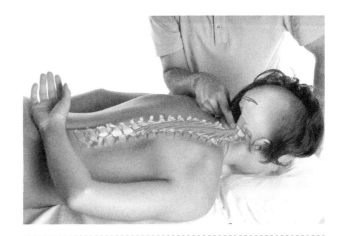

FIGURE 8-10 Palpation of the right semispinalis as the client extends the head and neck.

TREATMENT CONSIDERATIONS

- The multifidus is credited, along with the transversus abdominis, as being one of the most important muscles of core stabilization.
- Because the multifidus attaches inferiorly to the iliac crest and sacrum, the transversospinalis group can help stabilize the sacroiliac joint.

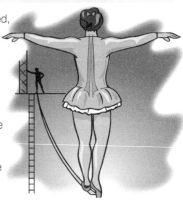

8

SPINE AND RIB CAGE
Interspinales; Intertransversarii

Pronunciation **IN-ter-spy-NA-leez • IN-ter-trans-ver-SA-ri-eye**

The interspinales and intertransversarii are small intrinsic muscles of the spine that are located between adjacent vertebrae, primarily in the lumbar and cervical regions. As their names indicate, the interspinales are located between the spinous processes, and the intertransversarii are located between the transverse processes (Figure 8-11).

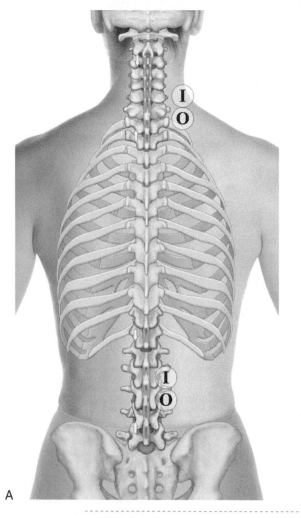

A

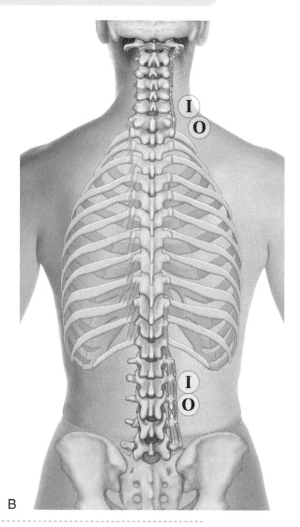

B

FIGURE 8-11 *A,* Posterior view of the right and left interspinales. *B,* Posterior view of the right intertransversarii. The levatores costarum have been ghosted in on the left. *O,* Origin; *I,* insertion.

WHAT'S IN A NAME?

The name, *interspinales,* tells us that these muscles are located between the spinous processes of the vertebrae.

The name, *intertransversarii,* tells us that these muscles are located between the transverse processes of the vertebrae.

✳ **Derivation:**
inter: L. between
spinales: L. refers to spinous processes
transversarii: L. refers to transverse processes

ATTACHMENTS

Interspinales

Origin (Proximal Attachment)

- Spinous process

Insertion (Distal Attachment)

- Spinous process directly superior

Intertransversarii

Origin (Proximal Attachment)

- Transverse process

Insertion (Distal Attachment)

- Transverse process directly superior

ACTIONS

Interspinales

- Extend the neck and trunk at the spinal joints.

Intertransversarii

- Laterally flex the neck and trunk at the spinal joints.

STABILIZATION

As a group, the interspinales and intertransversarii stabilize the cervical and lumbar spinal joints.

INNERVATION

- Spinal nerves

PALPATION

Interspinales

1. The client is seated. Place your palpating finger pads in the spaces between the spinous processes in the lumbar region. Place your resistance hand on the client's upper trunk (Figure 8-12).
2. Ask the client to flex slightly forward. Feel for the interspinous muscles between the spinous processes.
3. From this position of flexion, ask the client to extend back to anatomic position, and feel for the contraction of the interspinales muscles. If desired, resistance can be given to the client's trunk extension with your resistance hand (Figure 8-13).
4. This procedure can be repeated for other interspinales muscles between other spinous processes.

Intertransversarii

1. The intertransversarii are small and very deep and therefore difficult to palpate and discern from adjacent musculature.

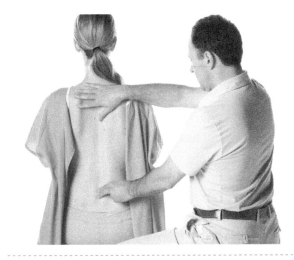

FIGURE 8-12 Starting position for seated palpation of the interspinales.

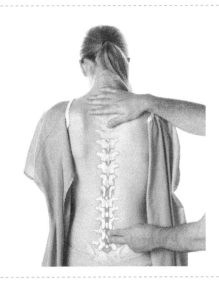

FIGURE 8-13 Palpation of the interspinales as the client extends the trunk back to anatomic position from a position of slight flexion.

TREATMENT CONSIDERATIONS

- The intertransversarii are considered to be primarily important as stabilizing postural muscles or as proprioceptive organs (not as movers of the spine), thereby providing precise monitoring of spinal joint positions.

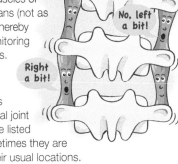

- The interspinales and intertransversarii vary in location. Sometimes they are found at spinal joint levels other than those listed in this textbook; sometimes they are absent at some of their usual locations.

- Essentially, the intertransversarii do not exist in the thoracic region. The levatores costarum and the intercostals are considered to be homologous with the two sets of intertransversarii in the thoracic region.

SPINE AND RIB CAGE: Serratus Posterior Group
Serratus Posterior Superior; Serratus Posterior Inferior

Pronunciation **ser-A-tus pos-TEE-ri-or sue-PEE-ri-or** • **ser-A-tus pos-TEE-ri-or in-FEE-ri-or**

The serratus posterior group is composed of two muscles: the serratus posterior superior and the serratus posterior inferior (Figure 8-14). These muscles attach to ribs. The serratus posterior superior is deep to the trapezius and rhomboids; the serratus posterior inferior is deep to the latissimus dorsi.

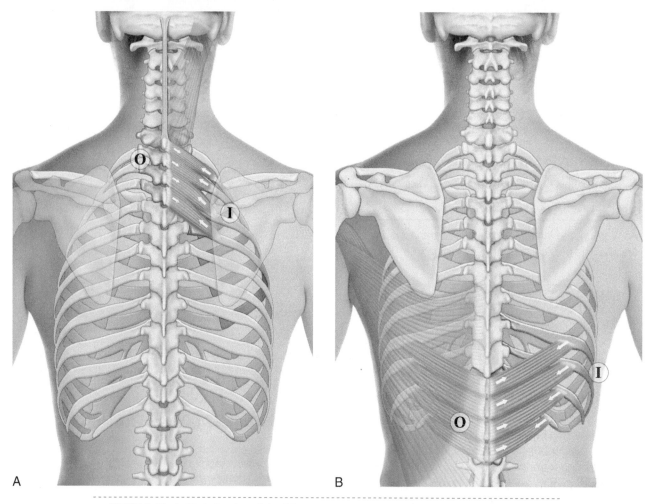

A   B

FIGURE 8-14 *A,* Posterior view of the right serratus posterior superior. The splenius capitis has been ghosted in on the right. *B,* Posterior view of the serratus posterior inferior bilaterally. The latissimus dorsi has been ghosted in on the left side. *O,* Origin; *I,* insertion.

WHAT'S IN A NAME?

The name, *serratus posterior,* tells us that these muscles have a serrated appearance and are posterior to the serratus anterior. The serratus posterior superior is superior to the serratus posterior inferior.

❊ **Derivation:**
serratus: L. notching
posterior: L. behind, toward the back
superior: L. above
inferior: L. below

ATTACHMENTS

Serratus Posterior Superior

Origin (Superior Attachment)

- Spinous processes of C7-T3

Insertion (Inferior Attachment)

- Ribs two through five

Serratus Posterior Inferior

Origin (Inferior Attachment)

- Spinous processes of T11-L2

Insertion (Superior Attachment)

- Ribs nine through twelve

ACTIONS

The serratus posterior muscles move ribs at the sternocostal and costospinal joints.

Serratus Posterior Superior

- Elevates ribs two through five.

Serratus Posterior Inferior

- Depresses ribs nine through twelve.

STABILIZATION

Stabilizes the rib cage.

INNERVATION

- Intercostal nerves (serratus posterior superior)
- Subcostal nerve and intercostal nerves (serratus posterior inferior)

PALPATION

The serratus posterior superior and inferior are thin muscles that are located deep to other muscles; therefore they are difficult to palpate and discern. If palpation is done, the client is prone.

Serratus Posterior Superior

1. Place your palpating finger pads in the region of the upper rhomboids.
2. Have the client take in a moderately deep breath. Feel for the contraction of the serratus posterior superior. Discerning the serratus posterior superior from the overlying rhomboids and trapezius is very challenging.

Serratus Posterior Inferior

1. Place your palpating finger pads in the upper lumbar region, lateral to the erector spinae.
2. Ask the client to exhale. Feel for the contraction of the serratus posterior superior by strumming perpendicular to its fibers. Discerning the serratus posterior inferior from the overlying latissimus dorsi is very challenging.

TREATMENT CONSIDERATIONS

- The serrated appearance of the serratus posterior superior and inferior comes from attaching onto separate ribs, which creates the notched look of a serrated knife.

- Stabilizing the lower ribs is an important function of the serratus posterior inferior. Its force of depression of the lower ribs stabilizes them from elevating when the diaphragm contracts and pulls superiorly on them.

SPINE AND RIB CAGE
Quadratus Lumborum (QL)

Pronunciation **kwod-RAY-tus lum-BOR-um**

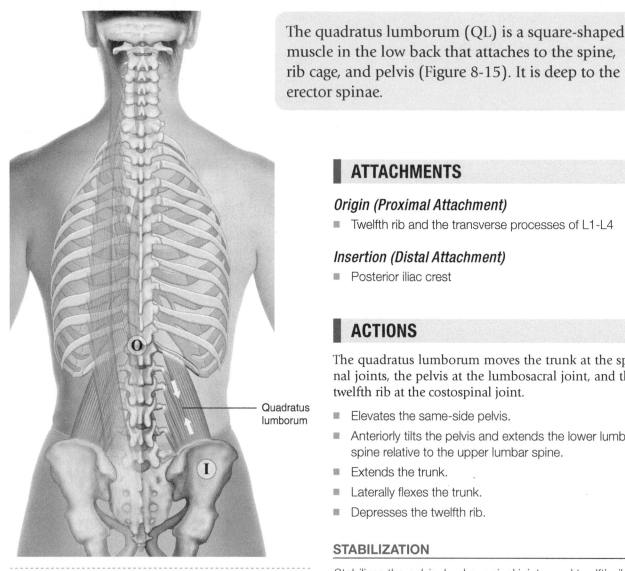

The quadratus lumborum (QL) is a square-shaped muscle in the low back that attaches to the spine, rib cage, and pelvis (Figure 8-15). It is deep to the erector spinae.

FIGURE 8-15 Posterior view of the quadratus lumborum bilaterally. The erector spinae group has been ghosted in on the left side. *O,* Origin; *I,* insertion.

ATTACHMENTS

Origin (Proximal Attachment)
- Twelfth rib and the transverse processes of L1-L4

Insertion (Distal Attachment)
- Posterior iliac crest

ACTIONS

The quadratus lumborum moves the trunk at the spinal joints, the pelvis at the lumbosacral joint, and the twelfth rib at the costospinal joint.

- Elevates the same-side pelvis.
- Anteriorly tilts the pelvis and extends the lower lumbar spine relative to the upper lumbar spine.
- Extends the trunk.
- Laterally flexes the trunk.
- Depresses the twelfth rib.

STABILIZATION

Stabilizes the pelvis, lumbar spinal joints, and twelfth rib.

INNERVATION

- Lumbar plexus

WHAT'S IN A NAME?

The name, *quadratus lumborum,* tells us that this muscle is shaped somewhat like a square and is located in the lumbar (i.e., lower back) region.

✳ **Derivation:**
quadratus: L. squared
lumborum: L. loin (low back)

PALPATION

1. The client is prone. Place your palpating finger pads just lateral to the lateral border of the erector spinae in the lumbar region.

   Note: Placing the fingers of other hand on the palpating fingers for extra support can be helpful.

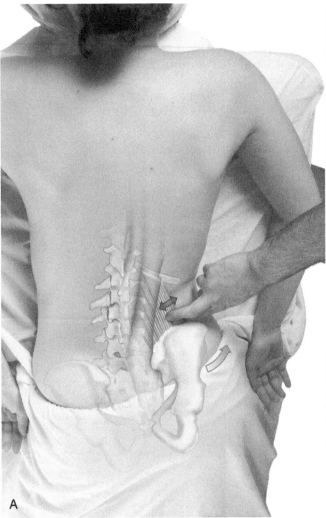

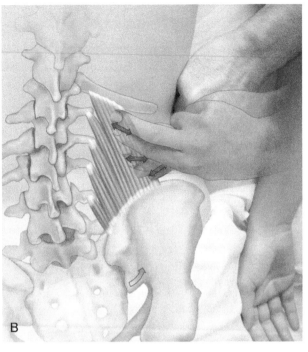

FIGURE 8-16 *A,* Palpation of the right quadratus lumborum as the client elevates the right side of the pelvis. The outline of the right erector spinae group has been ghosted in. *B,* Once the quadratus lumborum has been located, palpate in all three directions toward the rib, transverse process, and iliac attachments.

2. First locate the lateral border of the erector spinae musculature. (To do so, ask the client to raise the head and upper trunk from the table.) Then place your palpating finger just lateral to the lateral border of the erector spinae.

3. Direct palpating pressure medially, deep to the erector spinae musculature, and feel for the quadratus lumborum.

4. To engage the quadratus lumborum, ask the client to elevate the pelvis on that side at the lumbosacral joint and feel for its contraction (Figure 8-16, *A*).

   Note: The pelvis should move along the plane of the table toward the head; in other words, the pelvis should not lift up in the air, away from the table.

5. Once located, palpate medially and superiorly toward the twelfth rib, medially and inferiorly toward the iliac crest, and directly medially toward the transverse processes of the lumbar spine (Figure 8-16, *B*).

TREATMENT CONSIDERATIONS

- When working on the quadratus lumborum, you can position the client either prone, supine, or side lying. However, because much of this muscle is deep to the massive erector spinae musculature, it must be accessed with palpatory pressure from lateral to medial (i.e., come in from the side).

- Keep in mind that the quadratus lumborum is not the only muscle in the lateral lumbar region and should not be blamed for all the pain in this area. The nearby erector spinae musculature is also likely to develop tension and pain.

- If the quadratus lumborum is tight, it can pull up on the pelvic bone, causing the iliac crest on that side to elevate. This elevation can be seen during the postural assessment examination.

- The quadratus lumborum is important for stabilizing the twelfth rib when the diaphragm contracts during inspiration. Stabilization increases the efficiency of the diaphragm during breathing.

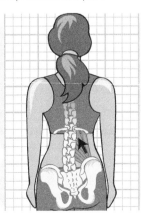

SPINE AND RIB CAGE: Intercostal Group
External Intercostals; Internal Intercostals

Pronunciation   **EKS-turn-al in-ter-KOS-tals • IN-turn-al in-ter-KOS-tals**

The intercostal group is composed of the external intercostals and the internal intercostals (Figure 8-17). These muscles are located in the anterior, lateral, and posterior thoracic region of the trunk. Depending on the specific location, they may be deep to other muscles or they may be superficial and easily palpable. The fiber directions of these two muscle groups are perpendicular to each other. The fiber direction of the external intercostals is the same as the fiber direction of the external abdominal oblique; the fiber direction of the internal intercostals is the same as the fiber direction of the internal abdominal oblique.

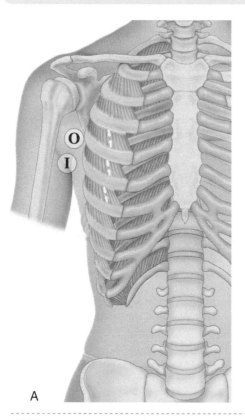
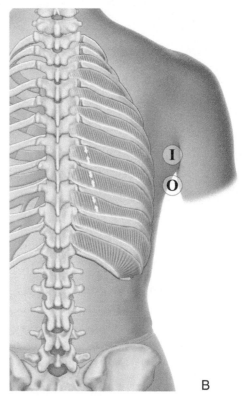

A   B

FIGURE 8-17 Views of the right intercostals. **A,** Anterior view of the external intercostals. **B,** Posterior view of the internal intercostals. *O,* Origin; *I,* insertion.

WHAT'S IN A NAME?

The name, *intercostals,* tells us that these muscles are located between the ribs in the intercostal spaces. The external intercostals are external (superficial) to the internal intercostals.

✴ **Derivation:**
inter: L. between
costals: L. refers to the ribs
external: L. outside
internal: L. inside

ATTACHMENTS

Origin/Insertion (Superior/Inferior Attachments)

- In the intercostal spaces of ribs one through twelve

ACTIONS

- The intercostals move the ribs at the sternocostal and costospinal joints and move the trunk at the spinal joints.

External Intercostals

- Elevate ribs two through twelve.
- Rotate the trunk contralaterally.

Internal Intercostals

- Depress ribs one through eleven.
- Rotate the trunk ipsilaterally.

STABILIZATION

Stabilize the rib cage.

INNERVATION

- Intercostal nerves

PALPATION

1. The client is side lying. Place your palpating finger pads in the intercostal spaces (between ribs) in the lateral trunk (Figure 8-18).

2. To locate an intercostal space, feel for the hard texture of the ribs in the lateral trunk and then drop your palpating fingers into the soft intercostal space between them.

3. Once located, palpate in the intercostal space as far posteriorly and anteriorly as possible. The presence of breast tissue in female clients makes it difficult to access fully the intercostals anteriorly.

   Note: Discerning between the external and internal intercostals is usually not possible.

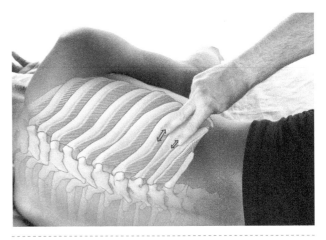

FIGURE 8-18 Palpation of right intercostal muscles between the ribs in the lateral trunk.

TREATMENT CONSIDERATIONS

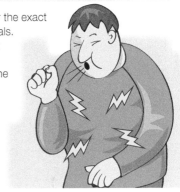

- Controversy exists over the exact actions of the intercostals. However, it is clear that they are involved in respiration. Therefore the intercostals should be addressed in any client who has a respiratory condition, especially a chronic one such as asthma, emphysema, or bronchitis, or simply a chronic cough.

- Athletes may also greatly benefit from having these muscles worked on because of the great demand for respiration during exercise.

- The intercostals are also involved in fixation (i.e., stabilization) of the rib cage during other movements of the body.

- Anteriorly the internal intercostals are located in the spaces between the costal cartilages; the external intercostals are not.

- The intercostal muscles are the meat that is eaten when one eats ribs or spare ribs.

SPINE AND RIB CAGE
Levatores Costarum

Pronunciation **le-va-TO-rez (singular: le-VAY-tor) kos-TAR-um**

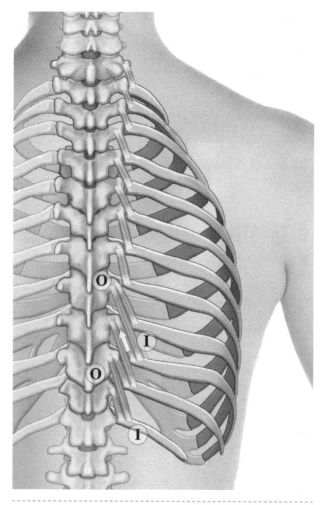

The levatores costarum are small muscles located in the thoracic region deep to the erector spinae musculature; they run from the vertebrae to the ribs. The lower levatores costarum have two slips of tissue at each level; the shorter ones are called *levatores costarum breves* and the longer ones are called *levatores costarum longi* (Figure 8-19).

FIGURE 8-19 Posterior view of the right levatores costarum. *O*, Origin; *I*, insertion.

WHAT'S IN A NAME?

The name, *levatores costarum,* tells us that these muscles elevate the ribs.

✳ **Derivation:**
   levator: L. lifter
   costarum: L. refers to the ribs

ATTACHMENTS

Origin (Superior Attachment)
■ Transverse processes of C7-T11

Insertion (Inferior Attachment)
■ Ribs one through twelve

ACTIONS

■ Elevate the ribs at the sternocostal and costospinal joints.

STABILIZATION

Stabilize the thoracic spinal joints and costospinal joints.

INNERVATION

■ Spinal nerves

PALPATION

1. The client is prone. Place your palpating finger pads on the erector spinae musculature over the angles of the ribs.

2. Ask the client to breathe in and out slowly and deeply. Try to feel for the contraction of the levatores costarum.

   Note: The levatores costarum are small and very deep. Palpating and discerning them from the adjacent musculature is extremely difficult, if not impossible.

TREATMENT CONSIDERATIONS

■ Some sources state that the primary function of the levatores costarum is to stabilize the spinal joints and ribs.

Notes

SPINE AND RIB CAGE
Subcostales; Transversus Thoracis

Pronunciation   **sub-kos-TAL-eez • trans-VER-sus thor-AS-is**

The subcostales and transversus thoracis are deep muscles, located on the internal side of the rib cage. The subcostales are located posteriorly; the transversus thoracis is located anteriorly (Figure 8-20).

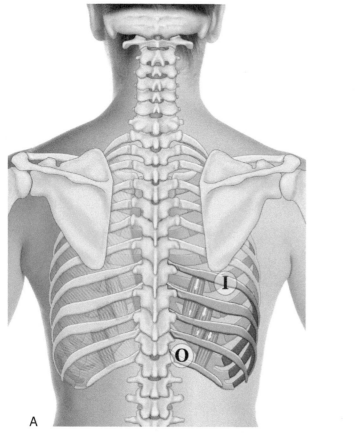

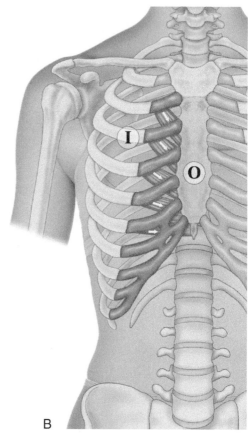

A

B

FIGURE 8-20 *A,* Posterior view of the subcostales bilaterally. The internal intercostals have been ghosted in on the left side. *B,* Anterior view of the right transverses thoracis. *O,* Origin; *I,* insertion.

WHAT'S IN A NAME?

The name, *subcostales,* tells us that these muscles are "under" (i.e., deep to) the ribs.

The name, *transversus thoracis,* tells us that this muscle runs transversely across the thoracic region.

✳ **Derivation:**
sub: L. under
costales: L. refers to the ribs
transversus: L. running transversely
thoracis: Gr. refers to the thorax (chest)

ATTACHMENTS

Subcostales

Origin (Inferior Attachment)
- Ribs ten through twelve

Insertion (Superior Attachment)
- Ribs eight through ten

Transversus Thoracis

Origin (Medial Attachment)

- Internal surfaces of the sternum, the xiphoid process, and the adjacent costal cartilages

Insertion (Lateral Attachment)

- Internal surface of costal cartilages two through six

ACTIONS

The subcostales and transversus thoracis move the ribs at the sternocostal and costospinal joints.

Subcostales

- Depress ribs eight through ten.

Transversus Thoracis

- Depresses ribs two through six.

STABILIZATION

Subcostales

- Stabilizes the lower ribs.

Transversus Thoracis

- Stabilizes the rib cage and sternum.

INNERVATION

- Intercostal nerves

PALPATION

The subcostales and transversus thoracis are deep to the rib cage and extremely challenging if not impossible to palpate and discern from adjacent musculature.

Subcostales

1. Place your palpating finger pads just lateral to the lateral border of the erector spinae in the posterior intercostal spaces between ribs eight to twelve. Feel for the subcostales deep to the intercostal musculature.

Transversus Thoracis

1. Place your palpating finger pads in the anteromedial intercostal spaces between ribs two to six, just lateral to the sternum, or immediately lateral to the xiphoid process of the sternum. Feel for the transversus thoracis.

TREATMENT CONSIDERATIONS

- The primary function of the subcostales might be to stabilize ribs eight through ten by stopping them from elevating, which could help stabilize the rib cage attachment of the diaphragm, enabling the diaphragm to pull more efficiently on its dome (central tendon). This function would make the subcostales important as accessory muscles of inspiration.

- Because a muscle cannot be palpated and discerned from adjacent musculature does not mean that pressure cannot be translated into it. Moderate-to-deeper pressure can be used successfully to work these muscles where the subcostales and transversus thoracis are accessible between the ribs.

8

8

SPINE AND RIB CAGE
Diaphragm

Pronunciation   **DI-a-fram**

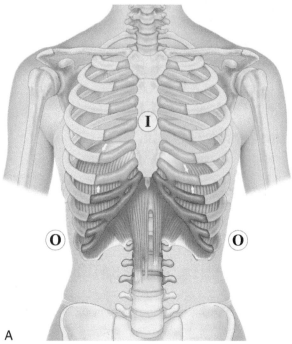

The diaphragm is a broad flat muscle that separates the thoracic cavity from the abdominal cavity. It attaches inferiorly and peripherally to the rib cage, and has an aponeurotic central tendon called *the dome* that is superiorly and centrally located (Figure 8-21). The diaphragm is the principle muscle of respiration. It contracts when we breathe in; it relaxes when we breathe out.

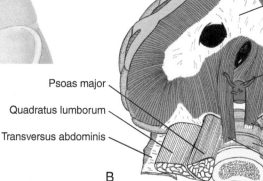

FIGURE 8-21 Views of the diaphragm. **A,** Anterior view. **B,** Inferior view. The psoas major, quadratus lumborum, and transversus abdominis are shown on the right side. *O,* Origin; *I,* insertion.

WHAT'S IN A NAME?

The name, *diaphragm,* tells us that this muscle is a partition (it separates the thoracic cavity from the abdominal cavity).

✳ **Derivation:**
diaphragm: Gr. partition

ATTACHMENTS

Origin (Inferior/Peripheral Attachment)
- Internal surfaces of the rib cage and sternum, and the spine

Insertion (Superior/Central Attachment)
- Central tendon (dome) of the diaphragm

ACTIONS

- Increases the volume of (i.e., expands) the thoracic cavity.

STABILIZATION

Stabilizes the trunk, including the joints of the lower rib cage and the thoracic and lumbar spinal joints.

INNERVATION

- Phrenic nerve

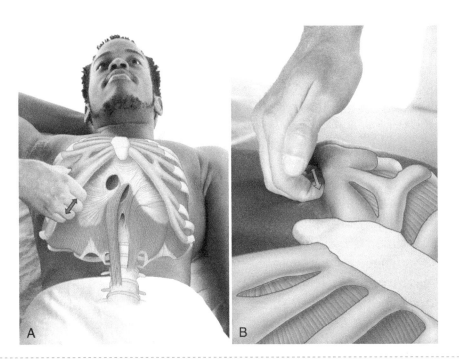

FIGURE 8-22 Palpation of the diaphragm. *A,* Palpation of the right side of the diaphragm as the client slowly exhales. *B,* Close-up showing palpation of the diaphragm by curling the fingers around the rib cage so that the finger pads are oriented against the muscle.

PALPATION

1. The client is supine with a roll under the knees to flex the thighs at the hip joint. Place your palpating fingers curled under the inferior margin of the anterior rib cage.

2. Ask the client to take in a deep breath and then slowly exhale. As the client exhales, curl your fingertips under (inferior and then deep to) the rib cage. Feel for the diaphragm on the internal surface of the rib cage with your finger pads (Figure 8-22).

3. Repeat this procedure anteriorly and posteriorly as far as possible on both sides of the rib cage.

   Note: Assessment of the diaphragm should only be made when it is totally relaxed, which occurs at the end of the exhalation.

TREATMENT CONSIDERATIONS

- When the diaphragm contracts, usually the rib cage attachment is more fixed; consequently, the central dome drops down. This increases the superior-to-inferior diameter of the thoracic cavity to enable the lungs to fill with air. Because this pushes the belly out, it is often called *belly breathing*. Once the dome cannot drop any 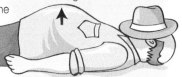 farther, the rib cage attachment lifts up, increasing the anterior-to-posterior diameter of the thoracic cavity to enable the lungs to further fill with air. Because this causes the rib cage to move outward, this is called *chest breathing*.

- A number of openings in the diaphragm allow passage of structures between the thoracic and abdominal cavities. The largest openings are for the esophagus, aorta, and inferior vena cava.

- The diaphragm is unusual in that it is under both conscious control and unconscious control. More specifically, contraction of the diaphragm is under constant unconscious regulation by the brainstem. However, we routinely override this brainstem control whenever we choose to sing, talk, sigh, hold our breath, or otherwise consciously change our breathing pattern.

- A *hiatal hernia* is when part of the stomach herniates (ruptures) through the diaphragm into the thoracic cavity.

- When the diaphragm contracts, the lungs inflate with air and the thoracic cavity becomes more rigid. Further, because the diaphragm drops down against the contents of the abdominal cavity, the abdominal cavity is also compressed, becoming more rigid. The result is that core stability is increased, including the thoracic and lumbar spinal joints. This is the reason why people intuitively take in and hold a deep breath when performing a joint action that requires great strength.

SPINE AND RIB CAGE: Anterior Abdominal Wall Muscles
Rectus Abdominis; External Abdominal Oblique; Internal Abdominal Oblique; Transversus Abdominis

Pronunciation   REK-tus ab-DOM-i-nis • EKS-turn-al ab-DOM-in-al o-BLEEK • in-TURN-al ab-DOM-in-al o-BLEEK • trans-VER-sus ab-DOM-i-nis

Four muscles make up the anterior abdominal wall: (1) rectus abdominis, (2) external abdominal oblique, (3) internal abdominal oblique, and (4) transversus abdominis (Figure 8-23). The rectus abdominis is superficial in the anteromedial abdominal wall. The other three are located in the anterolateral abdominal wall (they also reach around as far as the posterior abdominal wall). Of these three, the external abdominal oblique is the most superficial; the internal abdominal oblique is deep to it; and the transversus abdominis is the deepest of the three.

FIGURE 8-23 *A,* Rectus abdominis—anterior view bilaterally. The external abdominal oblique has been ghosted in on the left. *B,* Right external abdominal oblique—anterior view. *C,* Right external abdominal oblique—right lateral view.

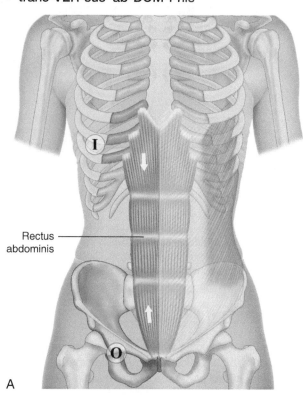

Rectus abdominis

A

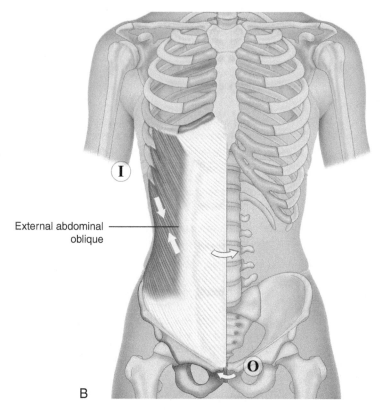

External abdominal oblique

B

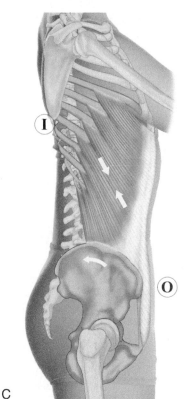

C

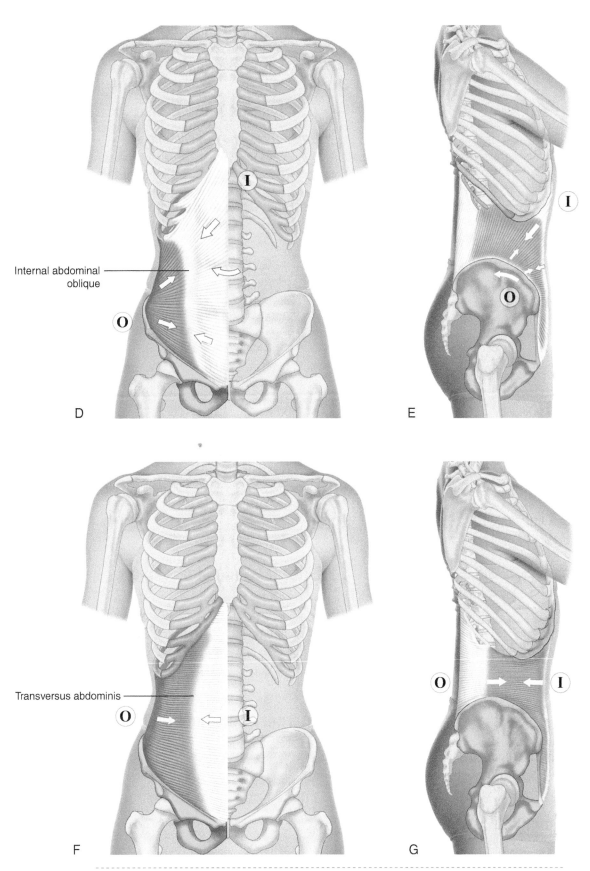

Internal abdominal oblique

D

E

Transversus abdominis

F

G

8

FIGURE 8-23, cont'd D, Right internal abdominal oblique—anterior view. **E,** Right internal abdominal oblique—right lateral view. **F,** Right transversus abdominis—anterior view. **G,** Right transversus abdominis—right lateral view. *O,* Origin; *I,* insertion.

Turn page to more.

WHAT'S IN A NAME?

The name, *rectus abdominis,* tells us that this muscle runs straight up the abdomen.

The name, *external abdominal oblique,* tells us that this muscle is located externally in the abdomen (superficial to the internal abdominal oblique) and its fibers are oriented obliquely.

The name, *internal abdominal oblique,* tells us that this muscle is located internally in the abdomen (deep to the external abdominal oblique) and its fibers are oriented obliquely.

The name, *transversus abdominis,* tells us that this muscle runs transversely across the abdomen.

✳ **Derivation:**
rectus: L. straight
oblique: L. slanting, diagonal
transversus: L. running transversely
abdominis: L. refers to the abdomen
external: L. outside
internal: L. inside

ATTACHMENTS

Rectus Abdominis

Origin (Proximal Attachment)
- Pubis

Insertion (Distal Attachment)
- Xiphoid process and the cartilage of ribs five through seven

External Abdominal Oblique

Origin (Proximal Attachment)
- Anterior iliac crest, pubic bone, and abdominal aponeurosis

Insertion (Distal Attachment)
- Lower eight ribs (ribs five through twelve)

Internal Abdominal Oblique

Origin (Proximal Attachment)
- Inguinal ligament, iliac crest, and thoracolumbar fascia

Insertion (Distal Attachment)
- Lower three ribs (ten through twelve) and the abdominal aponeurosis

Transversus Abdominis

Origin (Proximal Attachment)
- Inguinal ligament, iliac crest, thoracolumbar fascia, and lower costal cartilages

Insertion (Distal Attachment)
- Abdominal aponeurosis

ACTIONS

- The muscles of the anterior abdominal wall move the trunk at the spinal joints and the pelvis at the lumbosacral joint.
- The rectus abdominis and the abdominal obliques all flex and laterally flex the trunk and also posteriorly tilt the pelvis.

Rectus Abdominis
- Flexes the trunk.
- Posteriorly tilts the pelvis and flexes the lower trunk relative to the upper trunk.
- Laterally flexes the trunk.

External Abdominal Oblique
- Flexes the trunk.
- Posteriorly tilts the pelvis and flexes the lower trunk relative to the upper trunk.
- Laterally flexes the trunk.
- Contralaterally rotates the trunk.

Internal Abdominal Oblique
- Flexes the trunk.
- Posteriorly tilts the pelvis and flexes the lower trunk relative to the upper trunk.
- Laterally flexes the trunk.
- Ipsilaterally rotates the trunk.

Transversus Abdominis
- Compresses abdominopelvic cavity.

STABILIZATION

Stabilize the lumbar spinal joints, pelvis, and rib cage.

INNERVATION

■ Intercostal nerves

PALPATION

All muscles of the anterior abdominal wall are palpated with the client prone with a small roll under the knees.

Rectus Abdominis

1. The client is supine with a small roll under the knees. Place your palpating finger pads just off center of the midline of the abdomen.
2. Ask the client to flex the trunk slightly at the spinal joints (slightly curl the trunk upward), and feel for the contraction of the rectus abdominis (Figure 8-24).
3. With the rectus abdominis contracted, strum laterally and medially (perpendicularly) across its fibers to locate its lateral and medial borders. Continue palpating to the superior attachment (origin) and then to the inferior attachment (insertion) by strumming perpendicularly across the fibers.

External Abdominal Oblique

1. Place your palpating finger pads on the anterolateral abdominal wall between the iliac crest and the lower ribs. (Be sure you are lateral to the rectus abdominis.)

2. Ask the client to rotate the trunk to the opposite side of the body (contralateral rotation) and slightly flex the trunk; feel for the contraction of the external abdominal oblique (Figure 8-25).
3. Feel for the diagonal orientation of the external abdominal oblique fibers by strumming perpendicular to them. Continue palpating the external abdominal oblique toward its superior and inferior attachments.

Internal Abdominal Oblique

1. Repeat the same procedure; this time, however, ask the client to ipsilaterally rotate the trunk and to flex the trunk slightly (Figure 8-26).

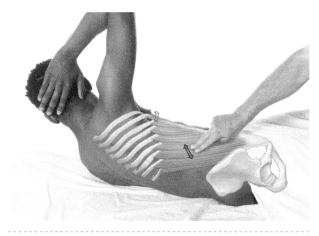

FIGURE 8-25 Palpation of the right external abdominal oblique as the client flexes and contralaterally (left) rotates the trunk against gravity.

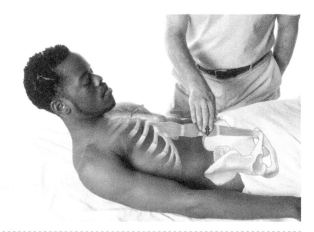

FIGURE 8-24 Palpation of the right rectus abdominis as the client flexes the trunk against gravity. Palpation should be done by strumming perpendicular to the fibers as shown.

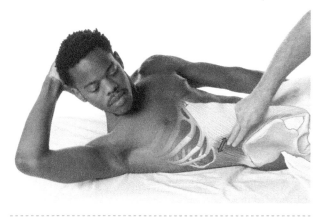

FIGURE 8-26 Palpation of the right internal abdominal oblique as the client flexes and ipsilaterally (right) rotates the trunk against gravity.

Turn page to 👁 more.

Transversus Abdominis

1. With palpating finger pads on the anterolateral abdomen, ask the client to compress the abdominal contents by forcefully breathing out. Feel for the contraction of the transversus abdominis.

   Note: The transversus abdominis is deep to the other anterolateral abdominal wall muscles and extremely difficult to discern from them because they also contract when compressing the abdominal contents.

TREATMENT CONSIDERATIONS

- All muscles of the abdominal wall compress against the abdominal contents and help create a flat abdomen.

- Stabilizing the lumbar spinal joints and the pelvis is stabilization of the *core of the body*. Although the transversus abdominis is best known for this function, the other abdominal muscles can assist.

- The abdominal aponeurosis is actually the midline aponeurosis of the three anterolateral abdominal wall muscles (external and internal abdominal obliques and the transversus abdominis). The abdominal aponeurosis is also known as the rectus sheath because it envelops or ensheathes the rectus abdominis.

- Three fibrous bands known as *tendinous inscriptions* transect the rectus abdominis muscles and divide each one into four sections or boxes. For this reason, the rectus abdominis muscles in a well-developed individual are often known as the *eight-pack (8-pack) muscle*. (Actually, it is more often incorrectly labeled the six-pack [6-pack] muscle, because six of the eight compartments are more visible.)

- If you were to put your hand into a coat pocket, your fingers would be pointing along the direction of the fibers of the external abdominal oblique on that side. For this reason, the external abdominal oblique muscles are sometimes called the *pocket muscles*.

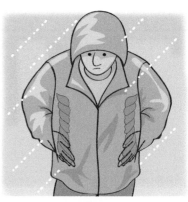

- The transversus abdominis is sometimes called the *corset* muscle because it wraps around the abdomen like a corset and, similar to a corset, it functions to hold in the abdomen.

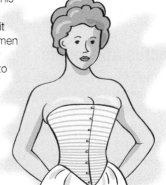

8

Notes

SPINE AND RIB CAGE: Splenius Group
Splenius Capitis; Splenius Cervicis

Pronunciation   **SPLEE-nee-us KAP-i-tis • SPLEE-nee-us SER-vi-sis**

Two splenius muscles are in the upper trunk and neck: (1) splenius capitis and (2) splenius cervicis. The splenius capitis attaches superiorly (inserts) onto the head; the splenius cervicis attaches superiorly (inserts) onto the cervical spine, hence their names (Figure 8-27). They are located deep to the trapezius and rhomboids; however, the splenius capitis is superficial in the posterior triangle of the neck (a triangular region bordered by the upper trapezius, sternocleidomastoid, and clavicle).

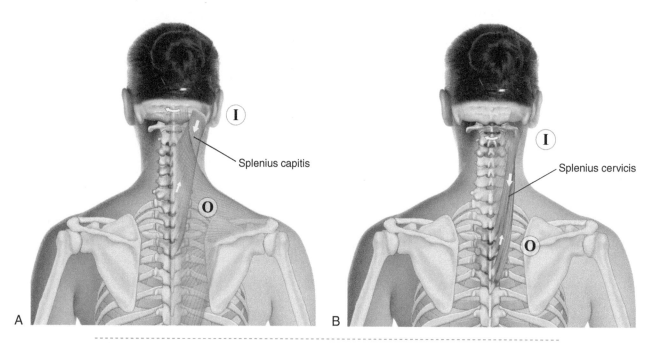

A   B

FIGURE 8-27 *A*, Posterior view of the right splenius capitis. The trapezius has been ghosted in. ***B*,** Posterior view of the right splenius cervicis. The splenius capitis has been ghosted in. *O*, Origin; *I*, insertion.

WHAT'S IN A NAME?

The name, *splenius capitis,* tells us that this muscle is shaped like a bandage (a narrow rectangle) and attaches onto the head.

    The name, *splenius cervicis,* tells us that this muscle is shaped like a bandage (a narrow rectangle) and attaches onto the cervical spine (the neck).

✳ **Derivation:**
splenius: Gr. bandage
capitis: L. refers to the head
cervicis: L. refers to the cervical spine

ATTACHMENTS

Splenius Capitis

Origin (Proximal Attachment)
- Nuchal ligament from C3-C6 and the spinous processes of C7-T4

Insertion (Distal Attachment)
- Mastoid process of the temporal bone and the occipital bone

Splenius Cervicis

Origin (Proximal Attachment)

- Spinous processes of T3-T6

Insertion (Distal Attachment)

- Transverse processes of C1-C3

ACTIONS

The splenius capitis and cervicis have the same actions on the neck at the spinal joints; the capitis also has these actions on the head at the atlanto-occipital joint.

Splenius Capitis

- Extends the head and neck.
- Laterally flexes the head and neck.
- Ipsilaterally rotates the head and neck.

Splenius Cervicis

- Extends the neck.
- Laterally flexes the neck.
- Ipsilaterally rotates the neck.

STABILIZATION

1. Both splenius muscles stabilize the cervical and upper thoracic vertebrae.
2. The splenius capitis also stabilizes the head.

INNERVATION

- Cervical spinal nerves

PALPATION

Splenius Capitis

1. The client is seated with the head and neck ipsilaterally rotated. Place your palpating finger pads at the upper aspect of the posterior triangle of the neck just inferior to the occiput and just posterior to the sternocleidomastoid muscle (see page 280). Place your resistance hand on the back of the client's head.
2. With the client's head and neck ipsilaterally rotated, resist the client from extending the head and neck at the spinal joints. Feel for the contraction of the splenius capitis (Figure 8-28).
3. Strum perpendicular to the fibers of the splenius capitis in the posterior triangle, working your way downward, until you reach the border of the upper trapezius.

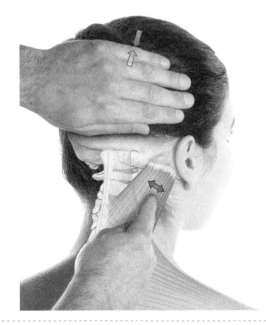

FIGURE 8-28 Palpation of the right splenius capitis in the posterior triangle of the neck as the client extends the head and neck against resistance. The upper trapezius has been ghosted in.

4. While asking the client to alternately extend the head and neck against gentle resistance and then relax, feel for the contraction and relaxation of the splenius capitis deep to the upper trapezius. Continue palpating the splenius capitis deep to the trapezius as far inferiorly as possible.

Splenius Cervicis

1. The splenius cervicis is deep to other musculature for its entire course; therefore palpating and discerning it can be difficult, especially from the splenius capitis.
2. If palpation is attempted, use the same protocol as that for the splenius capitis and feel for the splenius cervicis immediately lateral to the splenius capitis.

TREATMENT CONSIDERATIONS

- The left and right splenius capitis muscles bilaterally form a V shape. Because of their V shape, the left and right splenius capitis muscles are sometimes known as the *golf tee* muscles.

- The splenius capitis and splenius cervicis often blend together. By definition, any fibers that attach superiorly onto the head are defined as *splenius capitis* and any fibers that attach superiorly onto the cervical spine are defined as *splenius cervicis*.

SPINE AND RIB CAGE: Suboccipital Group
Rectus Capitis Posterior Major; Rectus Capitis Posterior Minor; Obliquus Capitis Inferior; Obliquus Capitis Superior

Pronunciation **REK**-tus **KAP**-i-tis pos-**TEE**-ri-or **MAY**-jor •
REK-tus **KAP**-i-tis pos-**TEE**-ri-or **MY**-nor •
ob-**LEE**-kwus **KAP**-i-tis in-**FEE**-ri-or • ob-**LEE**-kwus **KAP**-i-tis sue-**PEE**-ri-or

The suboccipital group is composed of four small deep muscles whose bellies are located directly inferior to the occiput, hence the name. These muscles are (1) rectus capitis posterior major, (2) rectus capitis posterior minor, (3) obliquus capitis inferior, and (4) obliquus capitis superior (Figure 8-29).

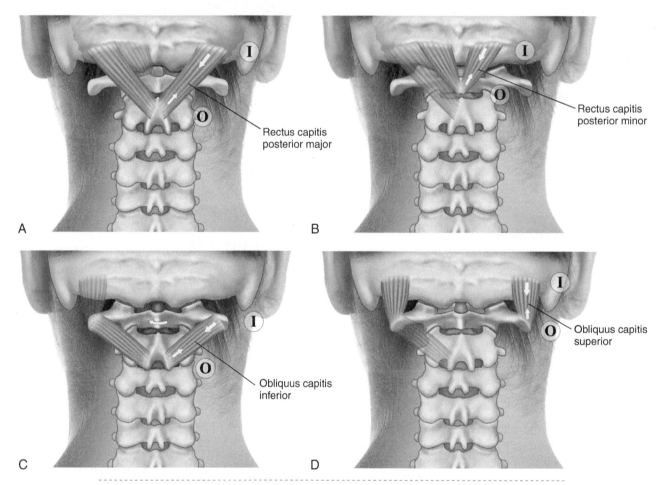

FIGURE 8-29 Posterior views bilaterally. **A,** The rectus capitis posterior major. The rectus capitis posterior minor has been ghosted in on the left. **B,** The rectus capitis posterior minor. The rectus capitis posterior major has been ghosted in on the left. **C,** The obliquus capitis inferior. The obliquus capitis superior has been ghosted in on the left. **D,** The obliquus capitis superior. The obliquus capitis inferior has been ghosted in on the left. *O,* Origin; *I,* insertion.

WHAT'S IN A NAME?

The names, *rectus capitis posterior major* and *minor*, tell us that they attach onto the head and that the fibers of these muscles run straighter than the two obliquus capitis suboccipital muscles. They also tell us that the major is larger than the minor.

The names, *obliquus capitis inferior* and *superior*, tell us that they attach onto or near the head and that the fibers of these muscles run obliquely in comparison to the two rectus capitis posterior suboccipital muscles. They also tell us that the inferior is located inferiorly to the superior.

❋ **Derivation:**
capitis: L. refers to the head
posterior: L. behind, toward the back
rectus: L. straight
obliquus: L. oblique/slanting/diagonal
major: L. larger
minor: L. smaller
inferior: L. below
superior: L. above

ATTACHMENTS

Rectus Capitis Posterior Major

Origin (Proximal Attachment)
- Spinous process of the axis (C2)

Insertion (Distal Attachment)
- Occiput

Rectus Capitis Posterior Minor

Origin (Proximal Attachment)
- Posterior tubercle of the atlas (C1)

Insertion (Distal Attachment)
- Occiput

Obliquus Capitis Inferior

Origin (Proximal Attachment)
- Spinous process of the axis (C2)

Insertion (Distal Attachment)
- Transverse process of the atlas (C1)

Obliquus Capitis Superior

Origin (Proximal Attachment)
- Transverse process of the atlas (C1)

Insertion (Distal Attachment)
- Occiput

ACTIONS

The suboccipital muscles move the head at the atlanto-occipital joint (AOJ) or move the atlas at the atlanto-axial joint (AAJ).

Rectus Capitis Posterior Major
- Extends the head at the AOJ.

Rectus Capitis Posterior Minor
- Protracts the head at the AOJ.

Obliquus Capitis Inferior
- Ipsilaterally rotates the atlas at the AAJ.

Obliquus Capitis Superior
- Protracts the head at the AOJ.

STABILIZATION

Suboccipital Group
1. Stabilizes the head and atlas at the AOJ.
2. Stabilizes the AAJ.

INNERVATION
- Suboccipital nerve

PALPATION

Rectus Capitis Posterior Major
1. The client is supine. Place your palpating finger pads just superior and slightly lateral to the spinous process of C2.
2. Find the spinous process of C2. Then palpate just superolateral to it and feel for the rectus capitis posterior major by strumming perpendicular to its fibers.
3. Continue strumming perpendicularly, following it superolaterally toward its occipital attachment (Figure 8-30).

Turn page to 👁 more.

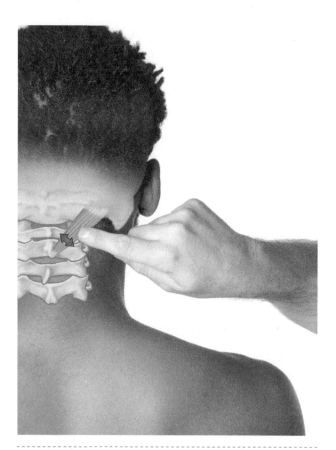

FIGURE 8-30 Palpation of the right rectus capitis posterior major between the spinous process of the axis (C2) and the occiput.

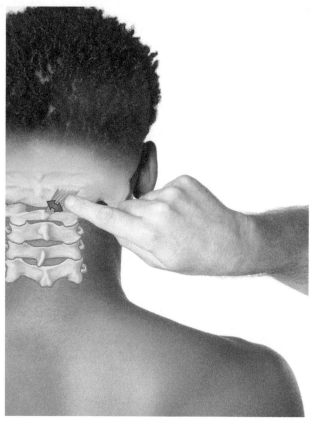

FIGURE 8-31 Palpation of the right rectus capitis posterior minor between the posterior tubercle of the atlas (C1) and the occiput.

Rectus Capitis Posterior Minor

1. Repeat the same steps but start just superolateral to the posterior tubercle of C1. Strum perpendicular to locate the rectus capitis posterior minor; then follow toward the occipital attachment (Figure 8-31). Asking the client to protract the head at the AOJ anteriorly to engage the muscle may be helpful.

Obliquus Capitis Inferior

1. Palpate between the spinous process of C2 and the transverse process of C1, strumming perpendicular to the fibers. Asking the client to rotate ipsilaterally the head against gentle resistance may be helpful to engage the muscle.

Obliquus Capitis Superior

1. This muscle is very challenging to palpate and discern from adjacent musculature. Feel for it just lateral to the superior attachment of the rectus capitis posterior major; if felt, try to continue palpating it inferiorly by strumming perpendicular to it.

TREATMENT CONSIDERATIONS

- As a group, the suboccipital muscles are generally thought to be primarily important as postural stabilization muscles, providing fine control of head posture. They are also rich in receptors for proprioception.

- The rectus capitis posterior minor has a fascial connective tissue attachment into the dura mater. Although tightness of any of the posterior cervical musculature may cause tension headaches, given this dura mater attachment, a tight rectus capitis posterior minor may be especially involved.

- Given their action of protraction of the head at the AOJ, a tight rectus capitis posterior minor and obliquus capitis superior can contribute to a posture of the head being held anteriorly; in other words, protracted.

- **A certain amount of caution must be exercised when palpating and pressing into the region known as the *suboccipital triangle* (bounded by the rectus capitis posterior major and the two obliquus capitis muscles), because of the presence of the vertebral artery and suboccipital nerve. The greater occipital nerve is also located nearby.**

Notes

SPINE AND RIB CAGE
Sternocleidomastoid (SCM)

Pronunciation   **STER-no-KLI-do-MAS-toyd**

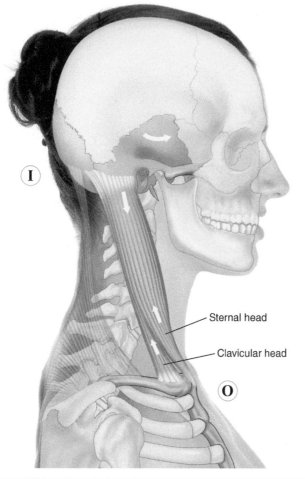

Sternal head

Clavicular head

FIGURE 8-32 Lateral view of the right sternocleidomastoid. The trapezius has been ghosted in. *O,* Origin; *I,* insertion.

The sternocleidomastoid (SCM) is a superficial muscle of the neck. It has two heads, a sternal head and clavicular head, which blend and attach superiorly onto the head (Figure 8-32).

ATTACHMENTS

Origin (Proximal Attachment)
- Sternal head: manubrium of the sternum
- Clavicular head: medial clavicle

Insertion (Distal Attachment)
- Mastoid process of the temporal bone

ACTIONS

The sternocleidomastoid moves the neck and head at the spinal joints.

- Flexes the lower neck.
- Extends the upper neck and head.
- Laterally flexes the neck and head.
- Contralaterally rotates the neck and head.

STABILIZATION

Stabilizes the cervical spinal joints.

INNERVATION

- Spinal accessory nerve (CN XI)

WHAT'S IN A NAME?

The name, *sternocleidomastoid,* tells us that this muscle attaches to the sternum, clavicle, and mastoid process of the temporal bone.

* **Derivation:**
sterno: Gr. refers to the sternum
cleido: Gr. refers to the clavicle
mastoid: Gr. refers to the mastoid process

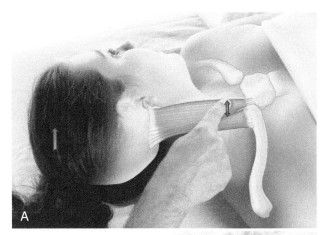

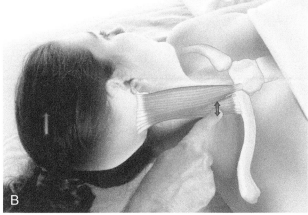

FIGURE 8-33 Supine palpation of the right SCM as the client raises the head and neck from the table. *A,* Palpation of the sternal head. *B,* Palpation of the clavicular head.

PALPATION

1. The client is supine with the head and neck contra-laterally rotated. Place your palpating finger pads just superior to the sternoclavicular joint.

2. Ask the client to lift the head and neck from the table. Look for the SCM to become visible (Figure 8-33).

   Note: The sternal head is usually more visible than the clavicular head.

3. Strumming perpendicular to the fibers, palpate superiorly toward the mastoid process attachment.

TREATMENT CONSIDERATIONS

- The SCM's major superior attachment is the mastoid process attachment of the temporal bone. However, it also has a thin aponeurotic attachment to the occipital bone.

- **The carotid sinus of the common carotid artery lies directly deep and medial to the SCM, midway up the neck. Because a neurologic reflex occurs to lower blood pressure when the carotid sinus is pressed, massage to this region must be done judiciously, especially with weak or older clients.**

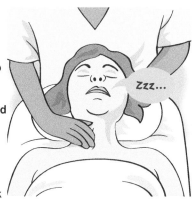

- The SCM and the scalenes are often injured as a result of car accidents. This trauma is usually called *whiplash* because the head and neck are forcefully thrown one way and then the other, similar to a whip being lashed. When the head and neck are thrown posteriorly, the anterior cervical musculature may be injured, causing it to spasm. When the head and neck are thrown anteriorly, the same trauma may occur to the posterior musculature.

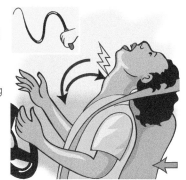

- The SCM forms a border of the posterior triangle of the neck and is, therefore, an excellent landmark for palpating other neck muscles. Locate the posterior (lateral) border of the SCM, the anterior border of the upper trapezius, and the clavicle; and then palpate in the tall narrow triangular space that is located between them.

8

SPINE AND RIB CAGE: Scalene Group
Anterior Scalene; Middle Scalene; Posterior Scalene

Pronunciation **an-TEE-ri-or SKAY-leen** • **MI-dil SKAY-leen** • **pos-TEE-ri-or SKAY-leen**

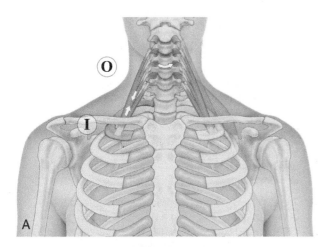

A

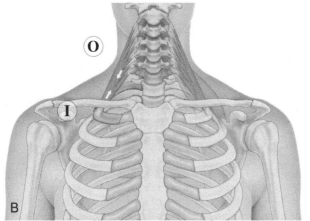

B

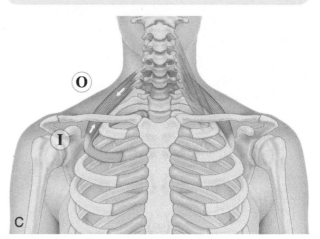

C

The scalene group is located in the antero-lateral neck and is composed of three muscles: the anterior, middle, and posterior scalenes (Figure 8-34). The spinal and rib attachments of the scalenes are deep to other structures, but much of the middle bellies of the scalene muscles are superficial in the posterior triangle of the neck between the sternocleidomastoid (SCM) and upper trapezius. The middle scalene is the largest of the three; the posterior scalene is the smallest.

FIGURE 8-34 *A,* Anterior view of the anterior scalene bilaterally. The other two scalenes have been ghosted in on the left side. *B,* Anterior view of the middle scalene bilaterally. The other two scalenes have been ghosted in on the left side. *C,* Anterior view of the posterior scalene bilaterally. The other two scalenes have been ghosted in on the left side. *O,* Origin; *I,* insertion.

WHAT'S IN A NAME?

The name, *scalene,* tells us that these muscles have a steplike or ladderlike shape.

The names *anterior, posterior,* and *middle,* tell us that the anterior scalene is the most anterior of the group; the posterior scalene is the most posterior of the group; and the middle scalene is between the other two.

✳ **Derivation:**
scalene: L. uneven, ladder
anterior: L. before, in front of
middle: L. middle (between)
posterior: L. behind, toward the back

ATTACHMENTS

Anterior Scalene and Middle Scalene

Origin (Proximal Attachment)
- Transverse processes of the cervical spine

Insertion (Distal Attachment)
- First rib

Posterior Scalene

Origin (Proximal Attachment)

- Transverse processes of the cervical spine

Insertion (Distal Attachment)

- Second rib

ACTIONS

The scalenes move the neck at the spinal joints and the ribs at the sternocostal and costospinal joints. All three scalenes laterally flex the neck and elevate the rib to which they attach; the anterior and middle scalenes also flex the neck.

Anterior Scalene and Middle Scalene

- Flex the neck.
- Laterally flex the neck.
- Elevate the first rib.

Posterior Scalene

- Laterally flexes the neck.
- Elevates the second rib.

STABILIZATION

1. Stabilize the cervical spinal joints.
2. Stabilize the first and second ribs.

INNERVATION

- Cervical spinal nerves

PALPATION

1. The client is supine. Locate the lateral border of the clavicular head of the SCM muscle (see Figure 8-33); then immediately drop off of it laterally onto the scalenes in the posterior triangle of the neck.
2. With your finger pads pressing into the scalene muscle group, ask the client to take in short, quick breaths through the nose and feel for the contraction of the scalene musculature (Figure 8-35).
3. Strumming perpendicular to the direction of the fibers, palpate as much of the scalenes in the posterior triangle of the neck as possible.
4. To palpate the origin (superior attachment) on the spine and the insertion (inferior attachment) on the ribs, slacken the SCM by passively laterally flexing the client's neck to the same side. For the spinal attachments, reach deep to the SCM toward

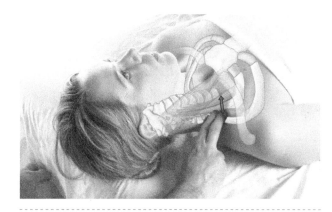

FIGURE 8-35 Palpation of the right scalenes as the client takes in short, quick breaths through the nose.

the transverse process attachments. For the rib attachments, with your finger pads oriented posteriorly, gently but firmly reach deep to the clavicle.

TREATMENT CONSIDERATIONS

- The brachial plexus of nerves and the subclavian artery run between the anterior and middle scalenes. If these muscles are tight, entrapment of these nerves and/or the artery can occur. When this happens, it is called *anterior scalene syndrome*, one of the four types of *thoracic outlet syndrome*. This condition can cause sensory symptoms (e.g., tingling, pain, numbness) and/or motor symptoms (e.g., weakness, partial paralysis) in the upper extremity.

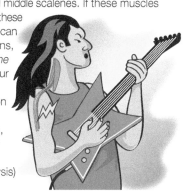

- **Very close to the superior attachment of the anterior scalene is the common carotid artery. Given the neurologic reflex that occurs to lower blood pressure when the carotid sinus of the common carotid artery is pressed, massage to this region must be done judiciously, especially with weak or older clients.**

- The SCM and the scalenes are often injured as a result of car accidents. This trauma is usually called *whiplash* because the head and neck are forcefully thrown one way and then the other, like a whip being lashed. When the head and neck are thrown posteriorly, the anterior cervical musculature may be injured, causing it to spasm. When the head and neck are thrown anteriorly, the same trauma may occur to the posterior musculature.

8

SPINE AND RIB CAGE: Suprahyoid Muscles
Digastric; Stylohyoid; Mylohyoid; Geniohyoid

Pronunciation   **di-GAS-trik • STI-lo-HI-oyd • MY-lo-HI-oyd • JEE-nee-o-HI-oyd**

The suprahyoids are named for attaching to and being located superior to the hyoid bone. The four suprahyoid muscles are the digastric, stylohyoid, mylohyoid, and geniohyoid (Figure 8-36). Other than a thin fascial muscle called the *platysma*, the suprahyoid group is superficial. Within this group, the geniohyoid is deep to the mylohyoid; and the digastric has two bellies, an anterior belly and a posterior belly. In addition, an infrahyoid group contains four muscles.

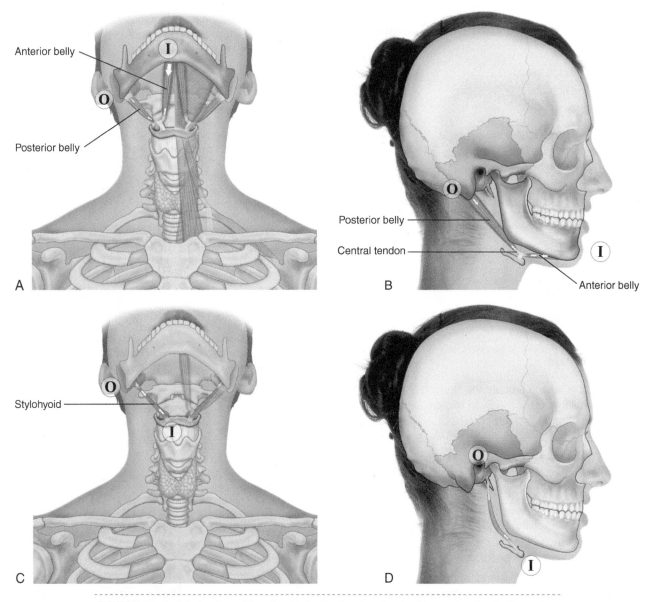

FIGURE 8-36 **A,** Anterior view of the digastric bilaterally with other hyoid muscles ghosted in on the client's left side. **B,** Right lateral view of the digastric. **C,** Anterior view of the stylohyoid bilaterally with the digastric ghosted in on the client's left side. **D,** Right lateral view of the stylohyoid.

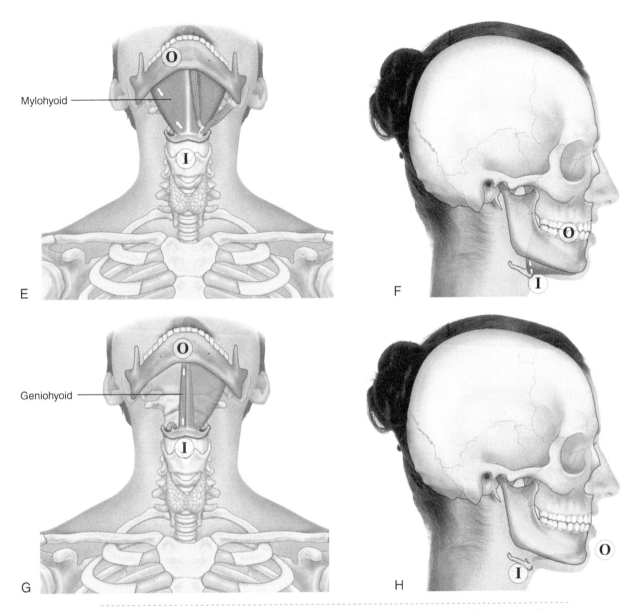

Mylohyoid

E

F

Geniohyoid

G

H

8

FIGURE 8-36, cont'd **E,** Anterior view of the mylohyoid bilaterally with the digastric shown on the client's left side. **F,** Right lateral view of the mylohyoid. **G,** Anterior view of the geniohyoid bilaterally with the mylohyoid ghosted in on the client's left side. **H,** Right lateral view of the geniohyoid. *O,* Origin; *I,* insertion.

WHAT'S IN A NAME?

The name, *digastric,* tells us that this muscle has two bellies (*gaster* means belly).

The name, *stylohyoid,* tells us that this muscle attaches from the styloid process (of the temporal bone) to the hyoid bone.

The name, *mylohyoid,* tells us that this muscle attaches to the hyoid bone. *Mylo,* referring to the molar teeth, tells us that this muscle also attaches close to the molar teeth.

The name, *geniohyoid,* tells us that this muscle attaches to the hyoid bone. *Genio,* referring to the chin, tells us that this muscle also attaches to the mandible.

❋ **Derivation:**
di: Gr. two
gastric: Gr. belly
hyoid: Gr. refers to the hyoid bone
stylo: Gr. refers to the styloid process
mylo: Gr. mill (refers to the molar teeth)
genio: Gr. chin

Turn page to 👁 more.

ATTACHMENTS

Digastric

Origin (Posterior Attachment)
- Temporal bone

Insertion (Anterior Attachment)
- Mandible

> Note: The digastric has an intermediate central tendon attached to the hyoid bone via a fascial sling of tissue.

Stylohyoid

Origin (Superior Attachment)
- Styloid process of the temporal bone

Insertion (Inferior Attachment)
- Hyoid

Mylohyoid

Origin (Superior Attachment)
- Inner surface of the mandible

Insertion (Inferior Attachment)
- Hyoid

Geniohyoid

Origin (Superior Attachment)
- Inner surface of the mandible

Insertion (Inferior Attachment)
- Hyoid

ACTIONS

The suprahyoid group moves the mandible at the temporomandibular joints (TMJs), the head and neck at the spinal joints, and the hyoid bone.
- Elevates the hyoid bone (all four).
- Depresses the mandible (all except the stylohyoid).
- Flexes the head and neck (all except the stylohyoid).

STABILIZATION

Stabilize the hyoid bone and TMJs.

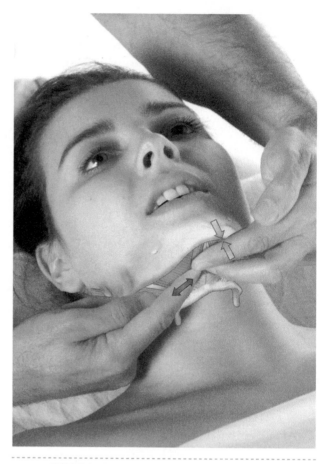

FIGURE 8-37 Palpation of the right suprahyoids.

INNERVATION

- Trigeminal nerve (cranial nerve [CN] V) and the facial nerve (CN VII) (digastric)
- Facial nerve (CN VII) (stylohyoid)
- Trigeminal nerve (CN V) (mylohyoid)
- Hypoglossal nerve (CN XII) (geniohyoid)

PALPATION

1. The client is supine. Place your palpating finger pads just inferior to the mandible, just off center. Place your resistance hand under the client's chin.
2. Ask the client to depress the mandible gently against resistance. Feel for the contraction of the suprahyoid muscles (Figure 8-37).
3. Continue palpating the suprahyoid muscles inferiorly toward the hyoid bone while resisting mandibular depression and strumming perpendicular to their fibers.

4. To palpate the stylohyoid and the posterior belly of the digastric, continue palpating laterally from the hyoid toward the mastoid process of the temporal bone, while resisting mandibular depression and strumming perpendicular to the fibers (Figure 8-38).

TREATMENT CONSIDERATIONS

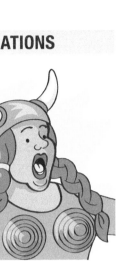

■ The external carotid artery lies inferior and deep to the stylohyoid and posterior belly of the digastric. Massage to this region must be judiciously done.

■ The digastric is the prime mover of depression of the mandible.

■ Tightness of the suprahyoid musculature can cause or aggravate TMJ dysfunction.

FIGURE 8-38 Palpation of the right stylohyoid and posterior belly of digastric (of the suprahyoid group).

SPINE AND RIB CAGE: Infrahyoid Muscles
Sternohyoid; Sternothyroid; Thyrohyoid; Omohyoid

Pronunciation   STER-no-HI-oyd • STER-no-THI-royd • THI-ro-HI-oyd • O-mo-HI-oyd

The infrahyoids are named for attaching to and being located inferior to the hyoid bone. The four infrahyoid muscles are the sternohyoid, sternothyroid, thyrohyoid, and omohyoid (Figure 8-39). Other than the sternocleidomastoid and a thin fascial muscle called the *platysma*, the infrahyoid group is superficial. Within this group, the sternothyroid and thyrohyoid are deep to the sternohyoid; and the omohyoid has two bellies, an inferior belly and a superior belly. In addition, a suprahyoid group contains four muscles.

8

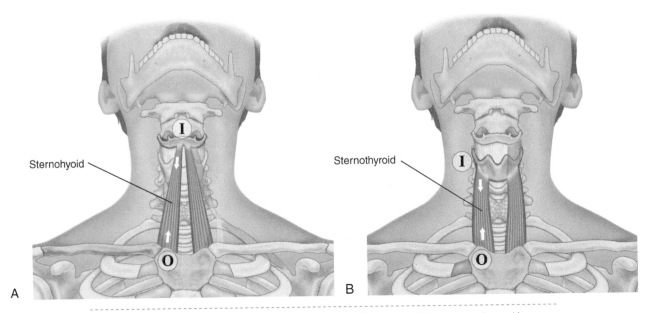

A

B

FIGURE 8-39 *A,* Anterior view of the sternohyoid bilaterally. The omohyoid has been ghosted in on the client's left side. *B,* Anterior view of the sternothyroid bilaterally. The thyrohyoid has been ghosted in on the client's left side.

Continued

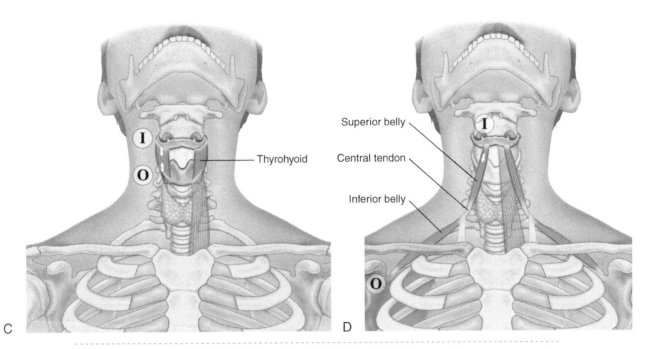

C

D

FIGURE 8-39, cont'd C, Anterior view of the thyrohyoid bilaterally. The sternothyroid has been ghosted in on the client's left side. **D,** Anterior view of the omohyoid. The sternohyoid has been ghosted in on the client's left side. *O,* Origin; *I,* insertion.

WHAT'S IN A NAME?

The name, *sternohyoid,* tells us that this muscle attaches from the sternum to the hyoid bone.

The name, *sternothyroid,* tells us that this muscle attaches from the sternum to the thyroid cartilage.

The name, *thyrohyoid,* tells us that this muscle attaches from the thyroid cartilage to the hyoid bone.

The name, *omohyoid,* tells us that this muscle attaches from the scapula (*omo* means shoulder, referring to the scapula) to the hyoid bone.

❋ **Derivation:**
  hyoid: Gr. refers to the hyoid
  thyroid/thyro: Gr. refers to the thyroid cartilage
  sterno: L. refers to the sternum
  omo: Gr. shoulder

ATTACHMENTS

Sternohyoid

Origin (Inferior Attachment)
■ Sternum

Insertion (Superior Attachment)
■ Hyoid

Sternothyroid

Origin (Inferior Attachment)
■ Sternum

Insertion (Superior Attachment)
■ Thyroid cartilage

Thyrohyoid

Origin (Inferior Attachment)
■ Thyroid cartilage

Insertion (Superior Attachment)
■ Hyoid

Omohyoid

Origin (Inferior Attachment)
■ Scapula

Insertion (Superior Attachment)
■ Hyoid

Note: The omohyoid has an intermediate central tendon attached to the clavicle via a fascial sling of tissue.

Turn page to ◉ more.

ACTIONS

The infrahyoid group moves the head and neck at the spinal joints and the hyoid bone.

- Depresses the hyoid bone and thyroid cartilage.
- Flexes the neck.

STABILIZATION

Stabilizes the hyoid bone and thyroid cartilage.

INNERVATION

- Cervical plexus (sternohyoid, sternothyroid, omohyoid)
- Hypoglossal nerve (CN XII) (thyrohyoid)

PALPATION

1. The client is supine. Place your palpating finger pads immediately inferior to the hyoid, just off center. Place your resistance hand under the client's chin.

2. Ask the client to depress the mandible gently at the TMJs against resistance. Feel for the contraction of the infrahyoid muscles by strumming perpendicular to their fibers (Figure 8-40).

3. Continue palpating them inferiorly toward the sternum while resisting mandibular depression and strumming perpendicular to their fibers.

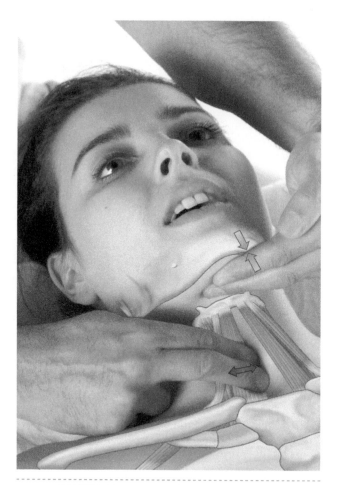

FIGURE 8-40 Palpation of the right infrahyoids.

TREATMENT CONSIDERATIONS

- The carotid sinus of the common carotid artery lies slightly lateral to the infrahyoid musculature. Because a neurologic reflex occurs to lower blood pressure when the carotid sinus is pressed, massage to this region must be judiciously done, especially with weak or older clients.

- The infrahyoid muscles can indirectly assist stabilization of the TMJs by stabilizing the hyoid bone when the suprahyoid muscles contract. With the hyoid stabilized, the suprahyoids can exert their pull on the mandible, thereby stabilizing the TMJs.

- The sternothyroid can play a role in stabilizing the hyoid bone by stabilizing the thyroid cartilage when the thyrohyoid contracts, which allows the contraction force of the thyrohyoid to be exerted on the hyoid bone.

- The infrahyoids play an important role in movement and stabilization of the hyoid bone when singing and playing wind and brass instruments.

- The thyrohyoid can be considered to be an upward continuation of the sternothyroid muscle.

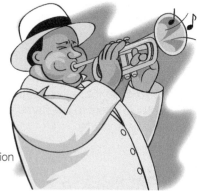

Notes

SPINE AND RIB CAGE: Prevertebral Group
Longus Colli; Longus Capitis; Rectus Capitis Anterior; Rectus Capitis Lateralis

Pronunciation   **LONG-us KOL-eye • LONG-us KAP-i-tis •**
REK-tus KAP-i-tis an-TEE-ri-or • REK-tus KAP-i-tis la-ter-A-lis

The prevertebral group is composed of four muscles located deep in the anterior neck. They are the longus colli, longus capitis, rectus capitis anterior, and rectus capitis lateralis (Figure 8-41). The longus colli is often described as having three parts: (1) *superior oblique part*, (2) *inferior oblique part*, and (3) *vertical part*.

8

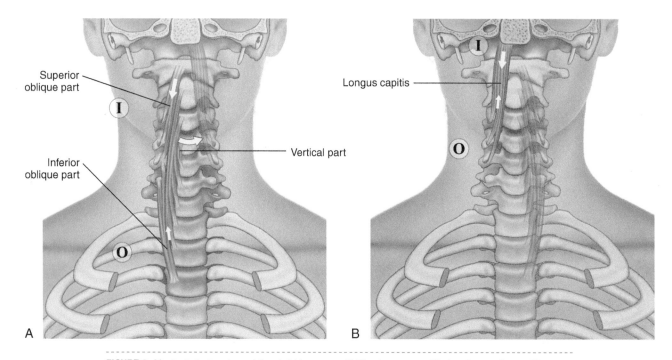

Superior oblique part

Inferior oblique part

Vertical part

Longus capitis

A

B

FIGURE 8-41   **A,** Anterior view of the right longus colli. The longus capitis has been ghosted in on the left. **B,** Anterior view of the right longus capitis. The longus colli has been ghosted in on the left.   *Continued*

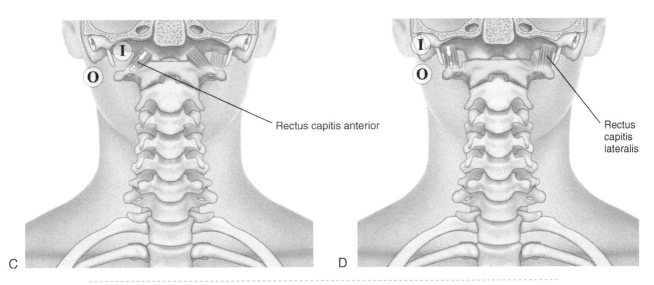

C

D

FIGURE 8-41, cont'd C, Anterior view of the rectus capitis anterior bilaterally. The rectus capitis lateralis has been ghosted in on the left. **D,** Anterior view of the rectus capitis lateralis bilaterally. The rectus capitis anterior has been ghosted in on the left. *O,* Origin; *I,* insertion.

WHAT'S IN A NAME?

The name, *longus colli,* tells us that this muscle is long and found in the neck.

The name, *longus capitis,* tells us that this muscle is long and attaches to the head.

The name, *rectus capitis anterior,* tells us that the fibers of this muscle run straight and attach to the head anteriorly (anterior to the rectus capitis lateralis).

The name, *rectus capitis lateralis,* tells us that the fibers of this muscle run straight and attach to the head laterally (lateral to the rectus capitis anterior).

❋ **Derivation:**
longus: L. long
colli: L. refers to the neck
capitis: L. refers to the head
rectus: L. straight
anterior: L. before, in front of
lateralis: L. refers to the side

ATTACHMENTS

Longus Colli

Origin (Inferior Attachment)
- Anterior bodies and transverse processes of cervical spine (C3-T3 vertebrae)

Insertion (Superior Attachment)
- Anterior arch (C1), anterior bodies and transverse processes of cervical spine (C2-C6)

Longus Capitis

Origin (Inferior Attachment)
- Transverse processes of the cervical spine (C3-C6)

Insertion (Superior Attachment)
- Occiput

Rectus Capitis Anterior

Origin (Inferior Attachment)
- Atlas (C1)

Insertion (Superior Attachment)
- Occiput

Rectus Capitis Lateralis

Origin (Inferior Attachment)
- Atlas (C1)

Insertion (Superior Attachment)
- Occiput

ACTIONS

The prevertebral muscles move the neck at the spinal joints and the head at the atlanto-occipital joint.

Longus Colli
- Flexes the neck.

Turn page to 👁 more.

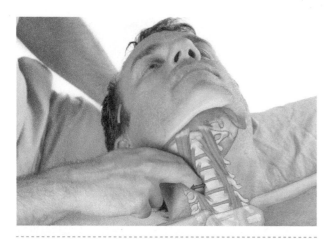

FIGURE 8-42 Palpation of the right longus colli and capitis as the client engages the muscles by lifting his head and neck into flexion.

Longus Capitis

■ Flexes the neck and head.

Rectus Capitis Anterior

■ Flexes the head.

Rectus Capitis Lateralis

■ Laterally flexes the head.

STABILIZATION

Stabilizes the cervical spinal joints and the head.

INNERVATION

■ Cervical spinal nerves

PALPATION

The prevertebral muscles are palpated with the client supine.

Longus Colli and Capitis

1. Locate the medial border of the sternal head of the sternocleidomastoid (SCM) muscle (see Fig. 8-33); then immediately drop off of it medially onto the longus muscles in the anterior neck.

2. Gently and slowly but firmly sink in posteriorly and slightly medially with your palpating finger pads toward the longus musculature (colli and capitis) on the anterior surface of the vertebral bodies and transverse processes of the cervical spine.

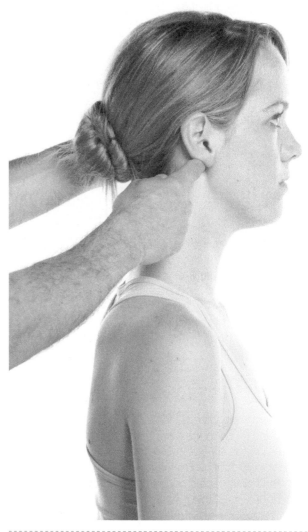

FIGURE 8-43 Palpation of the right rectus capitis lateralis superior to the transverse process of the atlas.

Note: If you feel a pulse under your fingers, you are on the common carotid artery. Either gently move it out of the way or move your fingers slightly to one side of it or the other, continuing to aim for the longus musculature. If necessary, the client's trachea can be gently displaced toward the other side of the body to allow for easier access to the longus muscles. Being gentle with displacing the trachea is important because many clients are sensitive to having their trachea touched or moved.

3. To confirm that you are on the longus musculature, ask the client to flex the head and neck at the spinal joints by lifting the head up from the table and feel for their contraction (Figure 8-42).

4. Once located, strum perpendicular to the fibers and palpate as far superiorly as possible and as far inferiorly as possible.

Rectus Capitis Lateralis

1. The rectus capitis lateralis is also quite deep but can sometimes be palpated and discerned from adjacent tissue. Place palpating finger pads immediately superior to the transverse process of the atlas (Figure 8-43).

   Note: The location of the transverse process of the atlas is immediately posterior to the ramus of the mandible and inferior to the ear.

2. Gently press into the small depression that can often be felt here, and feel for the rectus capitis lateralis.

   Note: Because the location of the facial nerve and styloid process is nearby, be careful to avoid pressing too forcefully.

Rectus Capitis Anterior

1. The rectus capitis anterior is extremely deep and is usually not palpable.

TREATMENT CONSIDERATIONS

- The longus colli and longus capitis are often injured in a whiplash accident, wherein the head and neck are forcefully thrown anteriorly and posteriorly (like a whip being lashed).

- The longus colli and longus capitis are also often aggravated when doing a lot of sit-ups, crunches, or curl-ups.

- The longus colli and other prevertebral muscles are important for stabilizing the neck and head while talking, swallowing, coughing, and sneezing. They also stabilize the neck during rapid arm movements. Talking, swallowing, coughing, and sneezing can exacerbate deep anterior neck pain in those who have a tight or injured longus colli.

- Clients with a tight longus colli and/or longus capitis often describe feeling as though they have a sore throat, especially when swallowing.

- **For many clients, the anterior neck can be an emotionally sensitive area of the body. Before placing your palpating hands there, let the client know that you will be working there and obtain verbal consent. The anterior neck can also be very physically sensitive because it has a number of fragile structures; therefore palpation into this region must be done carefully. When palpating, sink into the tissue slowly and gently, but with pressure that is firm enough to reach the longus musculature.**

REVIEW QUESTIONS

Circle or fill in the correct answer for each of the following questions. More study resources, including audio pronunciations of muscle names, are provided on the Evolve website at http://evolve.elsevier.com/Muscolino/knowthebody.

8

1. **What are the four muscles of the suboccipital group?**

    _____

    _____

    _____

    _____

2. **What are the three subgroups of the transverso-spinalis group?**

    _____

    _____

    _____

3. **What are the four suprahyoid muscles?**

    _____

    _____

    _____

    _____

4. **Which one of the following muscles flexes the trunk at the spinal joints?**
    a. Erector spinae
    b. External abdominal oblique
    c. Semispinalis
    d. Digastric

5. **Which of the following muscles attach onto the mastoid process of the temporal bone?**
    a. Sternocleidomastoid (SCM) and splenius capitis
    b. Rectus capitis posterior major and obliquus capitis inferior
    c. Anterior scalene and interspinales
    d. Erector spinae and transversospinalis

6. **Which of the following muscles are involved in respiration?**
    a. Rectus abdominis and obliquus capitis inferior
    b. Longus colli and digastric
    c. Serratus posterior superior and serratus posterior inferior
    d. Scalenes and splenius capitis

7. **What are the attachments of the quadratus lumborum?**
    a. Spinous processes of the lumbar spine to ribs eight through ten
    b. Iliac crest to the spinous processes of the lumbar spine
    c. Transverse processes of the lumbar spine to the scapula
    d. Iliac crest to the transverse processes of the lumbar spine and the twelfth rib

8. **Which one of the following muscles is the deepest muscle in the anterolateral abdominal wall?**
    a. External abdominal oblique
    b. Transversus abdominis
    c. Internal abdominal oblique
    d. Rectus abdominis

9. **The brachial plexus of nerves is located between which of the following muscles?**
    a. Anterior scalene and middle scalene
    b. Splenius capitis and splenius cervicis
    c. Middle scalene and posterior scalene
    d. Erector spinae and transversospinalis

10. **Which one of the following muscle groups attaches from a transverse process inferiorly to a spinous process superiorly?**
    a. Transversospinalis
    b. Erector spinae
    c. Scalenes
    d. External intercostals

CASE STUDY 1

A 52-year-old man is experiencing a bilateral mid-to-low back pain that extends to his upper gluteal region on both sides. He is approximately 20 pounds overweight but otherwise appears to be in good health. He admits to little regular physical activity in the last few years outside of the occasional round of golf. The pain he is experiencing started 1 week earlier after helping a friend load a moving truck. He was sore and stiff for the following 2 to 3 days and took an over-the-counter (OTC) pain medication. The OTC medication reduced the sharp pain to a manageable dull pain, but the stiffness remained. The client says he re-experiences sharp pain if he attempts to lift anything over 15 to 20 pounds. For example, when he removes a full trash bag from the trash can, sharp pain develops in his low back.

Postural analysis against a grid chart shows that the client's lumbar spine is hyperlordotic, and his thoracic region is slightly hyperkyphotic. During active range-of-motion (ROM) testing, the client is asked to stand with his hands by his sides, feet shoulder-width apart, and flex the trunk as far as possible. The client is only able to flex the trunk 30 degrees before sharp pain develops, causing him to flex his knees to regain balance. When asked to rotate the trunk in each direction, stiffness and dull pain prevent him from rotating beyond 20 degrees in each direction. Flexion of each thigh at the hip joint causes pain in the lumbosacral region, as does flexion of the arms at the glenohumeral joints. On a pain scale of 0 to 10, his pain reaches a threshold of 7 with these motions. The client remarks that he now has more muscle tightness after testing than before.

QUESTIONS

1. **Which major muscles are likely involved?**

   _____

   _____

   _____

2. **Why did flexion of the arms at the glenohumeral joints cause low back pain?**

   _____

   _____

   _____

3. **Why would flexion of the thigh at the hip joint cause pain in the lumbosacral region?**

   _____

   _____

   _____

4. **What would be recommended treatment options?**

   _____

   _____

   _____

8

CASE STUDY 2

While taking the history of a new client, Susan, a 30-year-old woman who had a baby 6 months earlier, recounts that she had a difficult pregnancy with multiple back strain issues that were treated with mild heat and massage. She experienced intense middle-to-low back pain during delivery, reaching a level of 8 on a pain scale of 0 to 10. Immediately after delivery, she had difficulty moving, bending over, and returning to a standing position. She said that she felt like she had been hit in the back with a bat. Pain was sharp if she was not careful when moving. After returning home from the hospital, Susan's back strain issues were treated with heat, massage therapy, and stretching, all of which gradually helped, bringing her pain level down to 2 or 3. Susan returned to work 3 months after delivery.

A month ago, Susan started attending yoga classes twice a week. The positions are difficult for her to attempt or hold for any length of time. She is also experiencing temporary stiffness and pain (reaching a level of 5 to 6), but she assumes this pain and stiffness are part of learning yoga. In the last week the soreness and stiffness have not subsided. When she picks up her child, pain develops once again in her low back. She returned to her physician and a magnetic resonance image (MRI) was ordered; the results were unremarkable. The physician suggested that she resume massage therapy and heat treatments. Pain medication was offered, but Susan declined because she is breast-feeding.

Postural analysis shows a slightly increased lumbar lordosis. Passive range-of-motion (ROM) testing produces a feeling of stiffness and pain. Flexion of the trunk produces dull pain in the lumbosacral region at a pain level of 4 on a scale of 0 to 10. Extension of the trunk produces a sharp pain at a level of 6. Left lateral flexion produces a pain level of 6 in the right low back, whereas right lateral flexion produces pain at a 4 level in the left lower back. What questions from the therapist would uncover additional information that might help explain what is contributing to the pain?

CHILD-RELATED QUESTIONS

1. When you pick up your child, do you bend from the back and reach over or do you bend at the knees?

_____

_____

_____

2. When you remove your child from the crib, do you lower the rail or reach over the rail?

_____

_____

_____

3. When you use the stroller, do you bend from the back or bend at the knees?

_____

_____

_____

4. When you hold your child, on what side of your body do you hold him or her?

_____

_____

_____

YOGA-RELATED QUESTIONS

1. During yoga class, do any of the positions or asanas produce immediate pain or stiffness?

_____

_____

_____

2. Do you feel looser or tighter directly after yoga class?

_____

_____

_____

3. Do you experience increased pain and/or stiffness later in the day on the days that you attend yoga class or upon awakening on the days after yoga class?

_____

_____

_____

_____

WORK-RELATED QUESTIONS

1. Does your job require any form of lifting?

_____

_____

_____

_____

2. Does your job require standing for any length of time?

_____

_____

_____

_____

3. What amount of stress is involved in your job?

_____

_____

_____

_____

Muscles of the Head

CHAPTER OUTLINE

The muscles addressed in this chapter are the muscles of the head. These muscles can be divided into muscles of mastication (chewing), muscles of the scalp, and muscles of facial expression.

Mastication is the act of chewing. Therefore the muscles of mastication are those that attach to and are involved in movement of the mandible at the temporomandibular joints (TMJs). The four major muscles of mastication are the temporalis, masseter, lateral pterygoid, and medial pterygoid.

Note: The eight muscles of the hyoid group are also involved in mastication; they are discussed in Chapter 7.

Muscles of the scalp and facial expression are superficial fascial muscles. The muscles of the scalp are involved in moving the scalp and the ear. Muscles of facial expression can be further subdivided into muscles of the eye, nose, and mouth. The contraction of these muscles is important for displaying emotions. Although some universality of facial expressions that display emotions are certainly apparent, variations are evident from one culture to another. Further, many of these muscles may act in concert with others to add to the spectrum of facial expressions. Some sources state that more than 1800 separate facial expressions can be created with combinations of the muscles of facial expression.

The companion CD at the back of this book allows you to examine the muscles of this body region, layer by layer, and individual muscle palpation technique videos are available in the Chapter 9 folder on the Evolve website.

OVERVIEW OF FUNCTION

The following general rules regarding actions can be stated for the functional groups of muscles of mastication at the TMJs:

- If a muscle attaches to the mandible and its other attachment is superior to the mandibular attachment, it can elevate the mandible at the TMJs.
- If a muscle attaches to the mandible and its other attachment is inferior to the mandibular attachment, it can depress the mandible at the TMJs.
- If a muscle attaches to the mandible and its other attachment is anterior to the mandibular attachment, it can protract the mandible at the TMJs.
- If a muscle attaches to the mandible and its other attachment is posterior to the mandibular attachment, it can retract the mandible at the TMJs.
- If a muscle attaches to the mandible and its other attachment is medial to the mandibular attachment, it can contralaterally deviate (do opposite side deviation of) the mandible at the TMJs.
- Reverse actions of the major muscles of mastication are unlikely because they would require movement of the entire head toward a fixed mandible (at the TMJs).

Superficial Right Lateral View of the Muscles of the Head

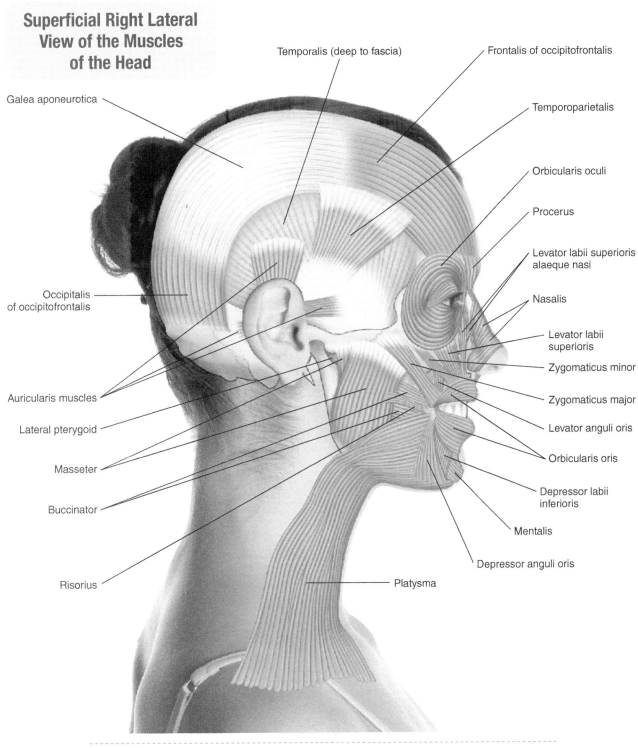

Galea aponeurotica

Temporalis (deep to fascia)

Frontalis of occipitofrontalis

Temporoparietalis

Orbicularis oculi

Procerus

Levator labii superioris alaeque nasi

Nasalis

Occipitalis of occipitofrontalis

Levator labii superioris

Zygomaticus minor

Zygomaticus major

Auricularis muscles

Lateral pterygoid

Levator anguli oris

Orbicularis oris

Masseter

Depressor labii inferioris

Buccinator

Mentalis

Depressor anguli oris

Risorius

Platysma

FIGURE 9-1 Superficial right lateral view of the muscles of the head.

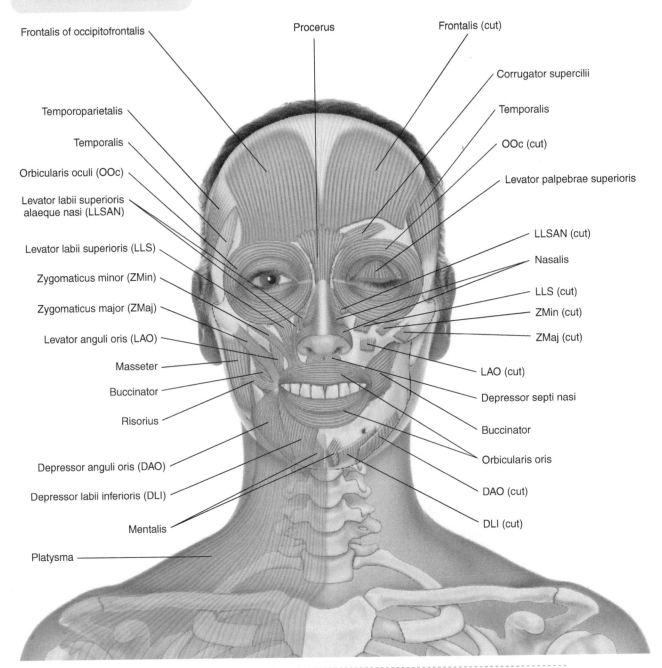

Frontalis of occipitofrontalis

Procerus

Frontalis (cut)

Corrugator supercilii

Temporoparietalis

Temporalis

Temporalis

OOc (cut)

Orbicularis oculi (OOc)

Levator palpebrae superioris

Levator labii superioris alaeque nasi (LLSAN)

LLSAN (cut)

Levator labii superioris (LLS)

Nasalis

Zygomaticus minor (ZMin)

LLS (cut)

Zygomaticus major (ZMaj)

ZMin (cut)

Levator anguli oris (LAO)

ZMaj (cut)

Masseter

LAO (cut)

Buccinator

Depressor septi nasi

Risorius

Buccinator

Orbicularis oris

Depressor anguli oris (DAO)

DAO (cut)

Depressor labii inferioris (DLI)

DLI (cut)

Mentalis

Platysma

FIGURE 9-2 Superficial anterior view of the muscles of the head. The platysma has been ghosted in. Note: Acronyms used on the person's left side are defined on the right side.

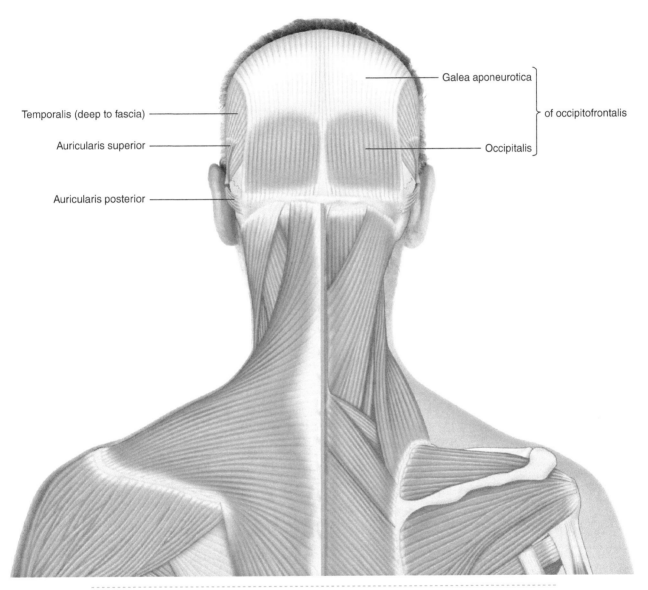

FIGURE 9-3 Superficial posterior view of the muscles of the head.

MUSCLES OF THE HEAD
Temporalis; Masseter

Pronunciation **tem-po-RA-lis • MA-sa-ter**

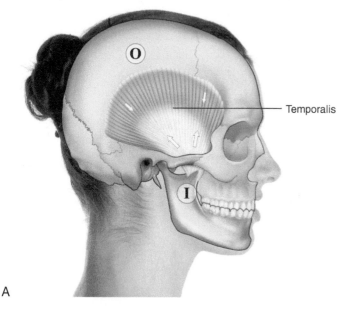

The temporalis and masseter are two of the four major muscles of mastication (chewing). The other two are the lateral and medial pterygoids discussed in the next layout. The temporalis and masseter are superficial muscles; the temporalis overlies the temporal bone and the masseter overlies the mandible (Figure 9-4). The masseter is usually divided into two layers: a *superficial layer* and a *deep layer*.

A

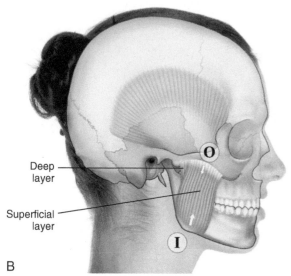

B

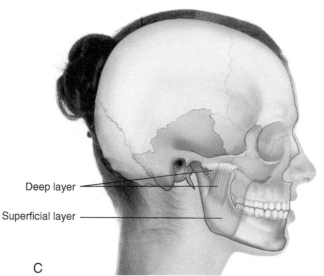

C

FIGURE 9-4 A, Lateral view of the right temporalis. **B,** Lateral view of the right masseter. The temporalis has been ghosted in. **C,** Lateral view of the right masseter. The superficial layer of the masseter has been ghosted in. *O,* Origin; *I,* insertion.

WHAT'S IN A NAME?

The name, *temporalis,* tells us that this muscle attaches onto the temporal bone.

The name, *masseter,* tells us that this muscle is involved with chewing.

✳ **Derivation:**
  temporalis: L. refers to the temple
  masseter: Gr. chewer

ATTACHMENTS

Temporalis

Origin (Superior Attachment)
- Temporal fossa

Insertion (Inferior Attachment)
- Coronoid process and the ramus of the mandible

9

Masseter

Origin (Superior Attachment)

- Inferior margins of both the zygomatic bone and the zygomatic arch of the temporal bone

Insertion (Inferior Attachment)

- Angle, ramus, and coronoid process of the mandible

ACTIONS

Both the temporalis and masseter move the mandible at the temporomandibular joints (TMJs).

- Elevate the mandible.

STABILIZATION

Stabilize the mandible at the TMJs.

INNERVATION

- Trigeminal nerve (cranial nerve [CN] V)

PALPATION

Both the temporalis and masseter are palpated with the client supine.

Temporalis

1. Place your palpating finger pads over the temporal fossa on the head (superior to the ear).
2. Ask the client to alternately contract and relax the temporalis; clenching the teeth and then relaxing the jaw will accomplish this. Feel for the contraction of the temporalis as the client clenches the teeth (Figure 9-5).
3. Once the contraction of the temporalis has been felt, palpate the entire muscle as the client continues to contract and relax it.

Masseter

1. Place your palpating finger pads between the zygomatic arch and the angle of the mandible.
2. Ask the client to alternately contract and relax the masseter; clenching the teeth and then relaxing the jaw will accomplish this. Feel for the contraction of the masseter as the client clenches the teeth (Figure 9-6).
3. Once the contraction of the masseter has been felt, palpate the entire muscle from the zygomatic arch to the angle of the mandible as the client continues to contract and relax it.

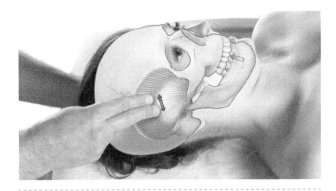

FIGURE 9-5 Palpation of the right temporalis as the client clenches the teeth.

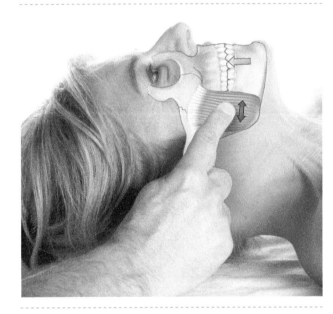

FIGURE 9-6 Palpation of the right masseter as the client clenches the teeth.

TREATMENT CONSIDERATIONS

- The temporalis muscle is deep to thick fibrous fascia called the *temporalis fascia*.

- A tight temporalis and masseter may be involved with tension headaches and with dysfunction of the temporomandibular joint (TMJ syndrome).

- The temporal fossa is much deeper in carnivores, allowing for a much thicker and stronger temporalis muscle, which contributes to the strength of a carnivore's bite.

- Proportional to its size, the masseter is stated by many sources to be the strongest muscle in the human body.

MUSCLES OF THE HEAD: Pterygoid Group
Lateral Pterygoid; Medial Pterygoid

Pronunciation   **LAT-er-al TER-i-goyd • MEE-dee-al TER-i-goyd**

The pterygoid group is composed of the lateral pterygoid and medial pterygoid muscles (Figure 9-7). The pterygoids are two of the four major muscles of mastication (chewing). The temporalis and masseter are the other two muscles and are discussed in the previous layout. Both pterygoids are deep to the mandible and best accessed from inside the mouth. The lateral pterygoid has two heads: a *superior head* and an *inferior head*.

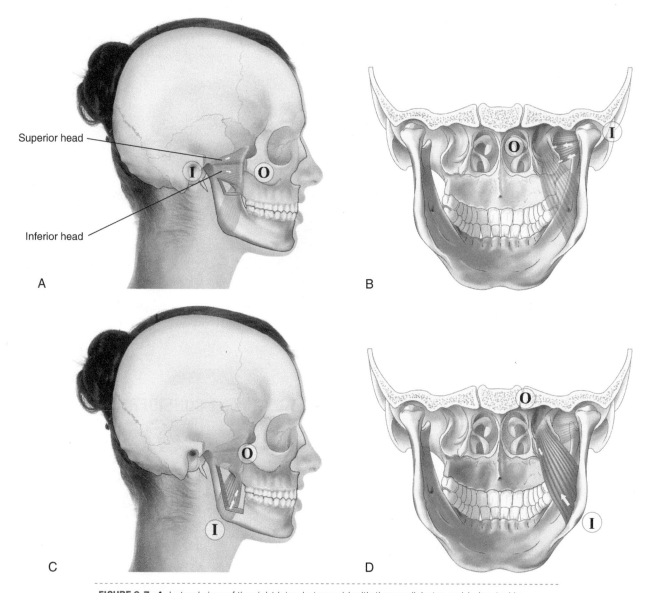

FIGURE 9-7 *A,* Lateral view of the right lateral pterygoid with the medial pterygoid ghosted in. The mandible has been partially cut away. ***B,*** Posterior view of the right lateral pterygoid with the medial pterygoid ghosted in. The cranial bones have been cut away. ***C,*** Lateral view of the right medial pterygoid with the lateral pterygoid ghosted in. The mandible has been partially cut away. ***D,*** Posterior view of the right medial pterygoid with the lateral pterygoid ghosted in. The cranial bones have been cut away. *O,* Origin; *I,* insertion.

WHAT'S IN A NAME?

The name, *pterygoid,* tells us that these muscles attach to the sphenoid bone (the pterygoid process). The lateral pterygoid is lateral to the medial pterygoid.

❋ **Derivation:**
pterygoid: Gr. wing shaped
lateral: L. side
medial: L. toward the middle

ATTACHMENTS

Lateral Pterygoid

Origin (Anterior/Medial Attachment)
- Sphenoid bone

Insertion (Posterior/Lateral Attachment)
- Neck of the mandible and the TMJ capsule

Medial Pterygoid

Origin (Anterior/Medial/Superior Attachment)
- Sphenoid bone

Insertion (Posterior/Lateral/Inferior Attachment)
- Internal surface of the angle of the mandible

ACTIONS

The pterygoids move the mandible at the TMJs.

Lateral Pterygoid
- Protracts the mandible.
- Contralaterally deviates the mandible.

Medial Pterygoid
- Elevates the mandible.
- Protracts the mandible.
- Contralaterally deviates the mandible.

STABILIZATION

Stabilizes the mandible at the TMJs.

INNERVATION

- Trigeminal nerve (cranial nerve [CN] V)

PALPATION

Both pterygoids are palpated with the client supine.

Lateral Pterygoid

1. Wearing either a glove or a finger cot, place your palpating finger inside the vestibule of the client's mouth (between the cheeks and the teeth) and run along the external surfaces of the upper teeth until you reach the back molars. Then press posteriorly and superiorly into a little pocket in the tissue between the gum above the upper teeth and the condyle of the mandible. You will be on the internal surface of the lateral pterygoid (Figure 9-8).

2. Now ask the client to gently either protract the mandible at the TMJs or deviate contralaterally the mandible slowly and carefully (deviate it to the opposite side of the body). Feel for the contraction of the lateral pterygoid (Figure 9-9).

9

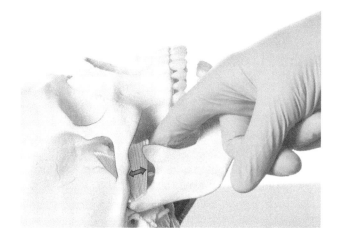

FIGURE 9-8 Supine palpation of the right lateral pterygoid shown with a skull.

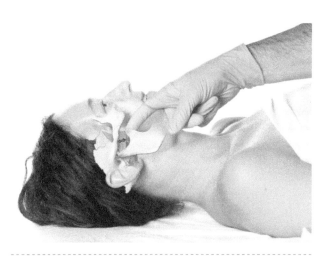

FIGURE 9-9 Supine palpation of the right lateral pterygoid as the client protracts the mandible.

Turn page to ◉ more.

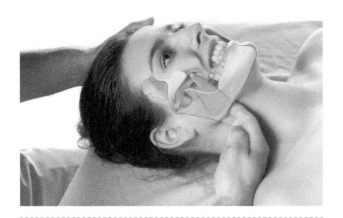

FIGURE 9-10 Palpation of the right medial pterygoid as the client clenches the teeth.

3. Once felt, palpate as much of the lateral pterygoid as possible, from the condyle of the mandible to the inside wall of the mouth (above the gum of the upper teeth).

Medial Pterygoid

1. From inside the mouth: Wearing either a glove or a finger cot, place your palpating finger along the internal surfaces of the lower teeth until you reach the back molars, then press posterolaterally until you reach the inside wall of the mouth.

2. Now ask the client to protract the mandible. Feel for the contraction of the medial pterygoid.

3. Once felt, palpate as much of the medial pterygoid as possible.

4. From outside the mouth: Curl your palpating fingers around to the inside surface of the angle of the mandible.

5. Ask the client to elevate the mandible at the TMJs by clenching the teeth. Feel for the contraction of the medial pterygoid (Figure 9-10).

TREATMENT CONSIDERATIONS

■ The direction of fibers of the medial pterygoid is essentially identical to the direction of the fibers of the masseter; in fact, these two muscles occupy the same position. The difference is that the masseter is external (superficial) to the mandible, and the medial pterygoid is internal (deep) to the mandible.

■ A tight lateral or medial pterygoid may be involved with dysfunction of the TMJ *(TMJ syndrome)*.

■ The lateral pterygoid functions to protract the mandible and the articular disc of the TMJ. It is important that the mandible and disc protract together when the jaw is opened. Therefore if the contraction of the lateral pterygoid is not precisely coordinated with the other muscles that move the mandible, the articular disc may become jammed between the two bones of the joint and dysfunction of the TMJ *(TMJ syndrome)* may occur.

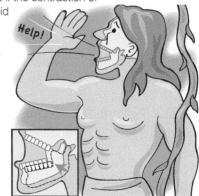

Notes

MUSCLES OF THE HEAD: Muscles of the Scalp
Occipitofrontalis; Temporoparietalis;
Auricularis Anterior; Auricularis Posterior; Auricularis Superior

Pronunciation   ok-SIP-i-to-fron-TA-lis • TEM-po-ro-pa-RI-i-TAL-is •
aw-RIK-u-la-ris an-TEE-ri-or • aw-RIK-u-la-ris pos-TEE-ri-or • aw-RIK-u-la-ris sue-PEE-ri-or

The muscles of the scalp are the occipitofrontalis (consisting of an occipitalis belly, a frontalis belly, and the intermediate galea aponeurotica), the temporoparietalis, and the three muscles of the auricularis group (auricularis anterior, auricularis posterior, and auricularis superior) (Figure 9-11). The occipitofrontalis and temporoparietalis are sometimes grouped together as the epicranius muscle. The muscles of the scalp are superficial fascial muscles.

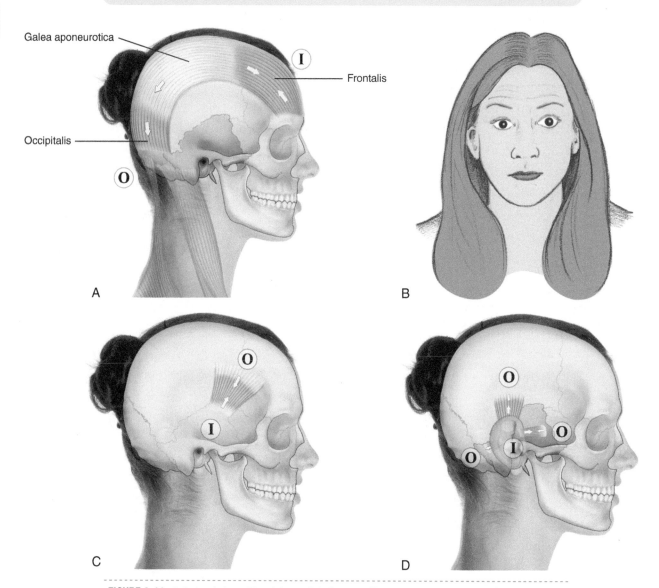

FIGURE 9-11 A, Lateral view of the right occipitofrontalis. The trapezius and sternocleidomastoid have been ghosted in. **B,** Expression of elevating the eyebrows created by the bilateral contraction of the occipitofrontalis. **C,** Lateral view of the right temporoparietalis. **D,** Lateral view of the right auricularis muscles. *O,* Origin; *I,* insertion.

The name, *occipitofrontalis,* tells us that this muscle lies over the occipital and frontal bones.

The name, *temporoparietalis,* tells us that this muscle lies over the temporal and parietal bones.

The name, *auricularis,* tells us that these muscles are involved with the ear. Anterior, superior, and posterior tell us their locations relative to the ear.

✳ Derivation:
occipitofrontalis: L. refers to the occiput and frontal bone
temporoparietalis: L. refers to the temporal and parietal bones
auricularis: L. ear
anterior: L. before, in front of
superior: L. upper, higher than
posterior: L. behind, toward the back

ATTACHMENTS

Occipitofrontalis

Origin (Posterior Attachment)
- Occipital bone and temporal bone

Insertion (Anterior Attachment)
- Fascia and skin overlying the frontal bone

    Note: The galea aponeurotica, a fibrous fascial aponeurosis, is intermediate between the occipital and frontal bellies of the occipitofrontalis.

Temporoparietalis

Origin (Superior Attachment)
- Lateral border of the galea aponeurotica

Insertion (Inferior Attachment)
- Fascia superior to the ear

Auricularis Group

Auricularis Anterior

Origin (Anterior Attachment)
- Galea aponeurotica

Insertion (Posterior Attachment)
- Anterior ear

Auricularis Superior

Origin (Superior Attachment)
- Galea aponeurotica

Insertion (Inferior Attachment)
- Superior ear

Auricularis Posterior

Origin (Posterior Attachment)
- Temporal bone

Insertion (Anterior Attachment)
- Posterior ear

9

ACTIONS

Occipitofrontalis
- Draws the scalp posteriorly (elevation of the eyebrow).

Temporoparietalis
- Elevates the ear.

Auricularis Group
- Draws the ear anteriorly (auricularis anterior).
- Elevates the ear (auricularis superior).
- Draws the ear posteriorly (auricularis posterior).

INNERVATION
- Facial nerve (cranial nerve [CN] VII)

Turn page to 👁 more.

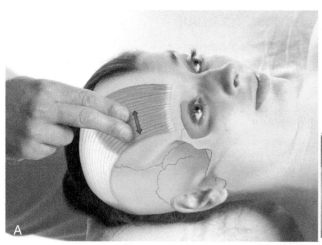

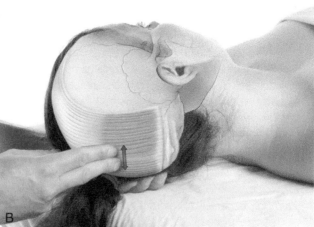

FIGURE 9-12 Palpation of the occipitofrontalis as the client engages it by raising the eyebrows. **A,** Palpation of the right frontalis belly of the occipitofrontalis. **B,** Palpation of the right and left occipitalis bellies of the occipitofrontalis muscles.

PALPATION

All three muscles and muscle groups are palpated with the client supine.

Occipitofrontalis

1. Place your palpating finger pads on the forehead of the client.
2. Ask the client to elevate the eyebrows. Feel for the contraction of the frontalis belly (Figure 9-12, *A*); once felt, palpate the entire frontalis.
3. Now palpate over the client's occipital bone, and ask the client to elevate the eyebrows. Feel for the contraction of the occipitalis belly (Figure 9-12, *B*); once felt, palpate the entire occipitalis.

Temporoparietalis

1. Place your palpating finger pads approximately 1 to 2 inches superior and slightly anterior to the ear.
2. Ask the client to elevate the ear. Feel for the muscle's contraction (Figure 9-13).

Auricularis group

1. Place your palpating finger pads either immediately anterior, superior, or posterior to the ear, and ask the client to move the ear in that direction, feeling for the contraction of that particular auricularis muscle.

Note: Many people cannot consciously control muscles that move their ears; therefore it is usually necessary to palpate the temporoparietalis and auricularis muscles by location while they are relaxed.

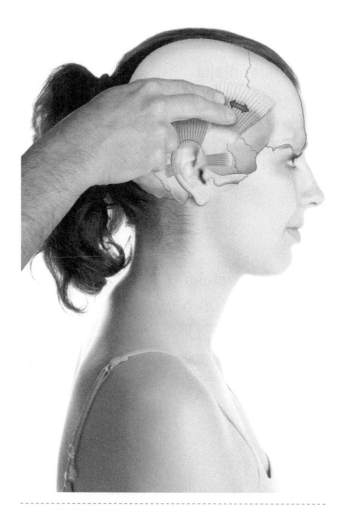

FIGURE 9-13 Palpation of the right temporoparietalis.

TREATMENT CONSIDERATIONS

■ Because the occipitofrontalis can elevate the eyebrow, it can also be considered to be a muscle of facial expression. Elevation of the eyebrows is associated with the expressions of surprise, shock, horror, fright, or recognition. It also often accompanies glancing upward.

■ The occipitofrontalis is a muscle like any other in the body, and moderate or even deeper work may be performed to benefit the client. Because tension headaches often involve the occipito-frontalis, this muscle should be evaluated in any client complaining of tension headaches.

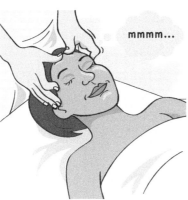

mmmm...

■ Although the temporoparietalis and auricularis muscles in humans are poorly formed and often nonfunctional, the analogous muscles in dogs (and many other animals) are highly developed. This is clear when one sees how a dog can direct its ears toward the location from which a sound originates.

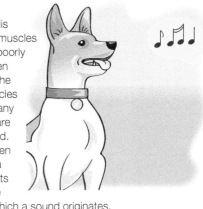

9

MUSCLES OF THE HEAD:
Muscles of Facial Expression—Eye
Orbicularis Oculi; Levator Palpebrae Superioris; Corrugator Supercilii

Pronunciation   or-BIK-you-la-ris OK-you-lie • LE-vay-tor pal-PEE-bree su-PEE-ri-OR-is •
KOR-u-gay-tor su-per-SIL-i-eye

The three muscles of facial expression of the eye are
the orbicularis oculi, levator palpebrae superioris, and
corrugator supercilii (Figure 9-14). The occipitofrontalis,
a muscle of the scalp presented in the last layout (see
page 310), can also be considered to be a muscle of facial
expression of the eye.

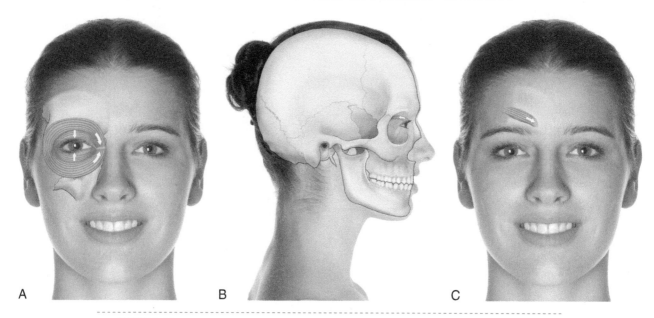

A   B   C

FIGURE 9-14 A, Anterior view of the right orbicularis oculi. **B,** Lateral view of the right levator
palpebrae superioris. **C,** Anterior view of the right corrugator supercilii.

WHAT'S IN A NAME?

The name, *orbicularis oculi,* tells us that this muscle
encircles the eye.
   The name, *levator palpebrae superioris,* tells us
that this muscle elevates the upper eyelid.
   The name, *corrugator supercilii,* tells us that this
muscle wrinkles the skin of the eyebrow.
✳ Derivation:
   orbicularis: L. small circle
   oculi: L. refers to the eye
   levator: L. lifter
   palpebrae: L. eyelid
   superioris: L. upper
   corrugator: L. to wrinkle together
   supercilii: L. refers to the eyebrow

ATTACHMENTS

Orbicularis Oculi

■ Encircles the eye (from the medial side of the eye, it
returns to the medial side of the eye)

Levator Palpebrae Superioris

■ Sphenoid bone to the upper eyelid

Corrugator Supercilii

■ Inferior frontal bone to the fascia and skin deep to the
eyebrow

ACTIONS

Orbicularis Oculi

- Closes and squints the eye (Figure 9-15).
- Expressions: wink, concern, perplexion

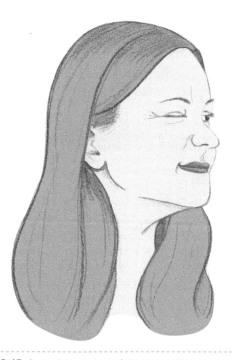

FIGURE 9-15 Anterolateral view of the expression created by the contraction of the right orbicularis oculi.

Levator Palpebrae Superioris

- Elevates the upper eyelid (Figure 9-16).
- Expressions: surprise, fear

Corrugator Supercilii

- Draws the eyebrow inferomedially (Figure 9-17).
- Expressions: anger, concern

INNERVATION

- Facial nerve (cranial nerve [CN] VII) (orbicularis oculi and corrugator supercilii)
- Oculomotor nerve (cranial nerve [CN] III) (levator palpebrae superioris)

PALPATION

Orbicularis Oculi

1. Gently place your palpating finger pad on the tissue around the client's eye, and ask the client to close the eye somewhat forcefully. Feel for the contraction of the orbicularis oculi (Figure 9-18).
2. Once felt, palpate the entire muscle as the client alternately contracts and relaxes it.

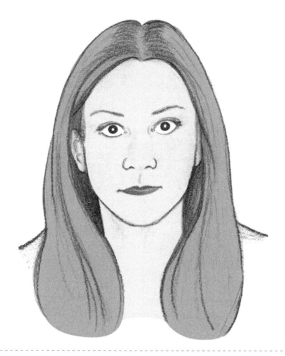

FIGURE 9-16 Anterior view of the expression created by the bilateral contraction of the levator palpebrae superioris.

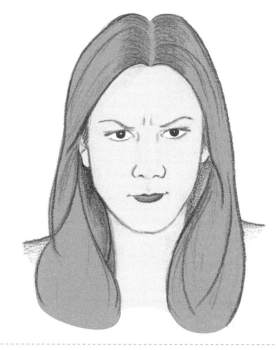

FIGURE 9-17 Anterior view of the expression created by the bilateral contraction of the corrugator supercilii.

Turn page to ◉ more.

Levator Palpebrae Superioris

1. Gently place your palpating finger pad on the client's upper eyelid, and ask the client to elevate the upper eyelid. Feel for the contraction of the levator palpebrae superioris (Figure 9-19).

2. Once felt, palpate as much of the muscle as possible as the client alternately contracts and relaxes it.

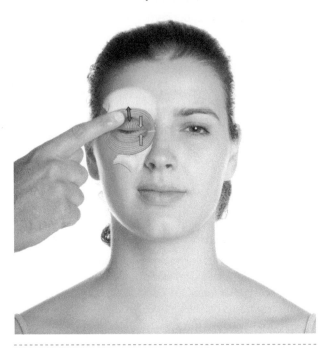

FIGURE 9-18 Palpation of the right orbicularis oculi as the client somewhat forcefully closes the eye as if to squint.

Corrugator Supercilii

1. Gently place your palpating finger pad on the medial portion of the client's eyebrow, and ask the client to frown, bringing the eyebrows down. Feel for the contraction of the corrugator supercilii (Figure 9-20).

   Note: The corrugator supercilii can also be easily palpated by squeezing the medial eyebrow between palpating finger pads while the client contracts it.

2. Once felt, palpate the entire muscle as the client alternately contracts and relaxes it.

TREATMENT CONSIDERATIONS

- The palpebral part of the orbicularis oculi is under both conscious and unconscious control and may contract reflexly to close the eye (for protection and as part of blinking).

- If the orbicularis oculi contracts forcefully, wrinkles that radiate out from the lateral eye will form; these wrinkles are called *crow's feet*.

- When the tissue located superior to the eye is pulled down around the eye by the contraction of the orbicularis oculi, it helps shield the eye from bright sunlight.

- When the corrugator supercilii contracts, it causes vertical wrinkles superior and medial to the eyes.

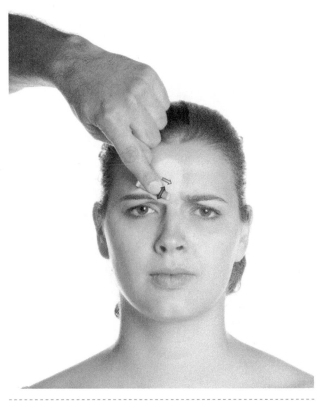

FIGURE 9-20 Palpation of the right corrugator supercilii as the client frowns.

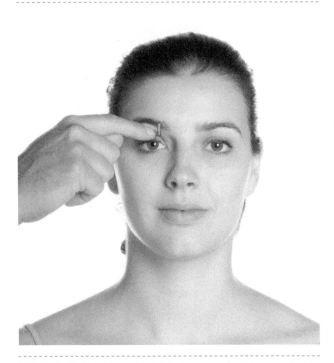

FIGURE 9-19 Palpation of the right levator palpebrae superioris in the upper eyelid as the client elevates the upper eyelid.

Notes

9

MUSCLES OF THE HEAD:
Muscles of Facial Expression—Nose
Procerus; Nasalis; Depressor Septi Nasi

Pronunciation   **pro-SAIR-rus • nay-SA-lis • dee-PRES-or SEP-ti NAY-zi**

Three muscles of facial expression of the nose are the procerus, nasalis, and depressor septi nasi (Figure 9-21). The levator labii superioris alaeque nasi presented in the next layout (see page 322) is a muscle of facial expression of both the mouth and the nose.

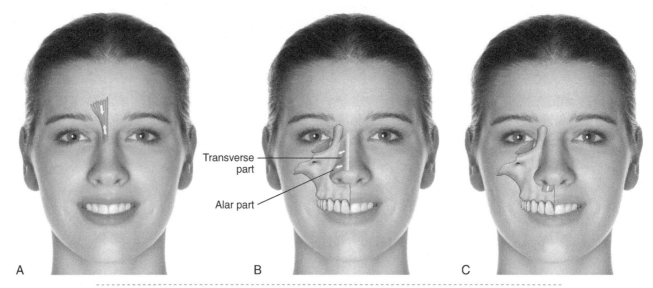

Transverse part

Alar part

A   B   C

FIGURE 9-21 *A,* Anterior view of the right procerus. ***B,*** Anterior view of the right nasalis. ***C,*** Anterior view of the right depressor septi nasi.

WHAT'S IN A NAME?

The name, *procerus,* tells us that this muscle helps create the expression of superiority of a nobleman or prince.

The name, *nasalis,* tells us that this muscle is involved with the nose.

The name, *depressor septi nasi,* tells us that this muscle depresses the nasal septum. (The septum is the midline cartilage of the nose.)

✳ **Derivation:**
procerus: L. chief noble, prince
nasalis: L. nose
depressor: L. depressor
septi: L. refers to the nasal septum
nasi: L. refers to the nose

ATTACHMENTS

Procerus
- Fascia and skin medial to the eyebrow *to the* fascia and skin over the nasal bone

Nasalis
- Maxilla *to the* cartilage of the nose and the opposite-side nasalis muscle

Depressor Septi Nasi
- Maxilla *to the* cartilage of the nose

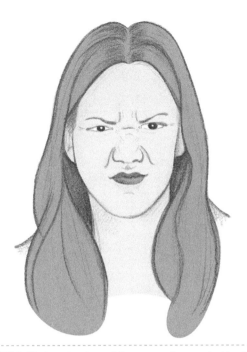

FIGURE 9-22 Anterior view of the expression created by the bilateral contraction of the procerus.

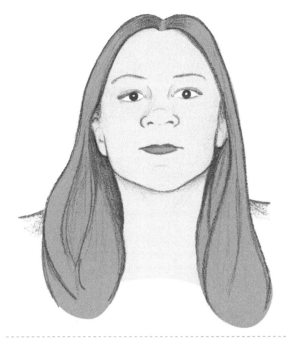

FIGURE 9-23 Anterior view of the expression created by the bilateral contraction of the alar part of the nasalis.

ACTIONS

Procerus
- Wrinkles the skin of the nose upward (Figure 9-22).
- Draws down the medial eyebrow.
- Expressions: superiority, disdain, frown

Nasalis
- Flares the nostril (alar part) (Figure 9-23).
- Constricts the nostril (transverse part) (Figure 9-24).
- Expressions: challenge, excitement, anger

Depressor Septi Nasi
- Constricts the nostril (see Figure 9-24).
- Expressions: disdain, coolness

INNERVATION

- Facial nerve (cranial nerve [CN] VII)

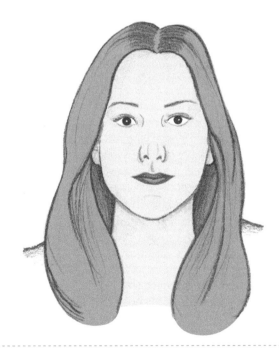

FIGURE 9-24 Anterior view of the expression created by the bilateral contraction of the transverse part of the nasalis or the depressor septi nasi.

Turn page to 👁 more.

9

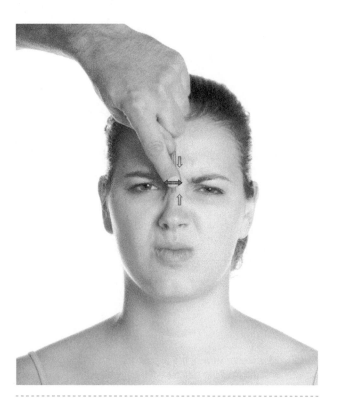

FIGURE 9-25 Palpation of the right procerus as the client makes a look of disdain.

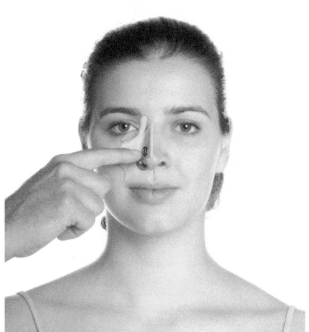

FIGURE 9-26 Palpation of the right nasalis as the client flares her nostril.

▎PALPATION

Procerus

1. Gently place your palpating finger pad(s) on the bridge of the client's nose, and ask the client to make a look of disdain, bringing the eyebrows down and/or wrinkling the skin of the nose upward. Feel for the contraction of the procerus (Figure 9-25).

2. Once felt, palpate the entire muscle as the client alternately contracts and relaxes it.

Nasalis

1. Gently place your palpating finger pad on the infero-lateral aspect of the client's nose, and ask the client to flare the nostril (as when taking in a deep breath). Feel for the contraction of the alar part of the nasalis (Figure 9-26).

2. Once felt, palpate the entire alar part of the muscle as the client alternately contracts and relaxes it.

3. To palpate the transverse part, palpate more superiorly on the nose and ask the client to constrict the nostril (as if pulling the middle of the nose down toward the mouth).

4. Once felt, palpate the entire transverse part of the muscle as the client alternately contracts and relaxes it.

Depressor Septi Nasi

1. Gently place your palpating finger pad directly inferior to the client's nose, and ask the client to constrict the nostril (as if pulling the middle of the nose down toward the mouth). Feel for the contraction of the depressor septi nasi (Figure 9-27).

2. Once felt, palpate the entire muscle as the client alternately contracts and relaxes it.

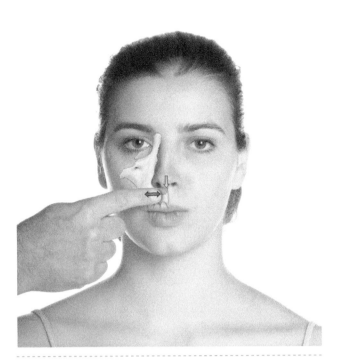

FIGURE 9-27 Palpation of the right depressor septi nasi as the client constricts her nostril.

TREATMENT CONSIDERATIONS

- The action of wrinkling the skin of the nose and/or drawing down the medial eyebrows can create the look of frowning or disdain that a person may make to convey an air of superiority (hence the name, *procerus*, meaning chief noble or prince).

- Bringing the medial eyebrows down is part of the facial expression of frowning, but it also helps shield the eyes from bright sunlight.

- The action of flaring the nostrils to increase the aperture for breathing in is also important for deep inspiration.

MUSCLES OF THE HEAD:
Muscles of Facial Expression—Mouth

Levator Labii Superioris Alaeque Nasi;
Levator Labii Superioris; Zygomaticus Minor;
Zygomaticus Major; Levator Anguli Oris; Risorius; Buccinator;
Depressor Anguli Oris; Depressor Labii Inferioris;
Mentalis; Orbicularis Oris; Platysma

Pronunciation le-VAY-tor LAY-be-eye soo-PEE-ri-o-ris a-LEE-kwe NAY-si •
le-VAY-tor LAY-be-eye soo-PEE-ri-O-ris • ZI-go-MAT-ik-us MY-nor •
ZI-go-MAT-ik-us MAY-jor • le-VAY-tor ANG-you-lie O-ris • ri-SO-ri-us • BUK-sin-A-tor •
dee-PRES-or ANG-you-lie O-ris • dee-PRES-or LAY-be-eye in-FEE-ri-O-ris •
men-TA-lis • or-BIK-you-LA-ris O-ris • pla-TIZ-ma

The twelve muscles of facial expression of the mouth are presented here. They are the levator labii superioris alaeque nasi (LLSAN), levator labii superioris, zygomaticus minor, zygomaticus major, levator anguli oris, risorius, buccinator, depressor anguli oris, depressor labii inferioris, mentalis, orbicularis oris, and platysma (Figure 9-28). Of these muscles, the platysma is primarily located in the neck but is classified as a muscle of facial expression because of its action upon the lower face. The LLSAN is a muscle of facial expression of the mouth and the nose; it has two parts, a medial slip and a lateral slip.

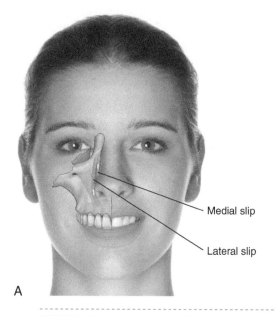

Medial slip

Lateral slip

A

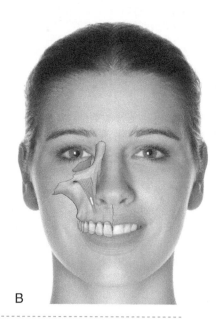

B

FIGURE 9-28 *A,* Anterior view of the right levator labii superioris alaeque nasi (LLSAN). The levator labii superioris and the orbicularis oris have been ghosted in. *B,* Anterior view of the right levator labii superioris. The LLSAN and the orbicularis oris have been ghosted in.

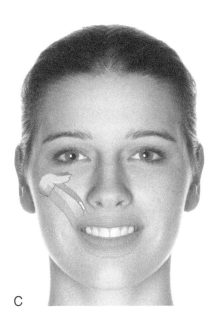

C

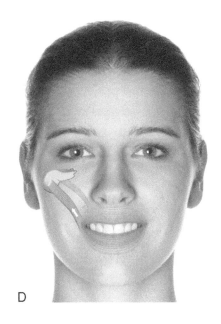

D

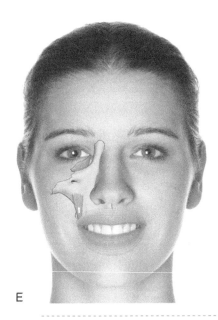

E

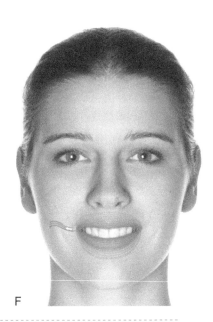

F

9

FIGURE 9-28, cont'd C, Anterior view of the right zygomaticus minor. The zygomaticus major and the orbicularis oris have been ghosted in. **D,** Anterior view of the right zygomaticus major. The zygomaticus minor and the orbicularis oris have been ghosted in. **E,** Anterior view of the right levator anguli oris. The orbicularis oris has been ghosted in. **F,** Anterior view of the right risorius. The orbicularis oris has been ghosted in.

Continued

Turn page to 👁 more.

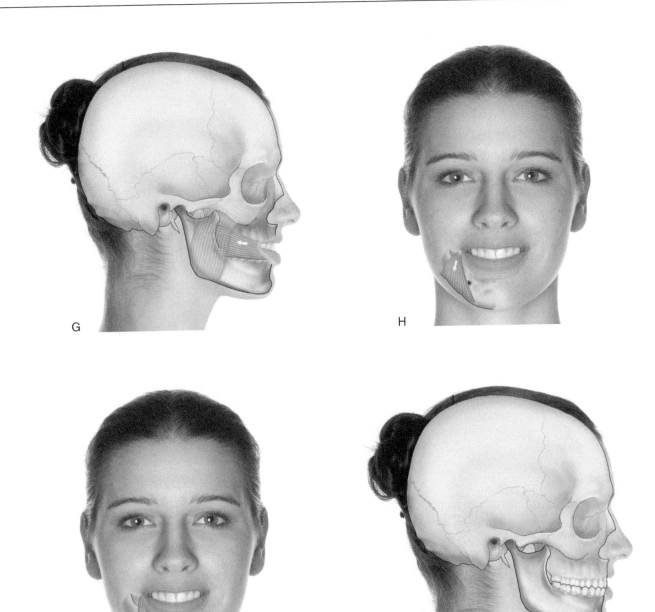

FIGURE 9-28, cont'd G, Right lateral view of the buccinator. The masseter has been ghosted in. *H,* Anterior view of the right depressor anguli oris. The orbicularis oris has been ghosted in. *I,* Anterior view of the right depressor labii inferioris. The orbicularis oris has been ghosted in. *J,* Right lateral view of the mentalis.

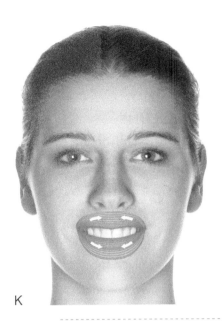

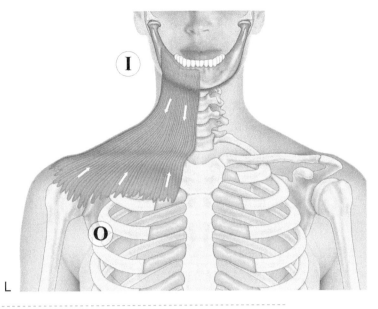

K

L

FIGURE 9-28, cont'd *K,* Anterior view of the orbicularis oris. *L,* Anterior view of the right platysma. *O,* Origin; *I,* insertion.

WHAT'S IN A NAME?

The name, *levator labii superioris alaeque nasi,* tells us that this muscle elevates the upper lip and is involved with the ala (cartilage of the nostril of the nose).

The name, *levator labii superioris,* tells us that this muscle elevates the upper lip.

The name, *zygomaticus minor,* tells us that this muscle attaches to the zygomatic bone and is smaller than the zygomaticus major.

The name, *zygomaticus major,* tells us that this muscle attaches to the zygomatic bone and is larger than the zygomaticus minor.

The name, *levator anguli oris,* tells us that this muscle elevates the angle of the mouth.

The name, *risorius,* tells us that this muscle is involved with laughing.

The name, *buccinator,* tells us that this muscle is found in the cheek region.

The name, *depressor anguli oris,* tells us that this muscle depresses the angle of the mouth.

The name, *depressor labii inferioris,* tells us that this muscle depresses the lower lip.

The name, *mentalis,* tells us that this muscle is related to the chin.

The name, *orbicularis oris,* tells us that this muscle encircles the mouth.

The name, *platysma,* tells us that this muscle is broad and flat in shape.

✳ **Derivation:**
levator: L. lifter
labii: L. refers to the lip
superioris: L. upper
alaeque: L. refers to the ala (alar cartilage)
nasi: L. refers to the nose
zygomaticus: Gr. refers to the zygomatic bone
minor: L. smaller
major: L. larger
anguli: L. refers to the angle (of the mouth)
oris: L. mouth
risorius: L. laughing
buccinator: L. trumpeter, refers to the cheek
depressor: L. depressor
inferioris: L. lower
mentalis: L. chin
orbicularis: L. small circle
platysma: Gr. broad, plate

Turn page to 👁 more.

ATTACHMENTS

Levator Labii Superioris Alaeque Nasi

- Maxilla *to the* upper lip and nose

Levator Labii Superioris

- Maxilla *to the* upper lip

Zygomaticus Minor

- Zygomatic bone *to the* upper lip

Zygomaticus Major

- Zygomatic bone *to the* angle of the mouth

Levator Anguli Oris

- Maxilla *to the* angle of the mouth

Risorius

- Fascia and skin superficial *to the* masseter to the angle of the mouth

Buccinator

- Maxilla and mandible *to the* lips

Depressor Anguli Oris

- Mandible *to the* angle of the mouth

Depressor Labii Inferioris

- Mandible *to the* lower lip

Mentalis

- Mandible *to the* fascia and skin of the chin

Orbicularis Oris

- Muscle that, in its entirety, surrounds the mouth

Platysma

- Subcutaneous fascia of the superior chest *to the* mandible and the subcutaneous fascia of the lower face

ACTIONS

Levator Labii Superioris Alaeque Nasi

- Elevates the upper lip (Figure 9-29).
- Flares the nostril.
- Expressions: anger, smugness, contempt

Levator Labii Superioris

- Elevates the upper lip (Figure 9-30).
- Expressions: disgust, smugness, contempt

Zygomaticus Minor

- Elevates the upper lip (Figure 9-31).
- Expressions: smile, smugness

Zygomaticus Major

- Elevates the angle of the mouth (Figure 9-32).
- Expressions: smile, laugh

Levator Anguli Oris

- Elevates the angle of the mouth (Figure 9-33 on page 328).
- Expressions: smile, sneer ("Dracula" expression)

Risorius

- Draws laterally the angle of the mouth (Figure 9-34 on page 328).
- Expressions: grin, smile, laugh

Buccinator

- Compresses the cheek against the teeth (Figure 9-35 on page 328).
- Expressions: pucker, exertion, sigh

Depressor Anguli Oris

- Depresses the angle of the mouth (Figure 9-36 on page 328).
- Expressions: sadness, uncertainty, dislike

Depressor Labii Inferioris

- Depresses the lower lip (Figure 9-37 on page 329).
- Expressions: sorrow, doubt, irony

Mentalis

- Elevates the lower lip (Figure 9-38 on page 329).
- Everts and protracts the lower lip.
- Expressions: doubt, pout, disdain

Orbicularis Oris

- Closes the mouth (Figure 9-39 on page 329).
- Protracts the lips.
- Expressions: puckering, whistling

Platysma

- Draws up the skin of the superior chest and neck, creating ridges of skin of the neck (Figure 9-40 on page 329).
- Expressions: disgust, disdain ("Creature from the Black Lagoon" expression)

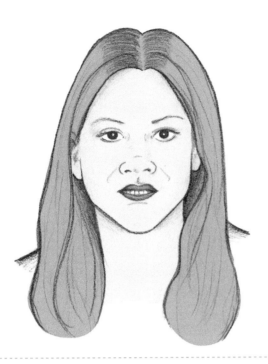

FIGURE 9-29 Anterior view of the expression created by the bilateral contraction of the LLSAN.

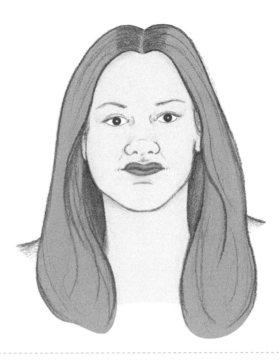

FIGURE 9-31 Anterior view of the expression created by the bilateral contraction of the zygomaticus minor.

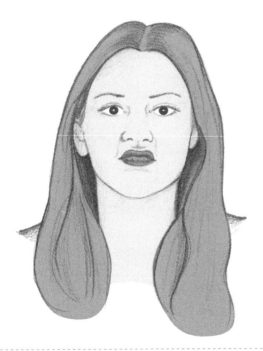

FIGURE 9-30 Anterior view of the expression created by the bilateral contraction of the levator labii superioris.

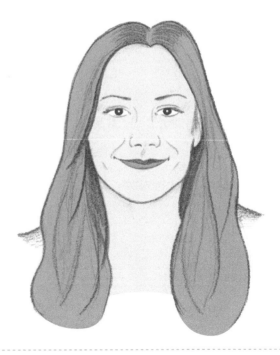

FIGURE 9-32 Anterior view of the expression created by the bilateral contraction of the zygomaticus major.

Turn page to 👁 more.

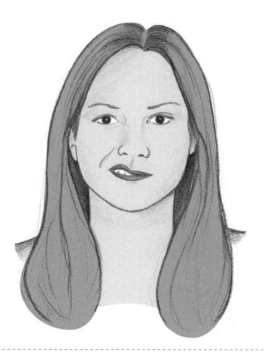

FIGURE 9-33 Anterior view of the expression created by the contraction of the right levator anguli oris.

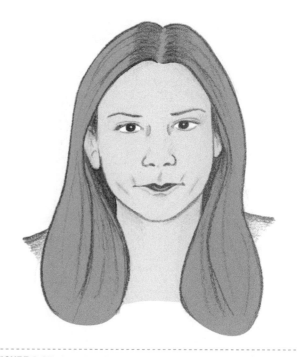

FIGURE 9-35 Anterior view of the expression created by the bilateral contraction of the buccinator.

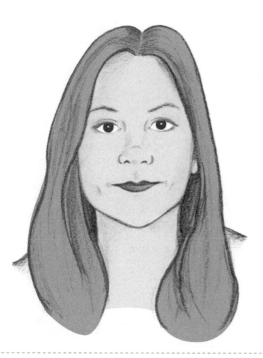

FIGURE 9-34 Anterior view of the expression created by the bilateral contraction of the risorius.

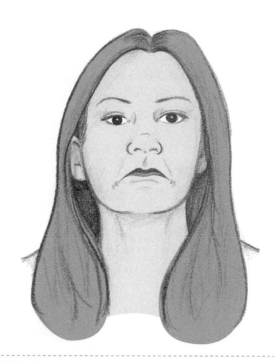

FIGURE 9-36 Anterior view of the expression created by the bilateral contraction of the depressor anguli oris.

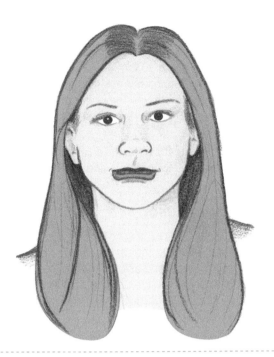

FIGURE 9-37 Anterior view of the expression created by the bilateral contraction of the depressor labii inferioris.

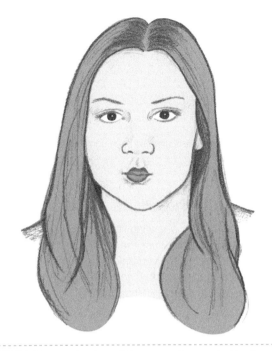

FIGURE 9-39 Anterior view of the expression created by the contraction of the orbicularis oris.

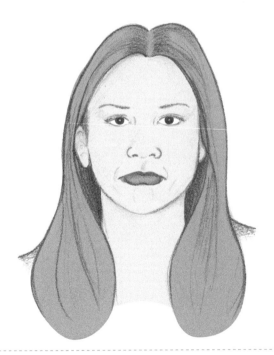

FIGURE 9-38 Anterior view of the expression created by the bilateral contraction of the mentalis.

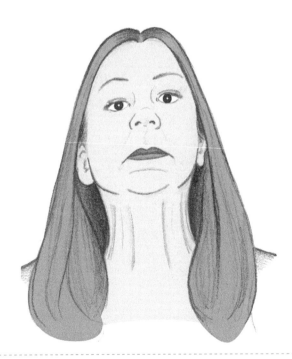

FIGURE 9-40 Anterior view of the expression created by the bilateral contraction of the platysma.

Turn page to ◉ more.

INNERVATION

■ Facial nerve (cranial nerve [CN] VII)

PALPATION

Note: The orbicularis oris has been ghosted in Figures 9-41 through 9-49.

Levator Labii Superioris Alaeque Nasi

1. Gently place your palpating finger pad just lateral to the client's nose, and ask the client to either elevate the upper lip to show you the upper gum or flare the nostril. Feel for the contraction of the levator labii superioris alaeque nasi (Figure 9-41).
2. Once felt, palpate the entire muscle as the client alternately contracts and relaxes it.

Levator Labii Superioris

1. Gently place your palpating finger pad approximately ½ inch lateral to the center of the upper lip at its superior margin, and ask the client to elevate the upper lip to show you the upper gum. Feel for the contraction of the levator labii superioris (Figure 9-42).
2. Once felt, palpate the entire muscle toward the eye as the client alternately contracts and relaxes it.

Zygomaticus Minor

1. Gently place your palpating finger pad approximately ½ to ¾ inch lateral to the center of the upper lip at its superior margin, and ask the client to elevate the upper lip to show you the upper gum. Feel for the contraction of the zygomaticus minor (Figure 9-43).
2. Once felt, palpate the entire muscle toward the zygomatic bone as the client alternately contracts and relaxes it.

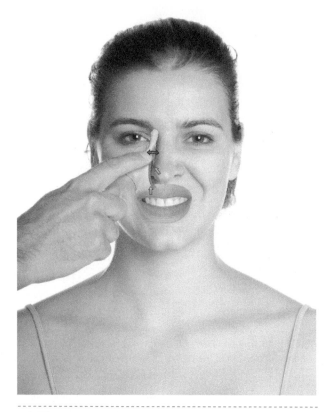

FIGURE 9-41 Palpation of the right levator labii superioris alaeque nasi as the client elevates the upper lip and flares the nostril.

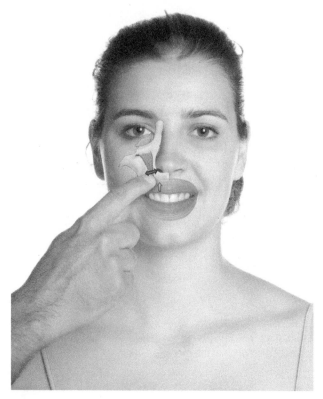

FIGURE 9-42 Palpation of the right levator labii superioris as the client elevates her upper lip.

Zygomaticus Major

1. Gently place your palpating finger pad immediately superolateral to the angle (corner) of the mouth, and ask the client to smile by drawing the corner of the mouth both superiorly and laterally. Feel for the contraction of the zygomaticus major (Figure 9-44).

2. Once felt, palpate the entire muscle toward the zygomatic bone as the client alternately contracts and relaxes it.

Levator Anguli Oris

1. Gently place your palpating finger pad immediately superior to the corner of the mouth, and ask the client to elevate the corner of the mouth directly superiorly as if to show you the canine tooth (making what could be described as a Dracula-like expression). Feel for the contraction of the levator anguli oris (Figure 9-45).

2. Once felt, palpate the entire muscle as the client alternately contracts and relaxes it.

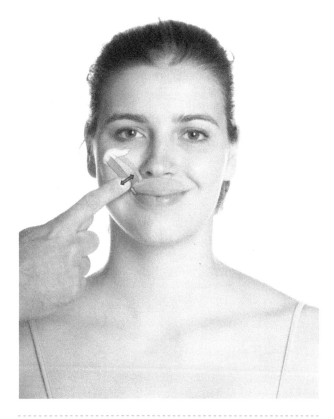

FIGURE 9-44 Palpation of the right zygomaticus major as the client smiles. The zygomaticus minor has been ghosted in.

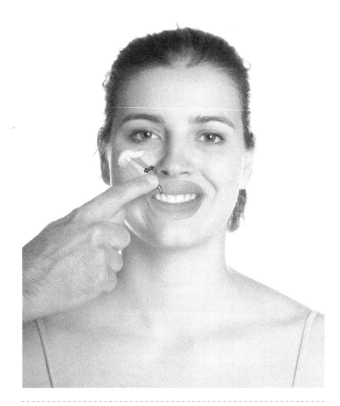

FIGURE 9-43 Palpation of the right zygomaticus minor as the client elevates her upper lip. The zygomaticus major has been ghosted in.

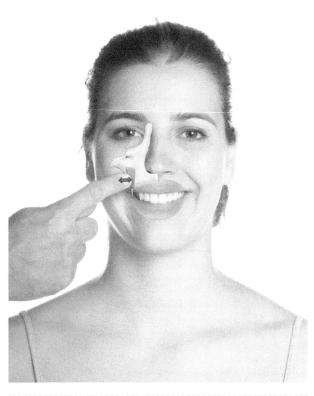

FIGURE 9-45 Palpation of the right levator anguli oris as the client elevates the corner of the mouth (making a Dracula-like expression).

Turn page to more.

▌ PALPATION—cont'd

Risorius

1. Gently place your palpating finger pad immediately lateral to the corner of the mouth, and ask the client to draw the corner of the mouth directly laterally. Feel for the contraction of the risorius (Figure 9-46).
2. Once felt, palpate the entire muscle as the client alternately contracts and relaxes it.

Buccinator

1. Gently place your palpating finger pad lateral and slightly superior to the corner of the mouth, and ask the client to take in a deep breath, purse the lips, and press the lips against the teeth as if expelling air while playing the trumpet. Feel for the contraction of the buccinator (Figure 9-47).
2. Once felt, palpate the entire muscle as the client alternately contracts and relaxes it.

Depressor Anguli Oris

1. Gently place your palpating finger pad slightly lateral and inferior to the corner of the mouth, and ask the client to frown by depressing and drawing the corner of the mouth laterally. Feel for the contraction of the depressor anguli oris (Figure 9-48).
2. Once felt, palpate the entire muscle as the client alternately contracts and relaxes it.

Depressor Labii Inferioris

1. Gently place your palpating finger pad inferior to the lower lip and slightly lateral to the midline, and ask the client to depress and slightly draw the lower lip laterally. Feel for the contraction of the depressor labii inferioris (Figure 9-49).
2. Once felt, palpate the entire muscle as the client alternately contracts and relaxes it.

Mentalis

1. Gently place your palpating finger pad approximately 1 inch inferior to the lower lip and slightly lateral to the midline, and ask the client to depress and stick out the lower lip as if pouting. Feel for the contraction of the mentalis (Figure 9-50).
2. Once felt, palpate the entire muscle as the client alternately contracts and relaxes it.

Orbicularis Oris

1. Wearing a finger cot or glove, gently place your palpating finger pad(s) on the tissue of the lips, and ask the client to pucker up the lips. Feel for the contraction of the orbicularis oris (Figure 9-51).
2. Once felt, palpate the entire muscle as the client alternately contracts and relaxes it.

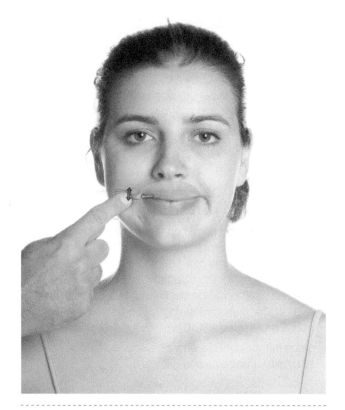

FIGURE 9-46 Palpation of the right risorius as the client draws the corner of the mouth laterally.

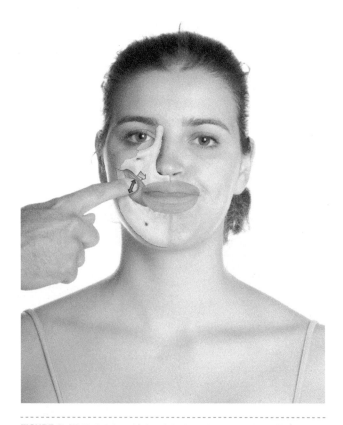

FIGURE 9-47 Palpation of the right buccinator as the client takes in a deep breath, purses the lips, and presses the lips against the teeth as if playing the trumpet.

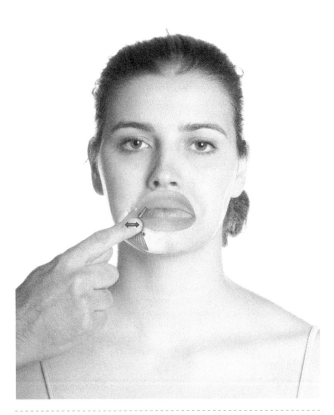

FIGURE 9-48 Palpation of the right depressor anguli oris as the client frowns. The orbicularis oris has been ghosted in.

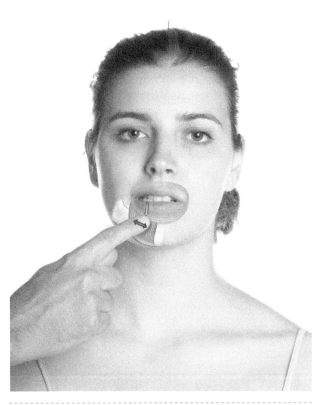

FIGURE 9-49 Palpation of the right depressor labii inferioris as the client depresses and draws the lower lip laterally. The orbicularis oris has been ghosted in.

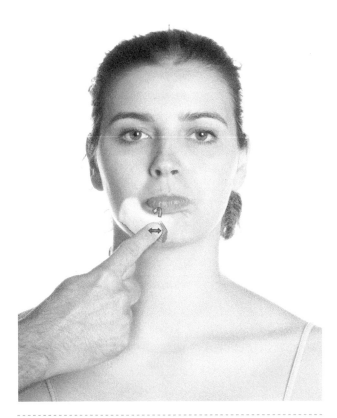

FIGURE 9-50 Palpation of the right mentalis as the client sticks out the lower lip as if pouting.

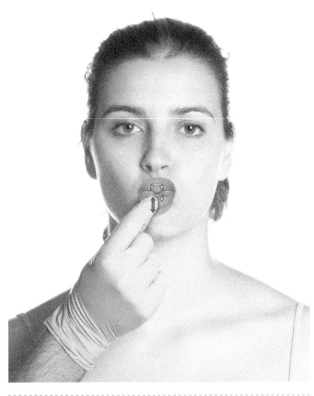

FIGURE 9-51 Palpation of the orbicularis oris on the right side as the client puckers the lips.

Turn page to 👁 more.

PALPATION—cont'd

Platysma

1. Place your palpating finger pads on the anterolateral neck, and ask the client to contract the platysma forcefully by depressing and drawing the lower lip laterally, while keeping the mandible fixed in a position of slight depression. Observe and feel for the ridges of skin of the neck caused by the contraction of the platysma (Figure 9-52).

2. Once felt, palpate the entire muscle as the client alternately contracts and relaxes it.

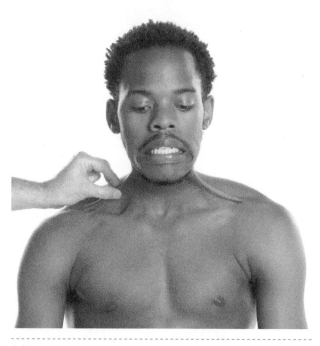

FIGURE 9-52 Anterior view of the right platysma contracted and being palpated.

TREATMENT CONSIDERATIONS

- Long-standing contraction of a facial expression muscle creates wrinkles in the skin of the face that run perpendicular to the direction of fibers of the underlying muscle. Botox injections remove these wrinkles because Botox paralyzes facial expression musculature. However, this paralysis also decreases the person's ability to create facial expressions to convey emotion.

- The levator anguli oris is also known as the *caninus*. This name is given because the contraction of the levator anguli oris can result in the teeth, especially the canine tooth, becoming visible. Bilateral contraction of this muscle can reproduce the typical Dracula expression wherein the canine teeth are exposed.

- The action of compressing the cheeks against the teeth by the two buccinators working bilaterally is important for forcefully expelling air from the mouth. The buccinator is the muscle that contracts when a musician blows air into a brass or woodwind instrument, whistles, or blows up a balloon.

- The actions of the mentalis of elevating, everting, and protracting the lower lip are also useful when drinking.

- The orbicularis oris in humans is particularly well developed. This is necessary for the intricacies of speech.

- The contraction of the orbicularis oris causes the lips to close and protrude as in puckering the lips for a kiss or whistling.

- The platysma in humans is considered to be a remnant of a broader fascial muscle called the *panniculus carnosus* found in four-legged mammals. The panniculus carnosus is what enables a horse to shake off flies from its skin, and it is the same muscle that enables a cat to raise the hair on its back.

- When the platysma contracts and the ridges or wrinkling of the skin of the neck occurs, it is reminiscent of the title character from the film *The Creature from the Black Lagoon*.

REVIEW QUESTIONS

Circle or fill in the correct answer for each of the following questions. More study resources, including audio pronunciations of muscle names, are provided on the Evolve website at http://evolve.elsevier.com/Muscolino/knowthebody.

1. **Name two of the major muscles of mastication.**

   _____

   _____

2. **Name two muscles of facial expression of the nose.**

   _____

   _____

3. **Name three muscles of facial expression of the eye.**

   _____

   _____

   _____

4. **Which of the following muscles can elevate the mandible at the TMJs?**
   a. Temporalis, masseter
   b. Medial pterygoid, lateral pterygoid
   c. Temporalis, occipitofrontalis
   d. Lateral pterygoid, temporoparietalis

5. **Which of the following muscles draws the scalp posteriorly?**
   a. Temporoparietalis
   b. Auricularis superior
   c. Occipitofrontalis
   d. Temporalis

6. **Which of the following muscles encircles the mouth?**
   a. Orbicularis oculi
   b. Zygomaticus minor
   c. Depressor anguli oris
   d. Orbicularis oris

7. **Which of the following muscles flares the nostril?**
   a. Depressor septi nasi
   b. Nasalis
   c. Levator labii superioris
   d. Platysma

8. **Which of the following muscles is located within the subcutaneous fascia of the superior chest?**
   a. Platysma
   b. Auricularis posterior
   c. Occipitofrontalis
   d. Masseter

9. **Which of the following muscles is a muscle of fascial expression of the mouth?**
   a. Procerus
   b. Zygomaticus minor
   c. Corrugator supercilii
   d. Nasalis

10. **Which of the following muscles attaches into the capsule of the TMJ?**
    a. Lateral pterygoid
    b. Medial pterygoid
    c. Masseter
    d. Temporalis

9

9

CASE STUDY 1

A 52-year-old male client, Robert, has recently been having pain and fatigue when chewing hard and/or crunchy foods such as steak, pretzels, and popcorn. Mild pain develops in his jaw and cheek as he chews. On a pain scale of 0 to 10, the pain intensity is approximately a 3 or 4. He experiences no pain when he is not chewing. Verbal history reveals no pathologic history or injury to the face or jaw structure. However, he recently visited his dentist for his biannual cleaning. The dentist told him that he showed minimal signs of teeth grinding and that an x-ray examination showed minor temporomandibular joint (TMJ) osteoarthritis; however, both are mild and not unusual for someone his age. Robert states that he does not think he clenches or grinds his teeth at night because his wife has never heard him do this. When asked about stress levels, Robert admits that his work has become more stressful lately, but he has taken up sailing to help alleviate the stress. Further questioning reveals that when sailing, Robert uses his mouth to hold the ropes as he pulls the sails.

Physical examination elicits tenderness and a pain intensity of approximately 4 when palpating between the zygomatic arch and the angle of the mandible, and a level 3 when palpating over the temporal fossa of the head. Palpating directly over the TMJ reveals a pain intensity of approximately 3.

QUESTIONS

1. **Why has holding ropes in his mouth created pain for Robert?**

_____

_____

_____

_____

_____

_____

2. **What treatment plan would most benefit Robert?**

_____

_____

_____

_____

_____

_____

_____

_____

CASE STUDY 2

A new client, Dolores, comes to see you for chronic headaches. She is a 42-year-old account executive, who admits to having a very stressful job and a long history of a tight neck and tension headaches. She has always received neck massage for her headaches, and it has always been successful—until now. The headache she is experiencing now began 6 days ago. It feels similar to all her previous headaches but has not been relieved with two neck massages received this week. She believes that the therapist she has gone to for years is very competent but has been unable to help her this time. Concerned, she visited her medical physician earlier today, who found no reason for her headaches; she was told to take an over-the-counter analgesic medication and return in 1 week if the headaches do not subside. She has come to you because she has heard that you work more thoroughly and clinically than many other massage therapists.

Your verbal history reveals that her current headache is indeed quite similar to and fits the pain pattern of all her previous headaches. She states that her massage therapist has always worked the posterior neck, with special attention to muscles that the therapist said were the upper trapezius and semispinalis capitis.

Upon physical examination, you palpate and discern that the upper trapezius and semispinalis capitis are only mildly tight. You palpate the entire posterior, lateral, and anterior cervical region and find no musculature that seems tight enough to justify Dolores' long-standing headaches. Dolores reports that with her usual headaches, when the therapist would press into the back of her neck, she would feel the headache pain refer into her head. However, with the present headache, when the therapist worked her neck and now when you are palpating into her neck, Dolores does not feel the pain refer into her head.

QUESTIONS

1. **Should you palpate and assess any other musculature? If so, what?**

_____

_____

_____

_____

_____

_____

_____

2. **If you find this musculature to be tight and a possible cause of Dolores' headaches, how should you proceed with treatment?**

_____

_____

_____

_____

_____

_____

_____

_____

_____

9

Muscles of the Pelvis and Thigh

The muscles of this chapter are involved with motions of the thigh or pelvis at the hip joint and/or motions of the leg or thigh at the knee joint. The psoas major also crosses the lumbar vertebral joints and can therefore move the spine. The bellies of the gluteal and deep lateral rotator groups and the iliacus are located on the pelvis. The bellies of the psoas major and minor are located in the abdomen. The bellies of the adductor, quadriceps femoris, and hamstring groups, as well as the tensor fasciae latae and sartorius, are located in the thigh.

As a general rule, muscles that move the hip joint have their origin (proximal attachment) on the pelvis and their insertion (distal attachment) on the thigh (or leg). These muscles move the thigh relative to the pelvis or the pelvis relative to the thigh. Muscles that move the knee joint have their origin (proximal attachment) on the pelvis or thigh and their insertion (distal attachment)

on the leg. These muscles move the leg relative to the thigh or the thigh relative to the leg.

The companion CD at the back of this book allows you to examine Chapter 10 muscles, layer by layer, and individual muscle palpation technique videos are available in the Chapter 10 folder on the Evolve website.

OVERVIEW OF FUNCTION: MUSCLES OF THE HIP JOINT

The following general rules regarding actions can be stated for the functional groups of muscles of the hip joint:
- If a muscle crosses the hip joint anteriorly with a vertical direction to its fibers, it can flex the thigh at the hip joint (standard action) by moving the anterior

surface of the thigh toward the anterior surface of the pelvis; or it can anteriorly tilt the pelvis at the hip joint (reverse action) by moving the anterior surface of the pelvis toward the anterior surface of the thigh.

- If a muscle crosses the hip joint posteriorly with a vertical direction to its fibers, it can extend the thigh at the hip joint (standard action) by moving the posterior surface of the thigh toward the posterior surface of the pelvis; or it can posteriorly tilt the pelvis at the hip joint (reverse action) by moving the posterior surface of the pelvis toward the posterior surface of the thigh.
- If a muscle crosses the hip joint laterally with a vertical direction to its fibers, it can abduct the thigh at the hip joint (standard action) by moving the lateral surface of the thigh toward the lateral surface of the pelvis; or it can depress (laterally tilt) the same-side pelvis at the hip joint (reverse action) by moving the lateral surface of the pelvis toward the lateral surface of the thigh.
- If a muscle crosses the hip joint medially, it can adduct the thigh at the hip joint by moving the medial surface of the thigh toward the medial surface of the pelvis (standard action); or it can elevate the same-side pelvis at the hip joint (reverse action) by moving the medial surface of the pelvis toward the medial surface of the thigh.
- Medial rotators of the thigh at the hip joint (standard action) wrap around the femur from medial to lateral, anterior to the hip joint. They can also ipsilaterally rotate the pelvis at the hip joint (reverse action).
- Lateral rotators of the thigh at the hip joint (standard action) wrap around the femur from medial to lateral, posterior to the hip joint. They can also contralaterally rotate the pelvis at the hip joint (reverse action).
- Reverse actions are common at the hip joint and tend to occur when the foot is planted on the ground, which causes the distal attachment to be fixed and therefore the proximal attachment to be mobile and move toward the distal attachment. The reverse actions wherein the pelvis moves at the hip joint are often as important as, if not more important than, the typically thought of standard mover actions of the thigh at the hip joint.

OVERVIEW OF FUNCTION: MUSCLES OF THE SPINAL JOINTS

The following general rules regarding actions can be stated for the functional groups of muscles of the spinal joints:

- If a muscle crosses the spinal joints anteriorly with a vertical direction to its fibers, it can flex the trunk, neck, and/or head at the spinal joints by moving the superior attachment (insertion) down toward the inferior attachment (origin) in front.

- If a muscle crosses the spinal joints posteriorly with a vertical direction to its fibers, it can extend the trunk, neck, and/or head at the spinal joints by moving the superior attachment down toward the inferior attachment in back.
- If a muscle crosses the spinal joints laterally, it can perform same-side lateral flexion of the trunk, neck, and/or head at the spinal joints by moving the superior attachment down toward the inferior attachment on that side of the body.
- Reverse actions occur by moving the pelvic or lower spine attachment (origin) toward the upper spine attachment (insertion). This movement usually occurs when a person is lying down.

OVERVIEW OF FUNCTION: MUSCLES OF THE KNEE JOINT

The following general rules regarding actions can be stated for the functional groups of muscles of the knee joint:

- If a muscle crosses the knee joint anteriorly with a vertical direction to its fibers, it can extend the leg at the knee joint by moving the anterior surface of the leg toward the anterior surface of the thigh.
- If a muscle crosses the knee joint posteriorly with a vertical direction to its fibers, it can flex the leg at the knee joint by moving the posterior surface of the leg toward the posterior surface of the thigh.
- If a muscle wraps around the knee joint, it can rotate the knee joint (the knee joint can only rotate if it is first flexed). Medial rotators attach to the medial side of the leg. The biceps femoris is the only lateral rotator and attaches to the lateral side of the leg.
- Reverse actions are common at the knee joint and tend to occur when the foot is planted on the ground, causing the distal attachment to be fixed and therefore the proximal attachment (the thigh) to be mobile and move toward the distal attachment (the leg).
- The reverse action of extension of the leg at the knee joint is extension of the thigh at the knee joint in which the anterior surface of the thigh moves toward the anterior surface of the leg.

> Note: This movement occurs every time we stand up from a seated position.

- The reverse action of flexion of the leg at the knee joint is flexion of the thigh at the knee joint in which the posterior surface of the thigh moves toward the posterior surface of the leg.
- The reverse action of medial rotation of the leg at the knee joint is lateral rotation of the thigh at the knee joint; the reverse action of lateral rotation of the leg at the knee joint is medial rotation of the thigh at the knee joint.

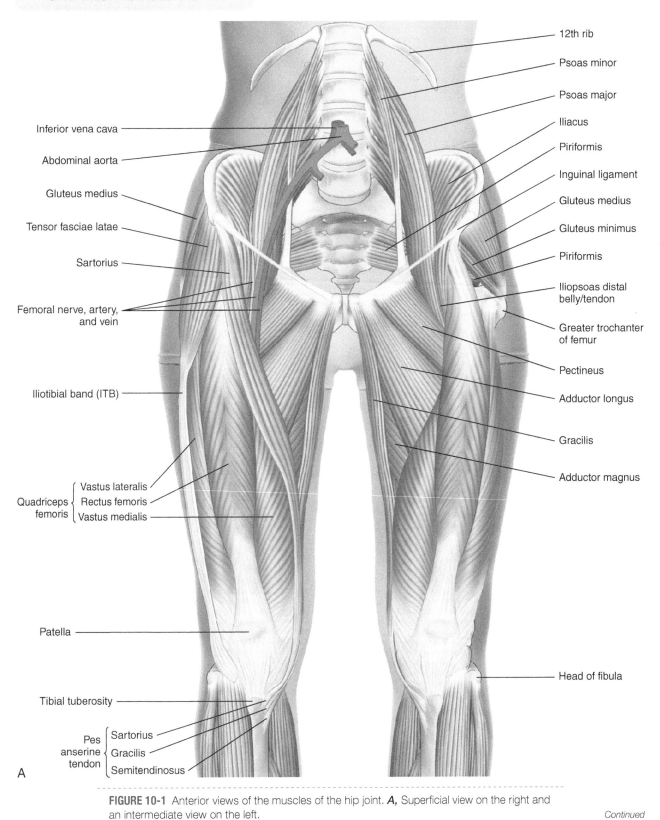

12th rib

Psoas minor

Psoas major

Iliacus

Piriformis

Inguinal ligament

Gluteus medius

Gluteus minimus

Piriformis

Iliopsoas distal belly/tendon

Greater trochanter of femur

Pectineus

Adductor longus

Gracilis

Adductor magnus

Head of fibula

Inferior vena cava

Abdominal aorta

Gluteus medius

Tensor fasciae latae

Sartorius

Femoral nerve, artery, and vein

Iliotibial band (ITB)

Quadriceps femoris { Vastus lateralis / Rectus femoris / Vastus medialis

Patella

Tibial tuberosity

Pes anserine tendon { Sartorius / Gracilis / Semitendinosus

A

FIGURE 10-1 Anterior views of the muscles of the hip joint. **A,** Superficial view on the right and an intermediate view on the left.

Continued

10

Anterior Views of the Muscles
of the Hip Joint—
Deep Views

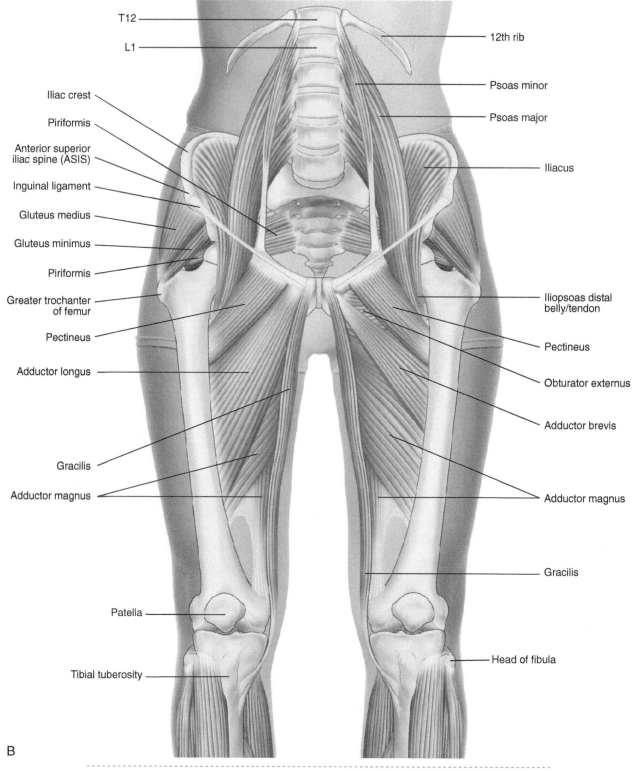

T12

L1

12th rib

Iliac crest

Piriformis

Anterior superior
iliac spine (ASIS)

Inguinal ligament

Gluteus medius

Gluteus minimus

Piriformis

Greater trochanter
of femur

Pectineus

Adductor longus

Gracilis

Adductor magnus

Patella

Tibial tuberosity

Psoas minor

Psoas major

Iliacus

Iliopsoas distal
belly/tendon

Pectineus

Obturator externus

Adductor brevis

Adductor magnus

Gracilis

Head of fibula

B

FIGURE 10-1, cont'd Anterior views of the muscles of the hip joint. **B,** Deep view on the right
and deeper view on the left.

10

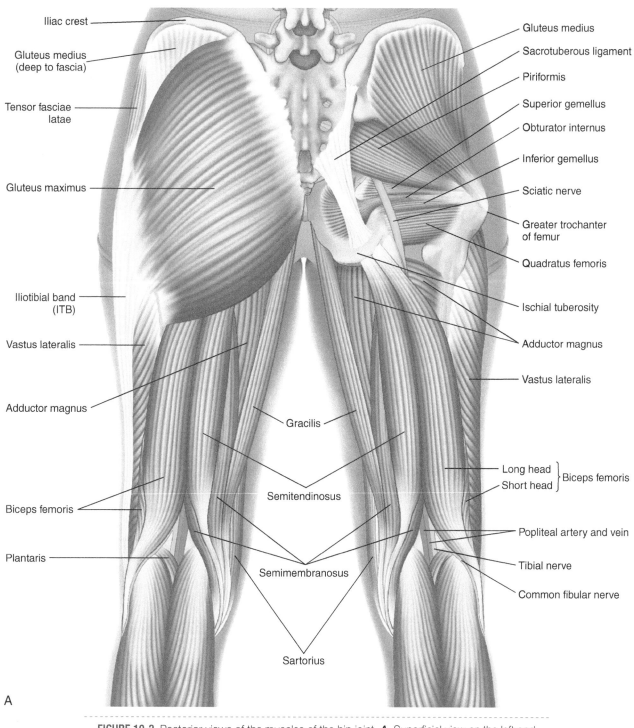

Iliac crest

Gluteus medius (deep to fascia)

Tensor fasciae latae

Gluteus maximus

Iliotibial band (ITB)

Vastus lateralis

Adductor magnus

Biceps femoris

Plantaris

Gluteus medius

Sacrotuberous ligament

Piriformis

Superior gemellus

Obturator internus

Inferior gemellus

Sciatic nerve

Greater trochanter of femur

Quadratus femoris

Ischial tuberosity

Adductor magnus

Vastus lateralis

Long head ⎫
Short head ⎬ Biceps femoris

Popliteal artery and vein

Tibial nerve

Common fibular nerve

Gracilis

Semitendinosus

Semimembranosus

Sartorius

A

FIGURE 10-2 Posterior views of the muscles of the hip joint. **A,** Superficial view on the left and an intermediate view on the right.

Continued

10

Posterior Views of the Muscles of the Hip Joint— Deep Views

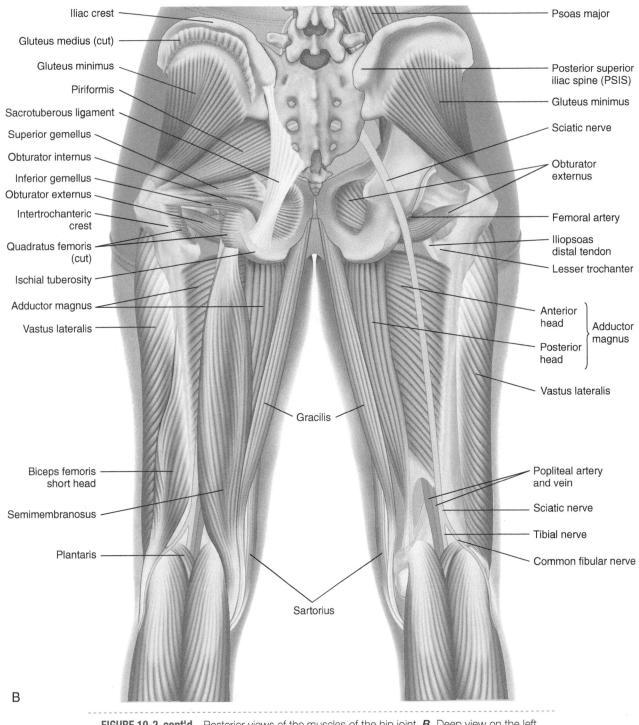

Iliac crest

Gluteus medius (cut)

Gluteus minimus

Piriformis

Sacrotuberous ligament

Superior gemellus

Obturator internus

Inferior gemellus

Obturator externus

Intertrochanteric crest

Quadratus femoris (cut)

Ischial tuberosity

Adductor magnus

Vastus lateralis

Psoas major

Posterior superior iliac spine (PSIS)

Gluteus minimus

Sciatic nerve

Obturator externus

Femoral artery

Iliopsoas distal tendon

Lesser trochanter

Anterior head

Posterior head

Adductor magnus

Vastus lateralis

Gracilis

Biceps femoris short head

Semimembranosus

Plantaris

Popliteal artery and vein

Sciatic nerve

Tibial nerve

Common fibular nerve

Sartorius

B

FIGURE 10-2, cont'd Posterior views of the muscles of the hip joint. **B,** Deep view on the left and deeper view on the right.

Medial and Lateral Views of the Muscles of the Right Hip Joint—Superficial Views

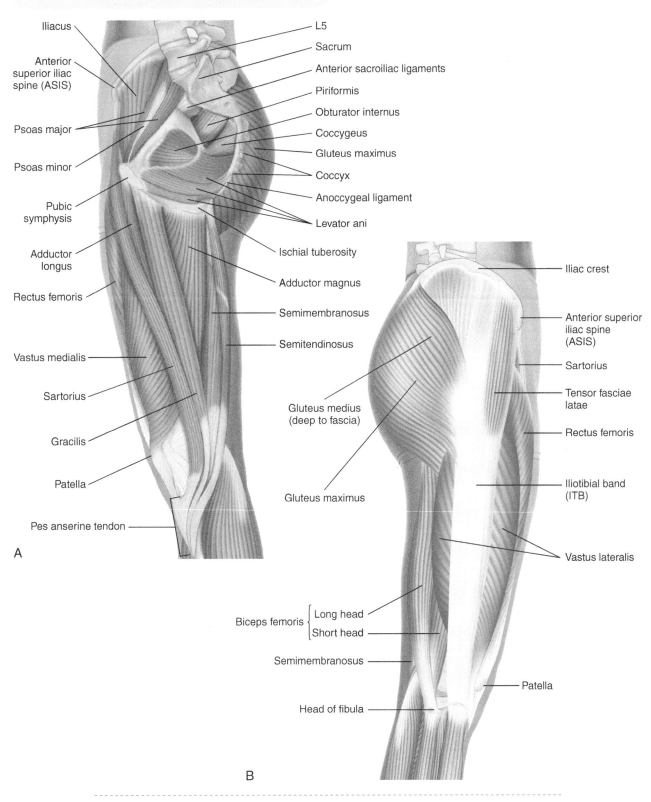

Iliacus
Anterior superior iliac spine (ASIS)
Psoas major
Psoas minor
Pubic symphysis
Adductor longus
Rectus femoris
Vastus medialis
Sartorius
Gracilis
Patella
Pes anserine tendon

L5
Sacrum
Anterior sacroiliac ligaments
Piriformis
Obturator internus
Coccygeus
Gluteus maximus
Coccyx
Anoccygeal ligament
Levator ani
Ischial tuberosity
Adductor magnus
Semimembranosus
Semitendinosus

A

Gluteus medius (deep to fascia)
Gluteus maximus

Iliac crest
Anterior superior iliac spine (ASIS)
Sartorius
Tensor fasciae latae
Rectus femoris
Iliotibial band (ITB)
Vastus lateralis

Biceps femoris { Long head
Short head
Semimembranosus
Head of fibula
Patella

B

FIGURE 10-3 *A,* Medial view of the muscles of the right hip joint—superficial. *B,* Lateral view of the muscles of the right hip joint—superficial.

MUSCLES OF THE PELVIS AND THIGH: Gluteal Group
Gluteus Maximus; Gluteus Medius; Gluteus Minimus

Pronunciation **GLOO-tee-us MAX-i-mus** •
GLOO-tee-us MEED-ee-us • **GLOO-tee-us MIN-i-mus**

10

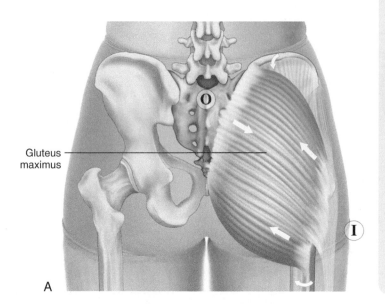

Gluteus
maximus

The gluteal group is composed of three muscles, the gluteus maximus, gluteus medius, and gluteus minimus. The gluteus maximus is the largest muscle in the human body and forms the contour of the buttock. It is superficial and covers much of the gluteus medius. The gluteus medius is deep to the gluteus maximus posteriorly and deep to the tensor fasciae latae anteriorly, but it is superficial laterally. It covers most all of the gluteus minimus. The gluteus minimus is the deepest and smallest of the group (Figure 10-4).

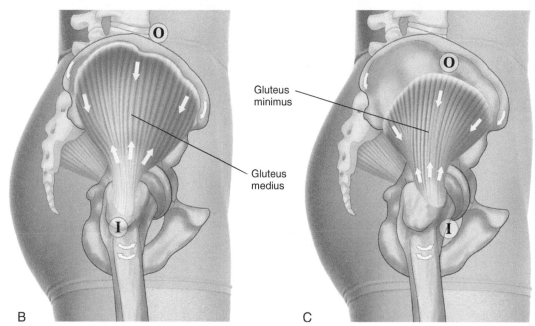

Gluteus
minimus

Gluteus
medius

FIGURE 10-4 **A,** Posterior view of the right gluteus maximus. The tensor fasciae latae, fascia over the gluteus medius, and iliotibial band have been ghosted in. **B,** Lateral view of the right gluteus medius. The piriformis has been ghosted in. **C,** Lateral view of the right gluteus minimus. The piriformis has been ghosted in. *O,* Origin; *I,* insertion.

WHAT'S IN A NAME?

The name, *gluteus maximus,* tells us that this muscle is located in the gluteal (buttock) region and is larger than the gluteus medius and gluteus minimus.

The name, *gluteus medius,* tells us that this muscle is located in the gluteal region and is smaller than the gluteus maximus and larger than the gluteus minimus.

The name, *gluteus minimus,* tells us that this muscle is located in the gluteal region and is smaller than the gluteus maximus and gluteus medius.

✳ **Derivation:**
gluteus: Gr. buttocks
maximus: L. greatest
medius: L. middle
minimus: L. least

ATTACHMENTS

Gluteus Maximus

Origin (Proximal Attachment)
- Posterior iliac crest, posterolateral sacrum, and coccyx

Insertion (Distal Attachment)
- Iliotibial band (ITB) and the gluteal tuberosity of the femur

Gluteus Medius and Minimus

Origin (Proximal Attachment)
- External ilium

Insertion (Distal Attachment)
- Greater trochanter of the femur

ACTIONS

All of the actions listed for the gluteal muscles occur at the hip joint. The standard actions (insertion/distal attachment moving toward origin/proximal attachment) move the thigh at the hip joint; the reverse actions (origin/proximal attachment moving toward insertion/distal attachment) move the pelvis at the hip joint.

Gluteus Maximus

- Extends the thigh.
- Laterally rotates the thigh.
- Abducts the thigh (upper fibers only).
- Adducts the thigh (lower fibers only).
- Posteriorly tilts the pelvis.
- Contralaterally rotates the pelvis.

Gluteus Medius and Minimus

- Abduct the thigh.
- Extend the thigh (posterior fibers only).
- Flex the thigh (anterior fibers only).
- Laterally rotate the thigh (posterior fibers only).
- Medially rotate the thigh (anterior fibers only).
- Depress the same-side pelvis.
- Posteriorly tilt the pelvis.
- Anteriorly tilt the pelvis.
- Contralaterally rotate the pelvis.

STABILIZATION

Stabilizes the thigh and pelvis at the hip joint.

INNERVATION

- Inferior gluteal nerve (gluteus maximus)
- Superior gluteal nerve (gluteus medius and minimus)

PALPATION

Gluteus Maximus

1. The client is prone. Place your palpating finger pads lateral to the sacrum. Place your resistance hand on the distal posterior thigh (if resistance is needed).
2. Ask the client to laterally rotate the thigh at the hip joint and then extend the laterally rotated thigh. Feel for the contraction of the gluteus maximus (Figure 10-5). Resistance can be added, if necessary.
3. With the muscle contracted, strum perpendicular to the fibers to discern the borders of the muscle.
4. Continue palpating the gluteus maximus laterally and inferiorly (distally) to its insertion (distal attachments) by strumming perpendicular to its fibers.

Turn page to 👁 more.

Gluteus Medius and Minimus

1. The client is side lying. Place your palpating finger pads just distal to the middle of the iliac crest, between the iliac crest and the greater trochanter of the femur. Place your resistance hand on the lateral surface of the distal thigh (if resistance is needed).

2. Palpating just distal to the middle of the iliac crest, ask the client to abduct the thigh at the hip joint. Feel

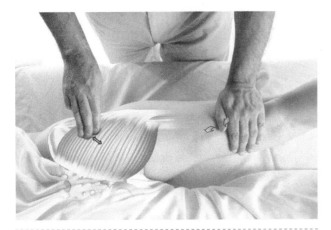

FIGURE 10-5 Palpation of the right gluteus maximus as the client extends and laterally rotates the thigh at the hip joint against resistance.

for the contraction of the middle fibers of the gluteus medius (Figure 10-6, *A*). If desired, resistance can be added to the client's thigh abduction with the resistance hand.

3. Strum perpendicular to the fibers, palpating the middle fibers of the gluteus medius distally toward the greater trochanter.

4. To palpate the anterior fibers, place your palpating hand immediately distal and posterior to the anterior superior iliac spine (ASIS), and ask the client to gently flex and medially rotate the thigh at the hip joint. Feel for the contraction of the anterior fibers of the gluteus medius (Figure 10-6, *B*). Discerning the anterior fibers from the more superficial tensor fasciae latae is difficult.

5. To palpate the posterior fibers, place your palpating hand over the posterior portion of the gluteus medius, and ask the client to gently extend and laterally rotate the thigh at the hip joint. Feel for the contraction of the posterior fibers of the gluteus medius (Figure 10-6, *C*). Discerning the posterior fibers from the more superficial gluteus maximus is difficult.

6. Palpating and discerning the gluteus minimus deep to the gluteus medius is difficult. The gluteus minimus is thickest anteriorly. To palpate the gluteus minimus, follow the same procedure as for the gluteus medius, and try to palpate deeper for the gluteus minimus.

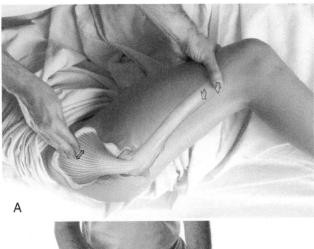

A

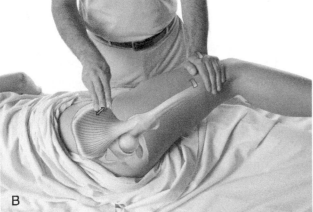

B

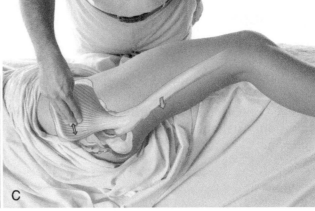

C

FIGURE 10-6 Side-lying palpation of the right gluteus medius. *A,* Palpation of the middle fibers of the right gluteus medius immediately distal to the middle of the iliac crest as the client attempts to abduct the thigh at the hip joint against resistance. *B,* Palpation of the anterior fibers of the gluteus medius as the client abducts and medially rotates the thigh. *C,* Palpation of the posterior fibers of the gluteus medius as the client abducts and laterally rotates the thigh.

10

TREATMENT CONSIDERATIONS

- Thinking of the gluteus maximus as the *speed skater's muscle* can be helpful. The gluteus maximus is powerful in extending, abducting, and laterally rotating the thigh at the hip joint, which are all actions that are necessary when speed skating.

- Usually a thick layer of fascia, called the *gluteal fascia* or the gluteal aponeurosis, overlies the gluteus medius muscle.

- Lateral rotation of the thigh at the hip joint by the gluteal muscles acts to prevent medial rotation of the thigh and entire lower extremity, including the talus at the subtalar joint. This lateral rotation can stabilize the subtalar joint and prevent excessive pronation (dropping of the arch) of the foot.

- When the gluteus medius is tight, it pulls on and depresses the pelvis toward the thigh on that side. This results in a *functional short leg* (as opposed to a *structural short leg* wherein the femur and/or the tibia on one side is actually shorter than on the other side). Further, depressing the pelvis on one side creates an unlevel sacrum for the spine to sit on, and a compensatory scoliosis must occur to return the head to a level position.

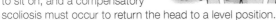

- When one foot is lifted off the floor, the pelvis should fall to that side because it is now unsupported. However, the gluteus medius and minimus on the support-limb (opposite) side, which contract and create a force of same-side depression of the pelvis, prevent the pelvis from falling to that side. Therefore the pelvis remains level. With every step a person takes, contraction of the gluteus medius on the support side occurs. You can easily feel this when walking or even walking in place.

- The gluteus medius and minimus contract to create a force of same-side pelvic depression when weight is simply shifted to one foot. Therefore the habitual practice of standing with all or most of the body weight on one side tends to cause the gluteus medius and minimus on that side to become overused and tight.

- The gluteus medius can be thought of as the "deltoid of the hip joint" because it performs all the same actions to the thigh at the hip joint as the deltoid does to the arm at the glenohumeral joint.

10

MUSCLES OF THE PELVIS AND THIGH:
Deep Lateral Rotator Group
Piriformis; Superior Gemellus; Obturator Internus; Inferior Gemellus; Obturator Externus; Quadratus Femoris

Pronunciation   **pi-ri-FOR-mis • su-PEE-ree-or jee-MEL-us • ob-too-RAY-tor in-TER-nus • in-FEE-ree-or jee-MEL-us • ob-too-RAY-tor ex-TER-nus • kwod-RATE-us FEM-o-ris**

The deep lateral rotator group is composed of six muscles that are located in the posterior pelvis, deep to the gluteus maximus. They are, from superior to inferior, the piriformis, which lies directly next to the gluteus medius, the superior gemellus, obturator internus, inferior gemellus, obturator externus, and quadratus femoris (Figure 10-7). The obturator externus is the only muscle of the deep lateral rotator group that is not visible in the second layer of the posterior pelvic muscles. It is either entirely covered or nearly entirely covered by the quadratus femoris. The quadratus femoris is a fairly massive muscle; it is often larger than the piriformis.

All muscles of this group laterally rotate the thigh at the hip joint when the pelvis is fixed and contralaterally rotate the pelvis at the hip joint when the thigh is fixed.

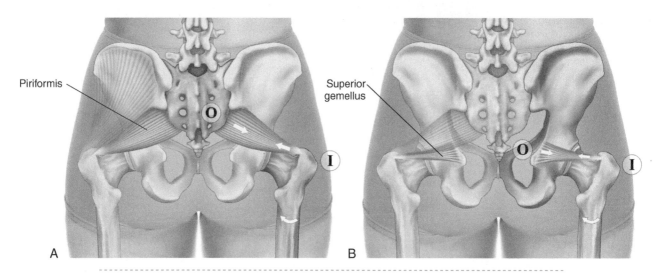

Piriformis

Superior gemellus

A

B

FIGURE 10-7 Posterior views of the deep lateral rotator group muscles. **A,** The piriformis has been drawn on both sides. The gluteus medius has been ghosted in on the left. **B,** The superior gemellus is shown on both sides. The piriformis has been ghosted in on the left.

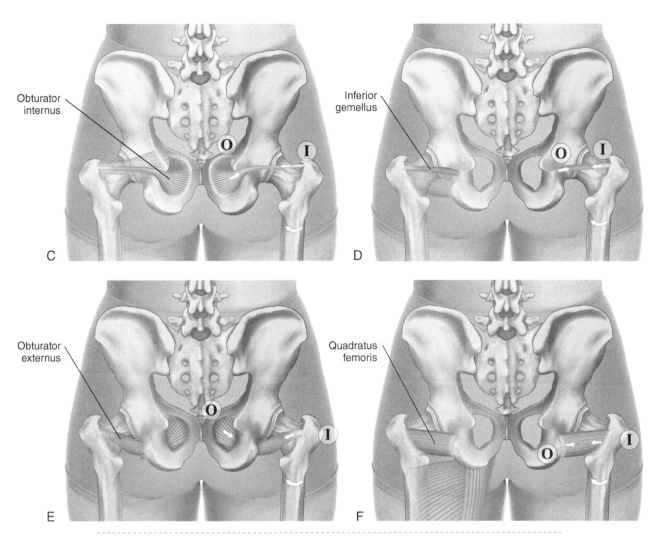

FIGURE 10-7, cont'd Posterior views of the deep lateral rotator group muscles. *C,* The obturator internus is shown on both sides. The superior gemellus and inferior gemellus have been ghosted in on the left. *D,* The inferior gemellus is shown on both sides. The quadratus femoris has been ghosted in on the left. *E,* The obturator externus is shown on both sides. The quadratus femoris has been cut and ghosted in on the left. *F,* The quadratus femoris is shown on both sides. The adductor magnus has been ghosted in on the left. *O,* Origin; *I,* insertion.

WHAT'S IN A NAME?

The name, *piriformis,* tells us that this muscle is shaped like a pear.

The name, *superior gemellus,* tells us that this muscle is the more superior muscle of a pair of similar muscles.

The name, *inferior gemellus,* tells us that this muscle is the more inferior muscle of a pair of similar muscles.

The name, *obturator internus,* tells us that this muscle attaches to the internal surface of the obturator foramen.

The name, *obturator externus,* tells us that this muscle attaches to the external surface of the obturator foramen.

The name, *quadratus femoris,* tells us that this muscle is square in shape and attaches to the femur.

❋ Derivation:
piriformis: L. pear shaped
gemellus: L. twin
obturator: L. to stop up, obstruct (refers to the obturator foramen)
superior: L. upper
inferior: L. lower
internus: L. inner
externus: L. outer
quadratus: L. squared
femoris: L. refers to the femur

Turn page to ◉ more.

ATTACHMENTS

Piriformis

Origin (Proximal Attachment)

■ Anterior sacrum

Insertion (Distal Attachment)

■ Greater trochanter of the femur

Superior Gemellus

Origin (Proximal Attachment)

■ Ischial spine

Insertion (Distal Attachment)

■ Greater trochanter of the femur

Obturator Internus

Origin (Proximal Attachment)

■ Internal surface of the pelvic bone surrounding the obturator foramen

Insertion (Distal Attachment)

■ Greater trochanter of the femur

Inferior Gemellus

Origin (Proximal Attachment)

■ Ischial tuberosity

Insertion (Distal Attachment)

■ Greater trochanter of the femur

Obturator Externus

Origin (Proximal Attachment)

■ External surface of the pelvic bone surrounding the obturator foramen

Insertion (Distal Attachment)

■ Trochanteric fossa of the femur

Quadratus Femoris

Origin (Proximal Attachment)

■ Ischial tuberosity

Insertion (Distal Attachment)

■ Intertrochanteric crest of the femur

ACTIONS

The standard actions (insertion/distal attachment moving toward origin/proximal attachment) move the thigh at the hip joint.

The reverse actions (origin/proximal attachment moving toward insertion/distal attachment) move the pelvis at the hip joint.

Piriformis

■ Laterally rotates the thigh.

■ Horizontally extends the thigh.

■ Medially rotates the thigh (if the thigh is first abducted to approximately 60 degrees or more).

■ Contralaterally rotates the pelvis.

Superior Gemellus, Obturator Internus, Inferior Gemellus, Obturator Externus, Quadratus Femoris

■ Laterally rotate the thigh.

■ Contralaterally rotate the pelvis.

STABILIZATION

1. All muscles of the deep lateral rotator group stabilize the thigh and pelvis at the hip joint.

2. The piriformis also stabilizes the sacrum at the sacroiliac and lumbosacral joints

INNERVATION

Piriformis

■ Nerve to piriformis (of the lumbosacral plexus)

Superior Gemellus, Obturator Internus

■ Nerve to obturator internus (of the lumbosacral plexus)

Inferior Gemellus, Quadratus Femoris

■ Nerve to quadratus femoris (of the lumbosacral plexus)

Obturator Externus

■ Obturator nerve

10

PALPATION

1. The client is prone with the leg flexed to 90 degrees at the knee joint. Place your palpating finger pads just lateral to the sacrum, halfway between the posterior superior iliac spine (PSIS) and the apex of the sacrum. Place the support/resistance hand on the medial surface of the distal leg, just proximal to the ankle joint.

2. Gently resist the client from laterally rotating the thigh at the hip joint, and feel for the contraction of the piriformis (Figure 10-8).

   Note: Lateral rotation of the client's thigh involves the client's foot moving medially toward the midline (and opposite side) of the body.

3. Continue palpating the piriformis laterally toward the superior border of the greater trochanter of the femur by strumming perpendicular to the fibers as the client alternately contracts (against resistance) and relaxes the piriformis.

4. To palpate the quadratus femoris, place your palpating finger pads just lateral to the lateral border of the ischial tuberosity, and place your support/resistance hand on the medial surface of the distal leg, just proximal to the ankle joint. Follow the same procedure as for the piriformis, and feel for the contraction of the quadratus femoris (Figure 10-9).

5. Continue palpating the quadratus femoris laterally toward the intertrochanteric crest by strumming perpendicular to the fibers as the client alternately contracts (against resistance) and relaxes the quadratus femoris.

6. To palpate the other deep lateral rotators, either find the piriformis and palpate inferior to it, or find the quadratus femoris and palpate superior to it. Follow the same procedure used to palpate the piriformis and quadratus femoris by giving gentle resistance to the client's lateral rotation of the thigh at the hip joint (Figure 10-10).

   Note: Discerning these muscles from each other is difficult.

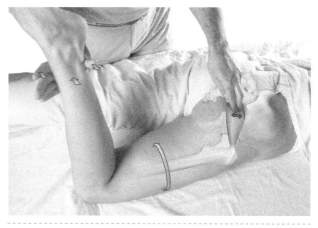

FIGURE 10-8 Palpation of the right piriformis as the client attempts to laterally rotate the thigh at the hip joint against gentle-to-moderate resistance.

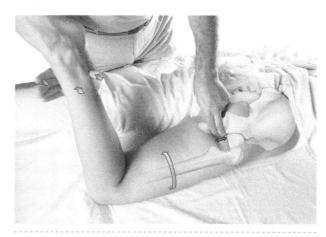

FIGURE 10-9 Palpation of the right quadratus femoris as the client attempts to laterally rotate the thigh at the hip joint against gentle-to-moderate resistance.

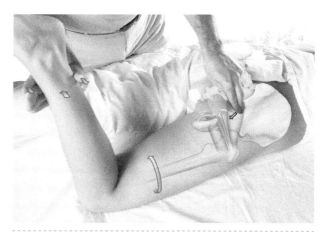

FIGURE 10-10 Palpation of the other deep lateral rotators by first locating the piriformis and then dropping inferiorly off it. This palpation is performed as the client attempts to laterally rotate the thigh against gentle-to-moderate resistance.

10

Turn page to 👁 more.

TREATMENT CONSIDERATIONS

■ Probably the most common method to stretch the piriformis is to have the client supine with the foot flat on the table (i.e., the thigh flexed at the hip joint and the leg flexed at the knee joint); then horizontally flex (horizontally adduct) the client's thigh toward the opposite side of the body.

■ The piriformis can change from being a lateral rotator of the thigh at the hip joint to a medial rotator of the thigh at the hip joint (if the thigh is first flexed at the hip joint); therefore the method of stretching the piriformis varies with the position of the client's thigh. If the client's thigh is flexed, lateral rotation must be used to stretch the piriformis. If the client's thigh were not flexed, medial rotation would be used. The thigh must be flexed to at least 60 degrees for the piriformis to become a medial rotator of the thigh.

■ The piriformis often protectively tightens when the client's sacroiliac joint is sprained.

■ The sciatic nerve normally exits from the pelvis between the piriformis and the superior gemellus. However, in approximately 10% to 20% of individuals, part or all of the sciatic nerve may pierce the piriformis muscle, exiting through the middle of it. Some sources believe this condition makes the sciatic nerve more susceptible to being compressed if the piriformis is tight; others do not. When the piriformis compresses the sciatic nerve, regardless of the relationship between the piriformis and the sciatic nerve, this condition is called *piriformis syndrome* and can result in symptoms of *sciatica*.

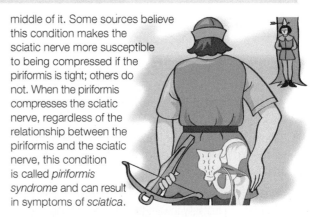

■ A force of lateral rotation of the thigh prevents medial rotation of the thigh and entire lower extremity (including the talus at the subtalar joint), if the foot overly pronates (and if the arch of the foot collapses).

■ **Be careful with pressure on the quadratus femoris because the sciatic nerve passes over this muscle.**

10

Notes

MUSCLES OF THE PELVIS AND THIGH
Tensor Fasciae Latae (TFL)

Pronunciation **TEN-sor FASH-ee-a LA-tee**

The tensor fasciae latae (TFL) is superficial and located anterolaterally on the proximal thigh (Figure 10-11).

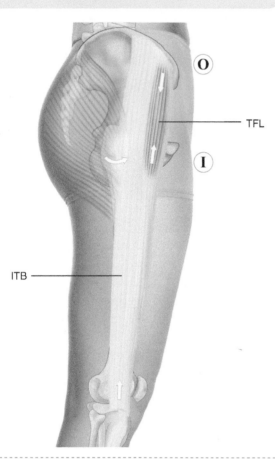

FIGURE 10-11 Lateral view of the right tensor fasciae latae (TFL). The gluteus maximus has been ghosted in. *ITB,* Iliotibial band. *O,* origin; *I,* insertion.

WHAT'S IN A NAME?

The name, *tensor fasciae latae,* tells us that this muscle tenses the fascia lata. The fascia lata is the broad covering of fascia that envelops the musculature of the thigh (the iliotibial band [ITB] is a thickening of the fascia lata).

* **Derivation:**
tensor: L. stretcher
fasciae: L. band/bandage
latae: L. broad, refers to the side

ATTACHMENTS

Origin (Proximal Attachment)
- Anterior superior iliac spine (ASIS)

Insertion (Distal Attachment)
- ITB

ACTIONS

The TFL moves the thigh and pelvis at the hip joint.
- Flexes the thigh.
- Abducts the thigh.
- Medially rotates the thigh.
- Anteriorly tilts the pelvis.
- Depresses the same-side pelvis.

STABILIZATION

- Stabilizes the thigh and pelvis at the hip joint.
- Stabilizes the knee joint via its attachment into the ITB.

INNERVATION

- Superior gluteal nerve

PALPATION

1. The client is supine with the thighs on the table and legs hanging off the table.

   Note: If this position is uncomfortable for the client, the foot of the lower extremity not being palpated can be placed on the table to stabilize the pelvis and low back.

2. Place your palpating finger pads just distal and lateral to the ASIS. Place the resistance hand on the distal anterolateral thigh.

3. Ask the client to medially rotate and flex the thigh at the hip joint. Feel for the contraction of the TFL. Resistance can be given with the resistance hand (Figure 10-12).

4. Continue palpating the TFL distally to its ITB attachment by strumming perpendicular to the fibers.

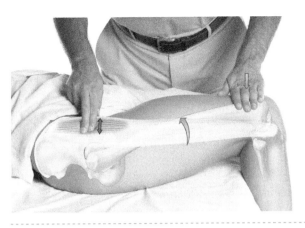

FIGURE 10-12 The right TFL is palpated by asking the client to medially rotate and flex the thigh at the hip joint.

TREATMENT CONSIDERATIONS

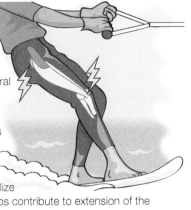

- If the TFL is tight, it can increase tension in the ITB, thereby increasing the likelihood of ITB friction syndrome at the greater trochanter or lateral condyle of the femur.

- Given that both the TFL and the gluteus maximus attach into the ITB and the ITB crosses the knee joint anteriorly, both of these muscles help stabilize the knee joint and perhaps contribute to extension of the knee joint as well.

10

MUSCLES OF THE PELVIS AND THIGH
Sartorius

Pronunciation **sar-TOR-ee-us**

The sartorius is the longest muscle in the body and is superficial for its entire course from the pelvis to the tibia. It crosses the hip joint anteriorly, crosses the knee joint posteriorly, and then returns anterior to attach to the proximal anterior tibia (Figure 10-13).

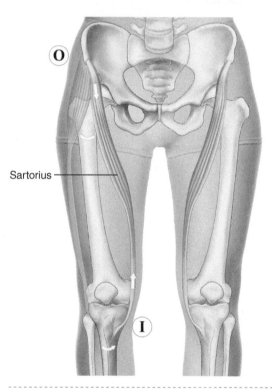

Sartorius

FIGURE 10-13 Anterior view of the right sartorius. The tensor fasciae latae and iliotibial band have been ghosted in. *O*, Origin; *I*, insertion.

WHAT'S IN A NAME?

The name, *sartorius,* tells us that this muscle performs the four actions necessary to create a cross-legged position that a *sartor* (Latin for *tailor*) sits in to do his or her work. These actions are flexion, abduction, and lateral rotation of the thigh at the hip joint and flexion of the leg at the knee joint.

✳ **Derivation:**
sartorius: L. tailor

ATTACHMENTS

Origin (Proximal Attachment)
- Anterior superior iliac spine (ASIS)

Insertion (Distal Attachment)
- Pes anserine tendon at the proximal anteromedial tibia

ACTIONS

The sartorius moves the thigh and pelvis at the hip joint and the leg at the knee joint.
- Flexes the thigh.
- Abducts the thigh.
- Laterally rotates the thigh.
- Anteriorly tilts the pelvis.
- Flexes the leg.

STABILIZATION

1. Stabilizes the thigh and pelvis at the hip joint.
2. Stabilizes the knee joint.

INNERVATION

- Femoral nerve

PALPATION

1. The client is supine with the thighs on the table and legs hanging off the table.

   Note: If this position is uncomfortable for the client, the foot of the lower extremity not being palpated can be placed on the table to stabilize the pelvis and low back.

2. Place your palpating finger pads just distal and medial to the ASIS. Place the resistance hand on the distal anteromedial thigh.

3. Ask the client to laterally rotate and flex the thigh at the hip joint. Feel for the contraction of the sartorius (Figure 10-14).

4. Continue palpating the sartorius toward its distal attachment by strumming perpendicular to the fibers.

10

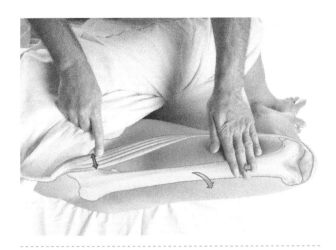

FIGURE 10-14 The proximal belly of the right sartorius engages and is easily palpable when the client laterally rotates and flexes the thigh at the hip joint. Note: The therapist usually palpates from the same side of the table but is shown here standing on the opposite side of the table for the purpose of this photograph.

TREATMENT CONSIDERATIONS

- The sartorius is one of three muscles that attach into the pes anserine tendon. *Pes anserine* means *goose foot*. The other two muscles that attach here are the gracilis and the semitendinosus.

- The medial border of the sartorius is the lateral border of the *femoral triangle* of the thigh. The femoral triangle is located between the medial borders of the sartorius and adductor longus and contains the femoral nerve, artery, and vein.

- The lateral femoral cutaneous nerve sometimes pierces the sartorius, which can lead to entrapment of this nerve, causing a condition known as *meralgia paresthetica*.

10

MUSCLES OF THE PELVIS AND THIGH: Iliopsoas
Iliacus; Psoas Major

Pronunciation   **I-lee-o-SO-as • i-lee-AK-us • SO-as MAY-jor**

The iliopsoas is composed of two muscles: the iliacus and psoas major. These two muscles have distinct origins (proximal attachments), but their distal bellies blend, and they have a common insertion (distal attachment) on the femur. The psoas major's belly lies deep in the posterior abdominal wall against the lumbar spine. The iliacus lies deep against the anterior (internal) surface of the pelvic bone. However, their distal belly is superficial immediately distal to the inguinal ligament (Figure 10-15).

10

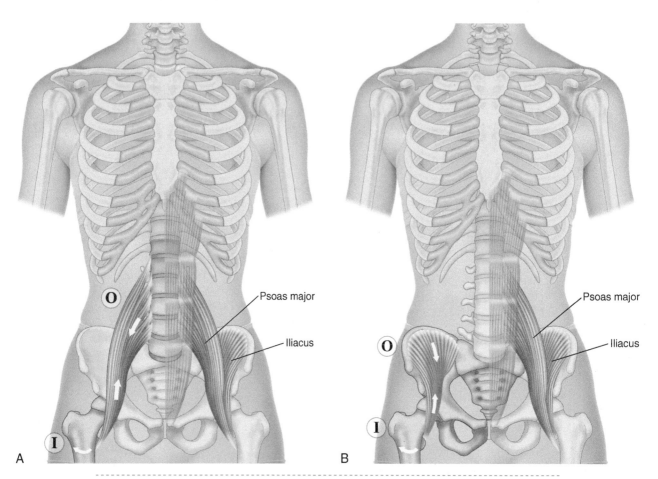

A

B

FIGURE 10-15 _A,_ Anterior view of the psoas major bilaterally. The left iliacus has been drawn in, and the rectus abdominis has been ghosted in. **_B,_** Anterior view of the iliacus bilaterally. The left psoas major has been drawn in, and the rectus abdominis has been ghosted in. _O,_ Origin; _I,_ insertion.

The name, *iliacus,* tells us that this muscle attaches onto the ilium.

The name, *psoas major,* tells us that this muscle is located in the loin (low back) area and is larger than the psoas minor.

✳ **Derivation:**
iliacus: L. refers to the ilium
psoas: Gr. loin (low back)
major: L. larger

ATTACHMENTS

Iliacus

Origin (Proximal Attachment)
■ Internal ilium

Insertion (Distal Attachment)
■ Lesser trochanter of the femur

Psoas Major

Origin (Proximal Attachment)
■ Anterolateral lumbar spine

Insertion (Distal Attachment)
■ Lesser trochanter of the femur

ACTIONS

Both the iliacus and psoas major move the thigh and pelvis at the hip joint. The psoas major also moves the trunk at the lumbar spinal joints.

Iliacus

■ Flexes the thigh.
■ Laterally rotates the thigh.
■ Anteriorly tilts the pelvis.

Psoas Major

■ Flexes the thigh.
■ Laterally rotates the thigh.
■ Anteriorly tilts the pelvis.
■ Flexes the trunk.

STABILIZATION

1. Both the iliacus and psoas major stabilize the thigh and pelvis at the hip joint.
2. The psoas major also stabilizes the lumbar spinal joints.

INNERVATION

■ Femoral nerve (iliacus)
■ Lumbar plexus (psoas major)

PALPATION

1. The client is seated with the trunk slightly flexed. Place your palpating finger pads anterolaterally on the client's abdominal wall, approximately halfway between the umbilicus and the anterior superior iliac spine (ASIS); ensure placement is lateral to the lateral border of the rectus abdominis.
2. Place the finger pads of your other hand over the fingers of your palpating hand to increase the strength and stability of the palpating fingers (Figure 10-16, *A*).
3. Ask the client to take in a deep but relaxed breath. As the client exhales, slowly (but firmly) sink in toward the belly of the psoas major by pressing diagonally in toward the spine. You may need to repeat this procedure two to three times before arriving at the psoas major.
4. To confirm that you are on the psoas major, ask the client to gently flex the thigh at the hip joint by lifting the foot slightly off the floor. Feel for the contraction of the psoas major.
5. Strum perpendicularly across the fibers to feel for the width of the muscle. Continue palpating the psoas major toward its superior vertebral attachment and inferiorly as far as possible within the abdominopelvic cavity.

   Note: The psoas major can also be palpated with the client supine with a roll under the knees (see Figure 10-16, *B*).

6. To palpate the iliacus, curl your fingers around the iliac crest with your finger pads oriented toward the internal surface of the ilium. Feel for the iliacus (Figure 10-17). To engage the iliacus, ask the client to flex the thigh at the hip joint by lifting the foot slightly off the floor.
7. The distal belly of the iliopsoas is also palpable in the proximal anterior thigh between the pectineus and the sartorius (Figure 10-18).

10

Turn page to 👁 more.

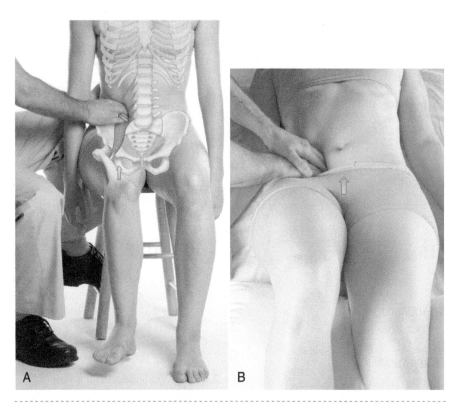

FIGURE 10-16 *A,* Palpation of the right psoas major as the client gently flexes the thigh at the hip joint by lifting her foot up slightly from the floor. *B,* The psoas major can also be palpated with the client supine or side lying. The disadvantage of the supine palpation position is that when the client flexes the thigh at the hip joint, the muscles of the abdominal wall may contract to stabilize the pelvis. This action can interfere with feeling the psoas major, located deep to these muscles. This action may also occur to some degree with the side-lying palpation position.

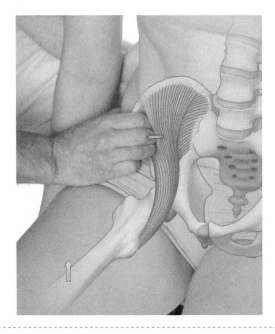

FIGURE 10-17 The right iliacus is palpated by curling the fingers around the iliac crest so that the finger pads are oriented against the muscle.

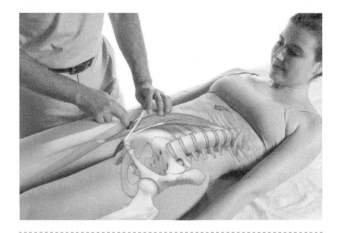

FIGURE 10-18 Palpation of the distal belly and tendon of the psoas major in the proximal thigh (immediately distal to the inguinal ligament) as the client flexes (curls) the trunk at the spinal joints against gravity. The sartorius has been ghosted in.

10

TREATMENT CONSIDERATIONS

- With regard to posture, a chronically tight iliopsoas anteriorly tilts the pelvis, causing the lumbar curve to increase (*hyperlordosis*, also known as *swayback*).

  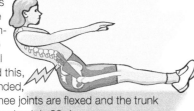

  Straight-legged sit-ups tend to strengthen the iliopsoas disproportionately in comparison to the anterior abdominal wall muscles. To avoid this, curl-ups are recommended, wherein the hip and knee joints are flexed and the trunk "curls" up (flexes) approximately 30 degrees.

- The roots of the lumbar plexus of nerves enter and pierce the psoas major muscle. Therefore a tight psoas major may entrap these nerves.

- Tenderloin (also known as *filet mignon*) is the psoas major of a cow.

- **You must be careful with palpation of the distal belly of the iliopsoas in the proximal thigh because the femoral nerve, artery, and vein lie over the iliopsoas and pectineus in the femoral triangle here.**

  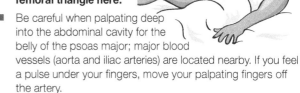

- Be careful when palpating deep into the abdominal cavity for the belly of the psoas major; major blood vessels (aorta and iliac arteries) are located nearby. If you feel a pulse under your fingers, move your palpating fingers off the artery.

- The psoas major is usually cited as a flexor of the lumbar spine because it crosses anteriorly to the axis of motion for the lumbar vertebrae. However, if the client has a hyperlordotic lumbar spine (swayback), the relationship of the psoas major's fibers relative to the joints can change such that it crosses posteriorly and is now an extensor.

10

MUSCLES OF THE PELVIS AND THIGH
Psoas Minor

Pronunciation **SO-as MY-nor**

The psoas minor is a small muscle that lies anteriorly on the belly of the psoas major in the abdominal cavity (Figure 10-19).

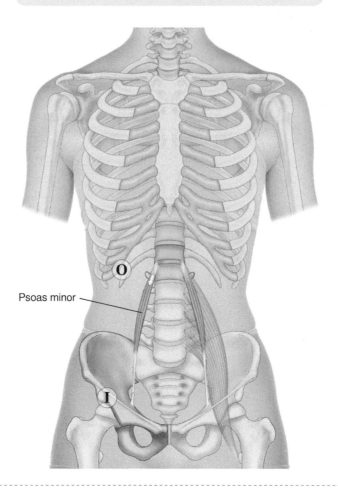

Psoas minor

FIGURE 10-19 Anterior view of the psoas minor bilaterally. The psoas major has been ghosted in on the left. *O*, Origin; *I*, insertion.

WHAT'S IN A NAME?

The name, *psoas minor,* tells us that this muscle is located in the low back area and is smaller than the psoas major.

❋ **Derivation:**
psoas: Gr. loin (low back)
minor: L. smaller

ATTACHMENTS

Origin (Proximal Attachment)
- Anterolateral bodies of T12 and L1

Insertion (Distal Attachment)
- Pubis

ACTIONS

The psoas minor moves the trunk at the spinal joints and the pelvis at the lumbosacral joint.

- Flexes the trunk.
- Posteriorly tilts the pelvis.

STABILIZATION

1. Stabilizes the lumbar spinal joints.
2. Stabilizes the pelvis.

INNERVATION

- L1 Spinal nerve

PALPATION

1. Locate the psoas major, and then feel for a small band of muscle that sits anteriorly on it. To discern these two muscles from each other, feel for a band of musculature on the psoas major that does not contract with flexion of the thigh at the hip joint.

TREATMENT CONSIDERATIONS

- The psoas minor is absent in approximately 40% of the population.

- A condition, called *psoas minor syndrome*, has been reported, in which the psoas minor in teenagers has not kept up with the growth of the trunk and pelvis and is, consequently, pulled taut and becomes painful.

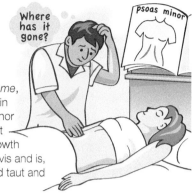

10

MUSCLES OF THE PELVIS AND THIGH: Adductor Group
Adductor Longus; Adductor Brevis; Adductor Magnus; Pectineus; Gracilis

Pronunciation **ad-DUK-tor LONG-us • ad-DUK-tor BRE-vis • ad-DUK-tor MAG-nus • pek-TIN-ee-us • gra-SIL-is**

The adductor group is composed of five muscles: the adductors longus, brevis, and magnus, and the pectineus and gracilis. All five muscles cross the hip joint and perform adduction of the thigh at the hip joint, hence the name of the group. The gracilis also crosses the knee joint. In lay terms, these muscles are referred to as *groin muscles*. The proximal aspects of the pectineus and adductor longus are superficial in the anteromedial thigh. The adductor brevis is deep to the longus. The gracilis is superficial for its entire course in the medial thigh. The adductor magnus has two heads, an anterior and posterior head, and is sandwiched between the other adductors anteriorly and the hamstrings posteriorly. A small portion of it is superficial in the medial thigh (Figure 10-20).

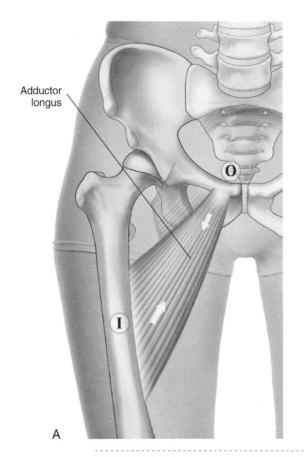

Adductor longus

A

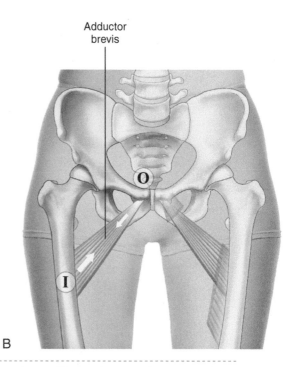

Adductor brevis

B

FIGURE 10-20 *A,* Anterior view of the right adductor longus. The pectineus has been cut and ghosted in. ***B,*** Anterior view of the right adductor brevis. The adductor longus has been cut and ghosted in on the left.

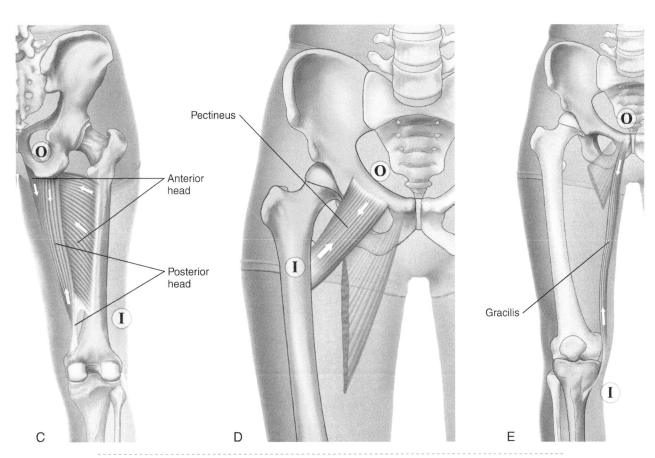

FIGURE 10-20, cont'd **C,** Posterior view of the right adductor magnus. **D,** Anterior view of the right pectineus. The adductor longus has been cut and ghosted in. **E,** Anterior view of the right gracilis. The adductor longus has been cut and ghosted in. *O,* Origin; *I,* insertion.

10

WHAT'S IN A NAME?

The name, *adductor longus,* tells us that this muscle is an adductor and longer than the adductor brevis.

The name, *adductor brevis,* tells us that this muscle is an adductor and shorter than the adductor longus.

The name, *adductor magnus,* tells us that this muscle is an adductor and larger than the adductor longus and adductor brevis.

The name, *pectineus,* means *comb.* The pectinus has a comblike appearance because its muscle fibers form a flat surface as they leave the pubic bone.

The name, *gracilis,* tells us that the shape of this muscle is slender and graceful.

❋ **Derivation:**
adductor: L. muscle that adducts a body part
longus: L. longer
brevis: L. shorter
magnus: L. great, larger
pectineus: L. comb
gracilis: L. slender, graceful

ATTACHMENTS

All five muscles of the adductor group originate on (attach proximally to) the pubic bone. The adductor magnus also attaches proximally to the ischium.

Adductors Longus and Brevis

Origin (Proximal Attachment)
- Pubis

Insertion (Distal Attachment)
- Linea aspera of the femur

Adductor Magnus

Origin (Proximal Attachment)
- Pubis and ischium

Insertion (Distal Attachment)
- Linea aspera of the femur

Turn page to ◉ more.

Pectineus

Origin (Proximal Attachment)
- Pubis

Insertion (Distal Attachment)
- Proximal posterior shaft of the femur

Gracilis

Origin (Proximal Attachment)
- Pubis

Insertion (Distal Attachment)
- Pes anserine tendon at the proximal anteromedial tibia

ACTIONS

The muscles of the adductor group move the thigh and pelvis at the hip joint. The gracilis also moves the leg and thigh at the knee joint.

Adductors Longus and Brevis, Pectineus, and Gracilis
- Adduct the thigh at the hip joint.
- Flex the thigh at the hip joint.
- Anteriorly tilt the pelvis at the hip joint.
- The gracilis also flexes the knee joint.

Adductor Magnus
- Adducts the thigh at the hip joint.
- Extends the thigh at the hip joint.
- Posteriorly tilts the pelvis at the hip joint.

STABILIZATION
1. All muscles of the adductor group stabilize the thigh and pelvis at the hip joint.
2. The gracilis also stabilizes the knee joint.

INNERVATION

- Obturator nerve (adductors longus and brevis; gracilis)
- Obturator nerve and sciatic nerve (adductor magnus)
- Femoral nerve (pectineus)

PALPATION

1. The palpation position for all of the muscles of the adductor group is to have the client supine with the thighs on the table and the legs hanging off the table.

   Note: If this position is uncomfortable for the client, the foot of the lower extremity not being palpated can be placed on the table to stabilize the pelvis and low back.

Adductors Longus and Brevis

1. The client is supine with the thighs on the table and legs hanging off the table.
2. The proximal tendon of the adductor longus is the most prominent tendon in the medial thigh and is usually easily palpable. To locate it, simply palpate along the pubic bone from lateral to medial until you encounter a prominent tendon. Place your palpating finger pads on the prominent tendon of the adductor longus in the proximal anterior thigh. Place the resistance hand on the distal anteromedial thigh, just proximal to the knee joint.
3. Ask the client to adduct the thigh at the hip joint against resistance. Feel for the tendon to tense (Figure 10-21).
4. Strum perpendicular to the tendon to palpate its width. Continue to palpate it distally as far as possible toward its linea aspera attachment.
5. The adductor brevis is difficult to palpate and discern from the adductor longus. Try to palpate it either deep to the adductor longus or between the adductor longus and adjacent gracilis (Figure 10-22).

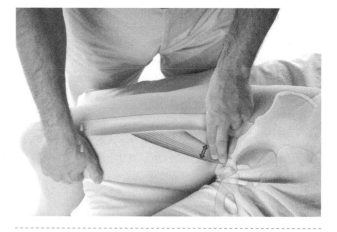

FIGURE 10-21 Engagement and palpation of the right adductor longus as the client adducts the thigh at the hip joint against resistance.

Pectineus

1. The client is supine with the thighs on the table and legs hanging off the table.

2. Place your palpating finger pads on the proximal tendon of the adductor longus. Now drop off of it anteriorly (laterally), and you will be on the pectineus. Staying close to the pubic bone is important. Place your resistance hand on the distal anteromedial thigh, just proximal to the knee joint.

3. Ask the client to adduct the thigh against resistance and feel for the pectineus to engage (Figure 10-23).

4. Once located, strum perpendicular to the fibers; continue palpating the pectineus distally as far as possible.

   Note: Other than the adductor brevis, the pectineus is the most challenging member of the adductor group to palpate and discern.

Gracilis

1. The client is supine with thighs on the table and legs hanging off the table.

2. Place your palpating finger pads on the proximal tendon of the adductor longus. Then drop just off of it posteriorly (medially), and you will be on the gracilis.

3. Ask the client to flex the leg at the knee joint against the table. Flexion of the leg at the knee joint will engage the gracilis but not the adductor longus and adductor magnus on either side of it, making it easy to discern the gracilis in the proximal thigh (Figure 10-24).

4. Once located, strum perpendicular to the fibers; continue palpating the gracilis distally to the tibia.

Adductor Magnus

1. The client is supine with the thighs on the table and the legs hanging off the table.

2. The adductor magnus is actually quite easily palpable in the proximal medial thigh between the gracilis and the hamstring muscles, where it is located in a depression between these muscles.

3. Locate the adductor magnus by first locating the gracilis and medial hamstrings, which contract with flexion of the leg at the knee joint performed by asking the client to press the leg against the table (Figure 10-25, A). Once you feel these muscles palpably harden with leg flexion, feel for the adductor magnus between them (it will stay relaxed and soft during this joint action) (Figure 10-25, B).

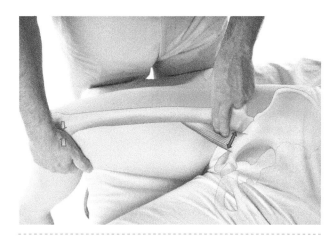

FIGURE 10-23 Engagement and palpation of the right pectineus as the client adducts the thigh against resistance.

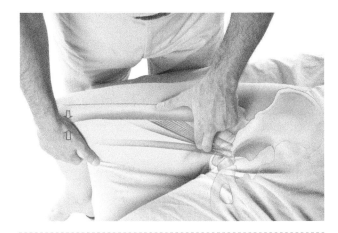

FIGURE 10-22 Palpation of the right adductor brevis proximally between the adductor longus (ghosted in) and gracilis as the client adducts the thigh against resistance.

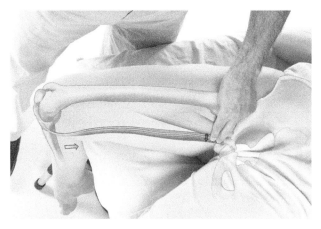

FIGURE 10-24 Engagement and palpation of the right gracilis as the client flexes the leg against the resistance of the table.

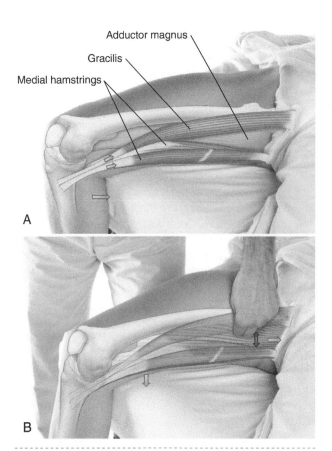

Adductor magnus

Gracilis

Medial hamstrings

A

10

B

FIGURE 10-25 Palpation of the right adductor magnus in the medial thigh between the gracilis and medial hamstrings. ***A,*** The gracilis and medial hamstrings engage when the client flexes the leg at the knee joint by pressing the leg against the table. ***B,*** Engagement and palpation of the adductor magnus occurs between these muscles as the client extends the thigh at the hip joint by pressing the thigh down against the table.

4. To engage the adductor magnus and confirm that you are on it, ask the client to extend the thigh at the hip joint against the resistance of the table (see Figure 10-25, *B*).

5. Continue palpating the adductor magnus distally as far as possible by strumming perpendicular to the fibers as the client alternately contracts and relaxes it.

TREATMENT CONSIDERATIONS

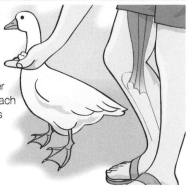

- The gracilis is one of three muscles that attach into the pes anserine tendon. *Pes anserine* means *goose foot*. The other two muscles that attach here are the sartorius and semitendinosus.

- The medial border of the adductor longus is the medial border of the femoral triangle of the thigh. The femoral triangle is located between the medial borders of the sartorius and adductor longus and contains the femoral nerve, artery, and vein.

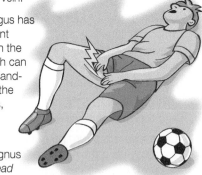

- The adductor longus has the most prominent proximal tendon in the groin region, which can serve as a useful landmark for locating the pectineus, gracilis, and adductor magnus.

- The adductor magnus has an *anterior head* and a *posterior head*, with a hiatus between them, through which the femoral artery and vein from the anterior thigh pass, becoming the popliteal artery and vein in the distal posterior thigh.

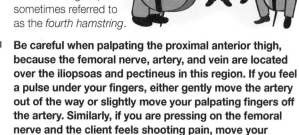

- Similar to the hamstring muscles, the adductor magnus attaches to the ischial tuberosity and can extend the thigh at the hip joint. For this reason, the adductor magnus (or more specifically, the posterior head of the adductor magnus) is sometimes referred to as the *fourth hamstring*.

- **Be careful when palpating the proximal anterior thigh, because the femoral nerve, artery, and vein are located over the iliopsoas and pectineus in this region. If you feel a pulse under your fingers, either gently move the artery out of the way or slightly move your palpating fingers off the artery. Similarly, if you are pressing on the femoral nerve and the client feels shooting pain, move your palpating fingers off the nerve.**

Notes

MUSCLES OF THE PELVIS AND THIGH: Quadriceps Femoris Group *(Quads)*
Rectus Femoris; Vastus Lateralis; Vastus Medialis; Vastus Intermedius

Pronunciation   REK-tus FEM-o-ris • VAS-tus lat-er-A-lis • VAS-tus mee-dee-A-lis • VAS-tus in-ter-MEE-dee-us

The quadriceps femoris group, or as they are usually known, the *quads,* are a group of four muscles that are superficial in the anterior thigh but reach around medially and laterally to attach posteriorly to the linea aspera of the femur. Therefore they envelop nearly the entire femur. The four muscles of the quads are the rectus femoris, vastus lateralis, vastus medialis, and the vastus intermedius (Figure 10-26). All four quads cross the knee joint; only the rectus femoris crosses the hip joint. The vastus lateralis is the largest of the four quadriceps femoris muscles.

10

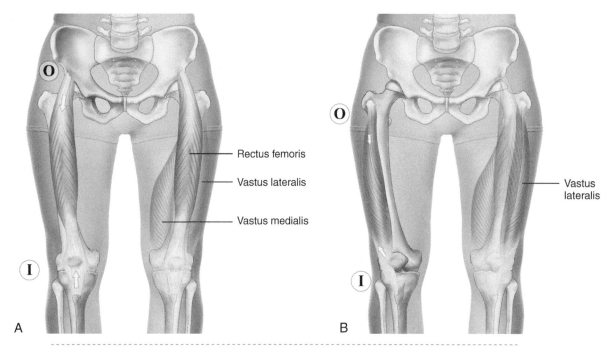

Rectus femoris
Vastus lateralis
Vastus medialis

Vastus lateralis

A   B

FIGURE 10-26 A, Anterior view of the rectus femoris bilaterally. The rest of the quadriceps femoris group has been ghosted in on the left. **B,** Anterior view of the vastus lateralis bilaterally. The rest of the quadriceps femoris group has been ghosted in on the left.

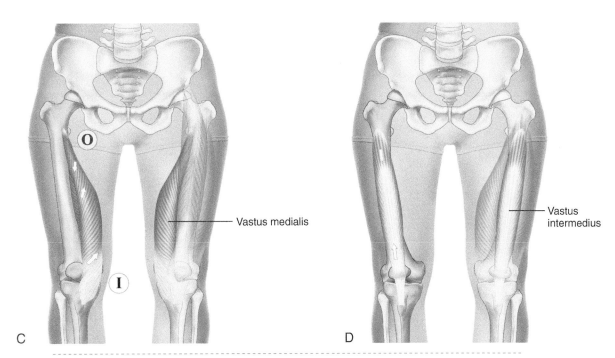

Vastus medialis

Vastus intermedius

C

D

FIGURE 10-26, cont'd C, Anterior view of the vastus medialis bilaterally. The rest of the quadriceps femoris group has been ghosted in on the left. **D,** Anterior view of the vastus intermedius bilaterally. The vastus lateralis and vastus medialis have been ghosted in on the left. *O,* Origin; *I,* insertion.

WHAT'S IN A NAME?

The name, *rectus femoris,* tells us that the fibers of this muscle run straight up and down (proximal to distal) on the femur.

The name, *vastus lateralis,* tells us that this muscle is vast in size and located laterally.

The name, *vastus medialis,* tells us that this muscle is vast in size and located medially.

The name, *vastus intermedius,* tells us that this muscle is vast in size and located between the two other vastus muscles.

✳ **Derivation:**
rectus: L. straight
femoris: L. refers to the femur
vastus: L. vast
lateralis: L. lateral
medialis: L. medial
inter: L. between
medius: L. middle

ATTACHMENTS

All four quads insert on (attach distally to) the tibial tuberosity via the patella and patellar ligament.

Rectus Femoris

Origin (Proximal Attachment)
■ Anterior inferior iliac spine (AIIS)

Insertion (Distal Attachment)
■ Tibial tuberosity via the patella and the patellar ligament

Vastus Lateralis and Vastus Medialis

Origin (Proximal Attachment)
■ Linea aspera of the femur

Insertion (Distal Attachment)
■ Tibial tuberosity via the patella and the patellar ligament

Vastus Intermedius

Origin (Proximal Attachment)
■ Anterior shaft and linea aspera of the femur

Insertion (Distal Attachment)
■ Tibial tuberosity via the patella and the patellar ligament

ACTIONS

All four quads move the leg or thigh at the knee joint. The rectus femoris also moves the thigh or pelvis at the hip joint.

- Extend the leg at the knee joint.
- Extend the thigh at the knee joint.

The rectus femoris also:

- Flexes the thigh at the hip joint.
- Anteriorly tilts the pelvis at the hip joint.

STABILIZATION

- All four quads stabilize the knee joint.
- The rectus femoris also stabilizes the pelvis and thigh at the hip joint.

INNERVATION

- Femoral nerve

PALPATION

The palpation position for all of the muscles of the quadriceps femoris group is to have the client supine with the thighs on the table and the legs hanging off the table.

> If this position is uncomfortable for the client, the foot of the lower extremity not being palpated can be placed on the table to stabilize the pelvis and low back.

1. The client is supine with the thighs on the table and the legs hanging off the table. Place your palpating finger pads midline on the anterior thigh. If resistance is necessary, place the resistance hand on the distal leg, just proximal to the ankle joint.

2. Ask the client to extend the leg at the knee joint. Feel for the contraction of the rectus femoris (Figure 10-27, *A*).

3. Continue palpating the rectus femoris distally to the tibial tuberosity and proximally toward the anterior inferior iliac spine (AIIS) by strumming perpendicular to it.

> Note: Palpating the origin (proximal attachment) at the AIIS is challenging.

4. For the vastus medialis, palpate in the anteromedial thigh, just proximal to the patella while the client extends the leg at the knee joint. Feel for its contraction. Then strum perpendicular to the muscle, and palpate as much of the vastus medialis as possible (Figure 10-27, *B*).

5. For the vastus lateralis, palpate in the anterolateral thigh, just proximal to the patella while the client extends the leg at the knee joint. Feel for its

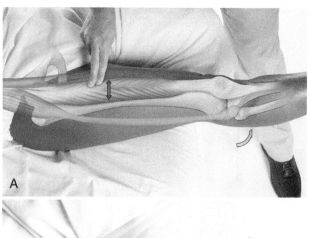

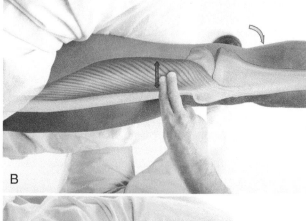

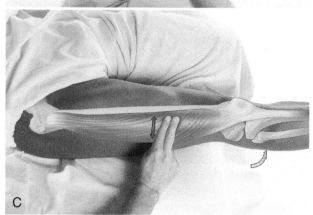

FIGURE 10-27 Anterior views of palpation of the quadriceps femoris muscles as the client extends the leg at the knee joint. *A,* Palpation of the rectus femoris. *B,* Palpation of the vastus medialis. *C,* Palpation of the vastus lateralis.

contraction. Then strum perpendicular to the fibers, and palpate the vastus lateralis in the anterolateral thigh, in the lateral thigh deep to the iliotibial band (ITB), and in the posterolateral thigh immediately posterior to the ITB (Figure 10-27, *C*).

6. The vastus intermedius is difficult to palpate and discern from the rectus femoris. If the rectus femoris can be lifted and/or moved aside, the distal vastus intermedius may be palpated deep to the rectus femoris when approached from either the medial or the lateral side. Make sure that the direction of your pressure is oriented toward the middle of the femur.

TREATMENT CONSIDERATIONS

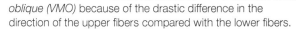

- Because of the difference in leverage, the rectus femoris is more powerful at the knee joint than at the hip joint.

- Pain attributed to the ITB is often caused by tightness of the vastus lateralis, which is deep to the ITB.

- Some sources refer to the upper fibers of the vastus medialis as the *vastus medialis longus (VML)* and the lower fibers as the *vastus medialis oblique (VMO)* because of the drastic difference in the direction of the upper fibers compared with the lower fibers.

- The most distal aspect of the vastus medialis is the bulkiest and may form a bulge in well-toned individuals.

- Strengthening the quadriceps femoris group is a major factor in knee joint stabilization or physical rehabilitation work.

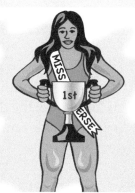

MUSCLES OF THE PELVIS AND THIGH
Articularis Genus

Pronunciation **ar-TIK-you-LA-ris JE-new**

The articularis genus is a very thin muscle that is located on the distal anterior femur deep to the quadriceps femoris musculature (Figure 10-28).

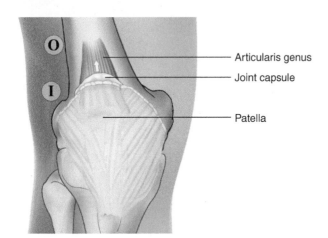

FIGURE 10-28 Anterior view of the right articularis genus. *O,* Origin; *I,* insertion.

WHAT'S IN A NAME?

The name, *articularis genus,* tells us that this muscle is involved with the knee joint.

* **Derivation:**
articularis: L. refers to a joint
genu: L. refers to the knee

ATTACHMENTS

Origin (Proximal Attachment)
■ Anterior distal femoral shaft

Insertion (Distal Attachment)
■ Knee joint capsule

ACTION

Tenses and pulls the knee joint capsule proximally.

STABILIZATION

Stabilizes the position of the knee joint capsule.

INNERVATION

■ Femoral nerve

PALPATION

■ The articularis genus is a small muscle deep to the rectus femoris and vastus intermedius and is extremely difficult, if not impossible, to palpate and distinguish from the adjacent musculature.

TREATMENT CONSIDERATIONS

■ The articularis genus works in concert with the quadriceps femoris musculature. When the quads contract and pull the patella proximally along the femur, the anterior genus contracts to pull the knee joint capsule proximally so that it does not become pinched between the patella and the femur.

Notes

MUSCLES OF THE PELVIS AND THIGH: Hamstring Group
Biceps Femoris; Semitendinosus; Semimembranosus

Pronunciation   **BY-seps FEM-o-ris • SEM-i-TEN-di-NO-sus • SEM-i-MEM-bra-NO-sus**

The hamstring group is composed of three muscles: biceps femoris, semitendinosus, and semimembranosus (Figure 10-29). The biceps femoris has two heads, a long head and a short head. The semitendinosus and semimembranosus are located medially and referred to as the medial hamstrings; the two heads of the biceps femoris are located laterally and referred to as the lateral hamstrings. Except at their origin (proximal attachment) at the ischial tuberosity where they are deep to the gluteus maximus, the hamstring group is superficial in the posterior thigh. Within the group, on the medial side, the semitendinosus is superficial to the semimembranosus; on the lateral side, the long head of the biceps femoris is superficial to the short head. The semimembranosus is the largest of the three hamstrings.

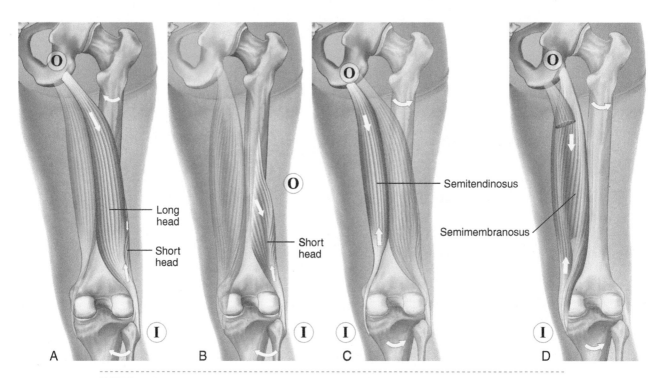

FIGURE 10-29 Posterior views of the right hamstrings. **A,** The long and short heads of the biceps femoris. The semitendinosus has been ghosted in. **B,** The short head of the biceps femoris. The semimembranosus has been ghosted in. **C,** The right semitendinosus. The biceps femoris has been ghosted in. **D,** The right semimembranosus. The proximal and distal tendons of the semitendinosus have been cut and ghosted in. *O,* Origin; *I,* insertion.

WHAT'S IN A NAME?

The name, *biceps femoris,* tells us that this muscle has two heads and lies over the femur.

The name, *semitendinosus,* tells us that this muscle has a long, slender (distal) tendon.

The name, *semimembranosus,* tells us that this muscle has a flattened, membranous (proximal) attachment.

❋ **Derivation:**
biceps: L. two heads
femoris: L. refers to the femur
semitendinosus: L. refers to its long tendon
semimembranosus: L. refers to its flattened, membranous tendon

ATTACHMENTS

All hamstrings (except for the short head of the biceps femoris) originate on (attach proximally to) the ischial tuberosity of the pelvic bone.

Biceps Femoris

Origin (Proximal Attachment)
- Ischial tuberosity (long head)
- Linea aspera (short head)

Insertion (Distal Attachment)
- Head of the fibula

Semitendinosus

Origin (Proximal Attachment)
- Ischial tuberosity

Insertion (Distal Attachment)
- Pes anserine tendon (at the proximal anteromedial tibia)

Semimembranosus

Origin (Proximal Attachment)
- Ischial tuberosity

Insertion (Distal Attachment)
- Posterior surface of the medial condyle of the tibia

ACTIONS

All hamstring muscles move the leg or thigh at the knee joint. All hamstring muscles (except the short head of the biceps femoris) move the thigh or pelvis at the hip joint.

- Flex the leg at the knee joint.
- Extend the thigh at the hip joint.
- Posteriorly tilt the pelvis at the hip joint.

STABILIZATION

1. Stabilize the thigh and pelvis at the hip joint.
2. Stabilize the knee joint.

INNERVATION

- Sciatic nerve

10

PALPATION

1. The client is prone with the leg partially flexed at the knee joint. Place your palpating finger pads just distal to the ischial tuberosity. Place the resistance hand around the distal leg, just proximal to the ankle joint.
2. Ask the client to try to flex the leg at the knee joint against gentle-to-moderate resistance. Feel for the contraction of the hamstrings.
3. Strumming perpendicular to the fibers, follow the biceps femoris toward the head of the fibula (Figure 10-30, *A*). Repeat this procedure from the ischial tuberosity to follow the medial hamstrings toward the medial side of the leg (Figure 10-30, *B*).

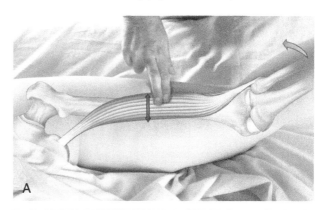

FIGURE 10-30 Palpation of the superficial hamstring muscles of the right thigh as the client attempts to flex the leg at the knee joint against resistance. *A,* Palpation of the long head of the biceps femoris on the lateral side. *Continued*

Turn page to ◉ more. ▶

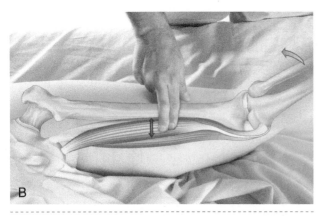

- The semimembranosus also attaches into the medial meniscus of the knee joint and facilitates the movement of the medial meniscus during knee flexion. This helps prevent impingement of the medial meniscus between the femur and tibia.

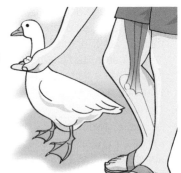

- The semitendinosus is one of three muscles that attach into the pes anserine tendon; *pes anserine* means *goose foot*. The other two muscles that attach here are the sartorius and the gracilis.

FIGURE 10-30, cont'd Palpation of the superficial hamstring muscles of the right thigh as the client attempts to flex the leg at the knee joint against resistance. *B,* Palpation of the semitendinosus on the medial side.

Note: The semimembranosus inserts on the posterior surface of the medial condyle of the tibia; the semitendinosus attaches anteriorly on the tibia at the pes anserine tendon.

TREATMENT CONSIDERATIONS

- The semitendinosus is named for its long distal tendon.

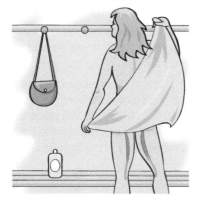

- The semimembranosus is named for its flattened, membranous proximal tendon.

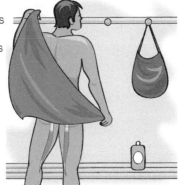

REVIEW QUESTIONS

Circle or fill in the correct answer for each of the following questions. More study resources, including audio pronunciations of muscle names, are provided on the Evolve website at http://evolve.elsevier.com/Muscolino/knowthebody.

1. **What are the three muscles of the hamstring group?**

   _____

   _____

   _____

2. **What are the four muscles of the quadriceps femoris group?**

   _____

   _____

   _____

   _____

3. **What are the three muscles of the gluteal group?**

   _____

   _____

   _____

4. **What is the only muscle of the deep lateral rotator group of the hip joint that attaches to the sacrum?**
   a. Quadratus femoris
   b. Obturator externus
   c. Piriformis
   d. Superior gemellus

5. **Which one of the following muscles is the lateral hamstring muscle?**
   a. Semitendinosus
   b. Rectus femoris
   c. Biceps femoris
   d. Semimembranosus

6. **What is the only quadriceps femoris muscle that crosses the hip joint?**
   a. Vastus lateralis
   b. Vastus medialis
   c. Vastus intermedius
   d. Rectus femoris

7. **What is the most inferior member of the deep lateral rotator group of the hip joint?**
   a. Piriformis
   b. Obturator internus
   c. Inferior gemellus
   d. Quadratus femoris

8. **Which of the following muscles can flex, abduct, and medially rotate the thigh at the hip joint?**
   a. Rectus femoris
   b. Sartorius
   c. TFL
   d. Piriformis

9. **Which of the following muscles can anteriorly tilt the pelvis at the hip joint?**
   a. Rectus femoris
   b. Gluteus maximus
   c. Piriformis
   d. Vastus medialis

10. **Which one of the following muscles attaches into the pes anserine tendon?**
    a. Sartorius
    b. TFL
    c. Rectus femoris
    d. Gluteus maximus

10

CASE STUDY 1

Julia, a 38-year-old woman and competitive cyclist, is experiencing pain on the lateral side of her right thigh from her greater trochanter to her knee joint. The pain is most intense when she is cycling and shortly thereafter. On a pain scale of 0 to 10, she rates the pain at a 6 or 7. She uses ice and heat to reduce pain and takes over-the-counter ibuprofen to manage the pain as needed.

Julia has had no traumatic injury to the region. She has trained for and competed in races for 7 years. Her weekly training regimen had always consisted of twice daily training, Monday through Thursday, resting on Friday, prolonged training on Saturday, and resting again on Sunday. Additionally, she has done weight training on Monday and Thursday. However, approximately 1 month earlier in preparation for an upcoming event, she recently decided to eliminate the second rest day on Sunday and replace it with a second long workout. Her lateral thigh pain began to develop 2 weeks ago and has progressively worsened.

On palpation, the tissue of the lateral thigh was found to be hard and taut. Further, palpation elicited pain at a level of approximately 4 to 7 in the middle of the lateral thigh.

10

QUESTIONS

1. **What soft tissue is likely dysfunctional?**

_____

_____

_____

_____

_____

_____

_____

2. **Why did Julia develop this problem now?**

_____

_____

_____

_____

_____

_____

_____

_____

_____

_____

CASE STUDY 2

A 46-year-old white-collar male client is experiencing sharp shooting sciatic pain that begins in his right gluteal region and shoots down his posterior thigh to the level of his knee joint. He also complains of a general feeling of stiffness in his right low back and buttock. No precipitating trauma occurred to begin this condition. Rather, the pain insidiously began approximately 4 weeks earlier and has been steadily increasing ever since.

He first visited his medical physician, who then referred him to an orthopedist. The orthopedist ordered a magnetic resonance image (MRI) of the lumbar spine, which showed negative for any involvement of the spine. Without a clear diagnosis, the orthopedist recommended a 2-week prescription of an antiinflammatory medication, which the client has declined to take.

On a pain scale of 0 to 10, the pain varies from a level of 2 to 7. Pain and stiffness are worst in the morning when he first awakes (pain level of 7). After taking a hot shower and stretching in the morning, the pain and stiffness largely subside and he feels pretty good (pain level of 2). However, as the day goes by, his pain level gradually increases until by the end of the day; he is back at a level of 7. He states that sitting aggravates the condition, and that driving is the worst.

When asked to identify the location of the pain, he points to the center of the right buttock as the location from which the sharp sciatic pain emanates. He also points to his right sacroiliac joint as another place where he feels pain; he states that here, the pain is more of a dull ache.

QUESTIONS

1. **What musculature should you assess? Why?**

_____

_____

_____

_____

_____

2. **Assuming the musculature you assess is tight, what modalities do you use to treat this client?**

_____

_____

_____

_____

_____

_____

3. **Do you suspect the involvement of any other condition?**

_____

_____

_____

_____

_____

_____

_____

4. **In addition to your in-session treatment, what home advice would you give this client?**

_____

_____

_____

_____

_____

_____

10

Muscles of the Leg and Foot

The muscles of this chapter are primarily involved with motions of the foot at the ankle and subtalar joints and/or the motions of the toes at the metatarsophalangeal (MTP) and interphalangeal (IP) joints.

As a rule, muscles that move the foot originate (attach proximally) and have their bellies in the leg. Leg muscles are usually divided into the four fascial compartments of the leg: anterior, lateral, superficial posterior, and deep posterior.

    The anterior compartment contains the tibialis anterior, extensor digitorum longus, extensor hallucis longus, and fibularis tertius.

    The lateral compartment contains the fibularis longus and fibularis brevis.

    The superficial posterior compartment contains the gastrocnemius, soleus, and plantaris.

    The deep posterior compartment contains the tibialis posterior, flexor digitorum longus, flexor hallucis longus, and popliteus. Some of these muscles are addressed in other chapters.

    The location by compartment helps determine the actions of these muscles. For example, all muscles of the anterior compartment perform dorsiflexion; all muscles of the lateral and posterior compartments perform plantarflexion; and all muscles of the lateral compartment perform eversion. The final determination of exactly what the actions of a muscle of the ankle and subtalar joints will be is where the distal tendon of that muscle crosses these joints (e.g., the belly of the tibialis anterior is located in the anterolateral leg, but its tendon crosses the subtalar joint medially; therefore it inverts the foot).

Muscles that move the toes are usually divided into long extrinsic foot muscles and short intrinsic foot muscles. Extrinsic foot muscles originate (attach proximally) in the leg or thigh and insert (attach distally) in the foot. Intrinsic foot muscles originate and insert (attach proximally and distally) in the foot; in other words, they are wholly located in the foot. The intrinsics of the foot are divided into dorsal and plantar muscles. Generally, dorsal muscles extend the toes; plantar muscles flex the toes. The plantar muscles are further divided into four layers, named Layers I through IV, from superficial to deep. The term *digitorum* refers to toes two through five; the term *hallucis* refers to the big toe.

The companion CD at the back of this book allows you to examine the muscles of this body region, layer by layer, and individual muscle palpation technique videos are available in the Chapter 11 folder on the Evolve website.

OVERVIEW OF FUNCTION: MUSCLES OF THE ANKLE AND SUBTALAR JOINTS

The following general rules regarding actions can be stated for the functional groups of muscles of the ankle and subtalar joints:

- If a muscle crosses the ankle joint anteriorly with a vertical direction to its fibers, it can dorsiflex the foot at the ankle joint by moving the dorsum of the foot toward the anterior (dorsal) surface of the leg.
- If a muscle crosses the ankle joint posteriorly with a vertical direction to its fibers, it can plantarflex the foot at the ankle joint by moving the plantar surface of the foot toward the posterior surface of the leg.
- If a muscle crosses the subtalar joint laterally, it can evert the foot at the subtalar joint by moving the lateral surface of the foot toward the lateral surface of the leg. Note: Eversion is the principle component of pronation.

- If a muscle crosses the subtalar joint medially, it can invert the foot at the subtalar joint by moving the medial surface of the foot toward the medial surface of the leg. Note: Inversion is the principle component of supination.
- Reverse actions occur when the foot is planted on the ground and the leg must move relative to the foot. The same terms can be used to describe these reverse actions. For example, when the anterior (dorsal) surface of the leg moves toward the dorsum of the foot, it is called dorsiflexion of the leg at the ankle joint.

OVERVIEW OF FUNCTION: MUSCLES OF THE TOES

The following general rules regarding actions can be stated for the functional groups of toe muscles:

- Toes two through five can move at three joints: the MTP, proximal interphalangeal (PIP), and distal interphalangeal (DIP) joints. The big toe (toe one) can move at two joints: the MTP and IP joints.
- To move a joint of the toe, the muscle must cross that joint; therefore knowing the attachments of the toe muscles determines which toe joints can be moved by that muscle.
- If a muscle crosses the joints of the toes on the plantar side, it can flex the toe at the joint(s) crossed; if a muscle crosses joints of the toes on the dorsal side, it can extend the toe at the joint(s) crossed.
- Reverse actions involve the origin (proximal attachment) moving toward the insertion (distal one). This occurs when the distal end of the foot is fixed, usually when the foot is planted on the ground (for example, when we toe-off during the gait cycle, the metatarsals of the toes extend toward the proximal phalanger, and therefore the foot extends toward the toes at the MTP joints).

**Anterior View
of the Muscles
of the Right Ankle
and Subtalar Joints**

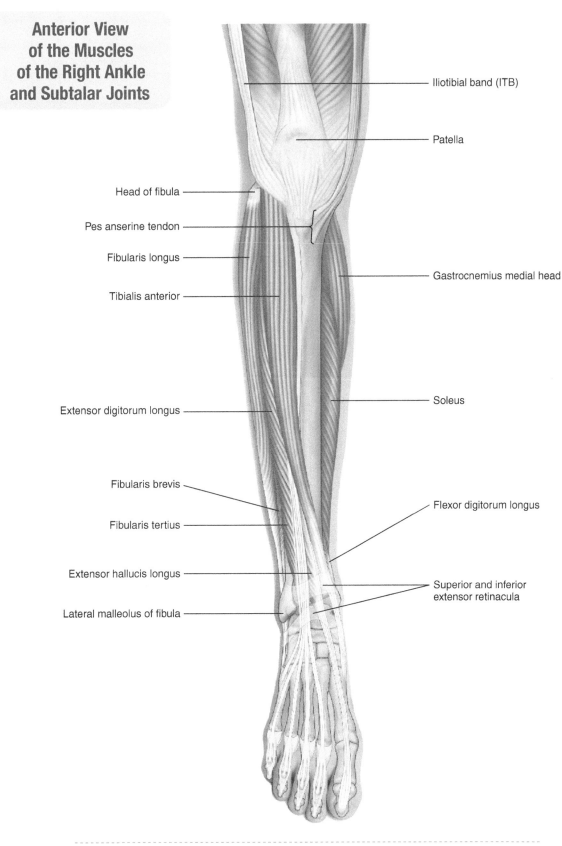

Iliotibial band (ITB)

Patella

Head of fibula

Pes anserine tendon

Fibularis longus

Tibialis anterior

Gastrocnemius medial head

Extensor digitorum longus

Soleus

Fibularis brevis

Fibularis tertius

Flexor digitorum longus

Extensor hallucis longus

Lateral malleolus of fibula

Superior and inferior
extensor retinacula

11

FIGURE 11-1 Anterior view of the muscles of the right ankle and subtalar joints.

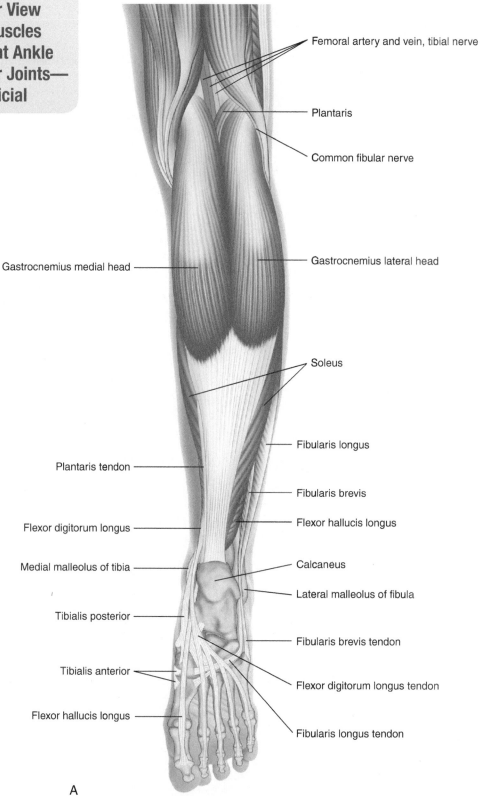

Posterior View of the Muscles of the Right Ankle and Subtalar Joints— Superficial

Femoral artery and vein, tibial nerve

Plantaris

Common fibular nerve

Gastrocnemius medial head

Gastrocnemius lateral head

Soleus

Fibularis longus

Plantaris tendon

Fibularis brevis

Flexor digitorum longus

Flexor hallucis longus

Medial malleolus of tibia

Calcaneus

Lateral malleolus of fibula

Tibialis posterior

Fibularis brevis tendon

Tibialis anterior

Flexor digitorum longus tendon

Flexor hallucis longus

Fibularis longus tendon

A

FIGURE 11-2 Posterior view of the muscles of the right ankle and subtalar joints. **A,** Superficial view.

Posterior View of the Muscles of the Right Ankle and Subtalar Joints—Deep

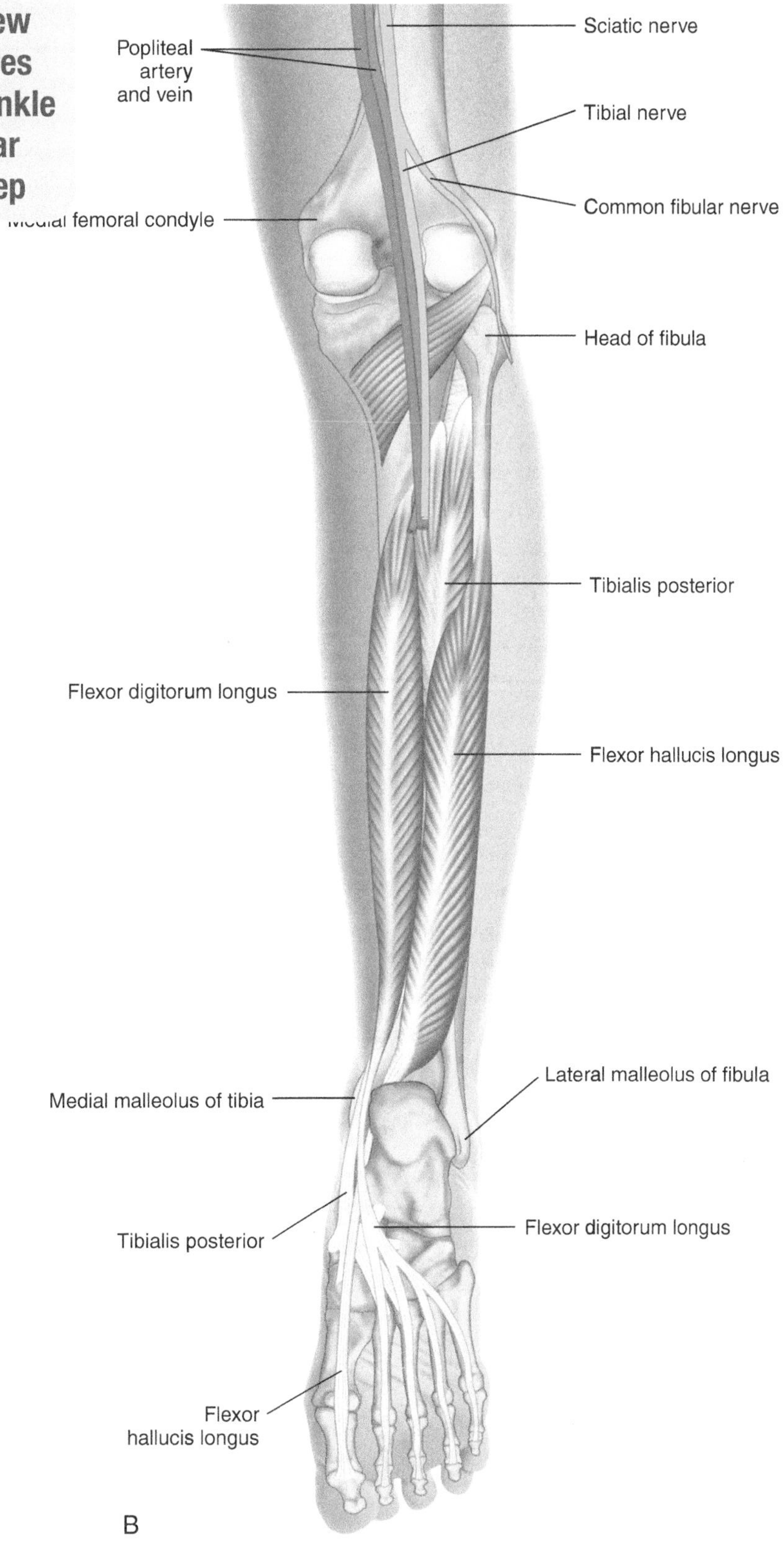

Sciatic nerve

Popliteal artery and vein

Tibial nerve

Common fibular nerve

Medial femoral condyle

Head of fibula

Tibialis posterior

Flexor digitorum longus

Flexor hallucis longus

Medial malleolus of tibia

Lateral malleolus of fibula

Tibialis posterior

Flexor digitorum longus

Flexor hallucis longus

B

FIGURE 11-2, cont'd   Posterior view of the muscles of the right ankle and subtalar joints. **B,** Deep view.

11

Lateral and Medial Views of the Muscles of the Right Ankle and Subtalar Joints

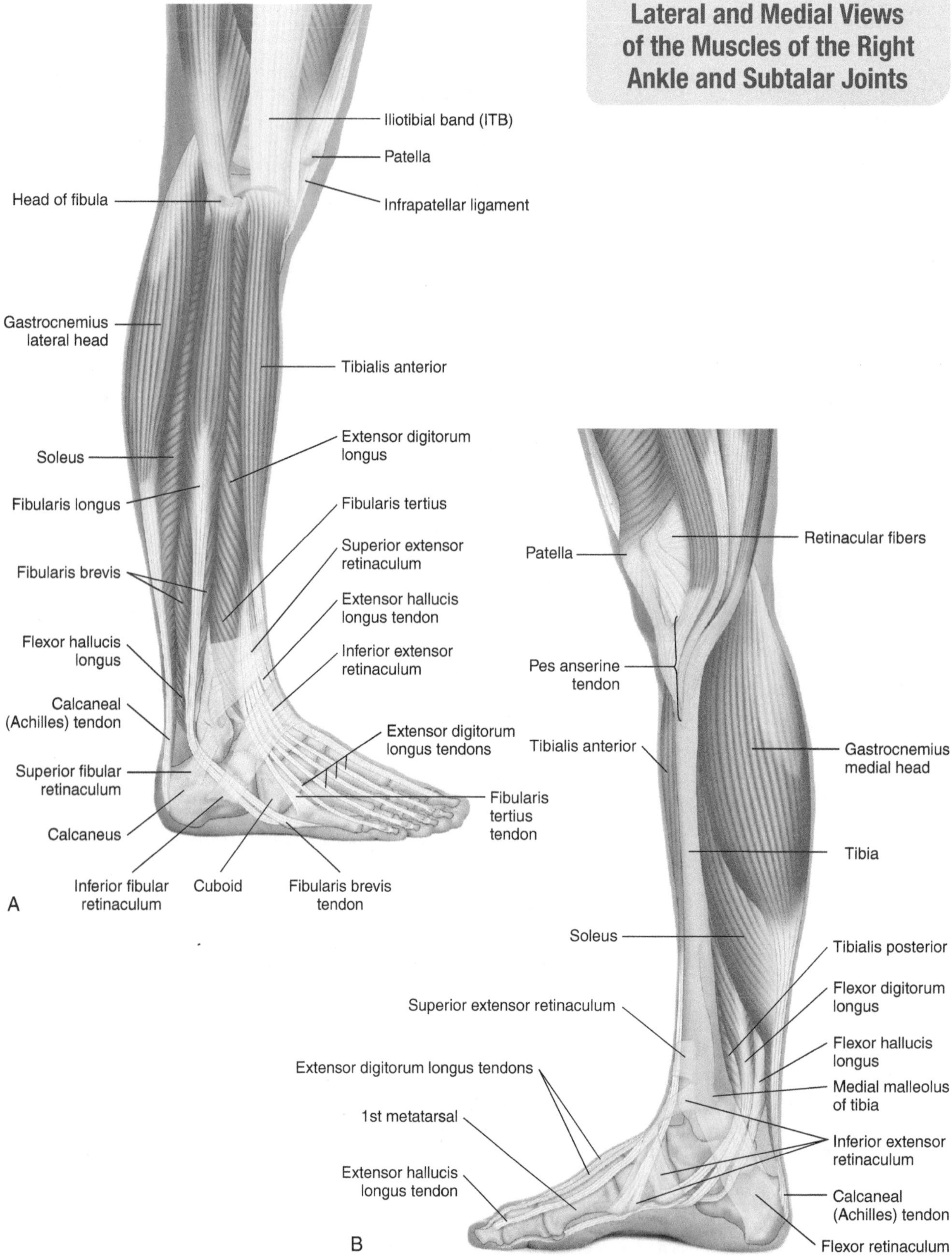

Iliotibial band (ITB)
Patella
Head of fibula
Infrapatellar ligament
Gastrocnemius lateral head
Tibialis anterior
Extensor digitorum longus
Soleus
Fibularis longus
Fibularis tertius
Fibularis brevis
Superior extensor retinaculum
Extensor hallucis longus tendon
Flexor hallucis longus
Inferior extensor retinaculum
Calcaneal (Achilles) tendon
Extensor digitorum longus tendons
Superior fibular retinaculum
Fibularis tertius tendon
Calcaneus
Inferior fibular retinaculum
Cuboid
Fibularis brevis tendon
A
Retinacular fibers
Patella
Pes anserine tendon
Tibialis anterior
Gastrocnemius medial head
Tibia
Soleus
Tibialis posterior
Flexor digitorum longus
Superior extensor retinaculum
Flexor hallucis longus
Extensor digitorum longus tendons
Medial malleolus of tibia
1st metatarsal
Inferior extensor retinaculum
Extensor hallucis longus tendon
Calcaneal (Achilles) tendon
B
Flexor retinaculum

FIGURE 11-3 ***A,*** Lateral view of the muscles of the right ankle and subtalar joints. ***B,*** Medial views of the muscles of the right ankle and subtalar joints—superficial.

Compartments of the Leg and Dorsal View of the Right Foot

ANTERIOR

Anterior Compartment

Tibia

Lateral Compartment

Fibula

Deep Posterior Compartment

MEDIAL

LATERAL

Superficial Posterior Compartment

POSTERIOR

Anterior Compartment:
Tibialis Anterior
Extensor Digitorum Longus
Extensor Hallucis Longus
Fibularis Tertius

Lateral Compartment:
Fibularis Longus
Fibularis Brevis

Superficial Posterior Compartment:
Gastrocnemius
Soleus
Plantaris

Deep Posterior Compartment:
Popliteus
Tibialis Posterior
Flexor Digitorum Longus
Flexor Hallucis Longus

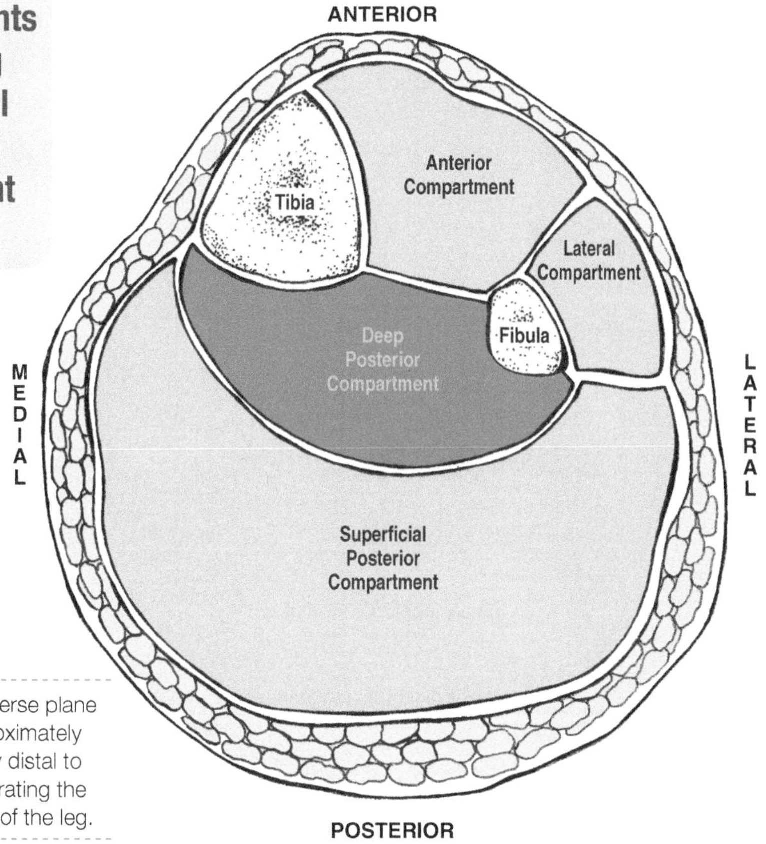

FIGURE 11-4 Transverse plane cross section (approximately one-third of the way distal to the knee joint), illustrating the four compartments of the leg.

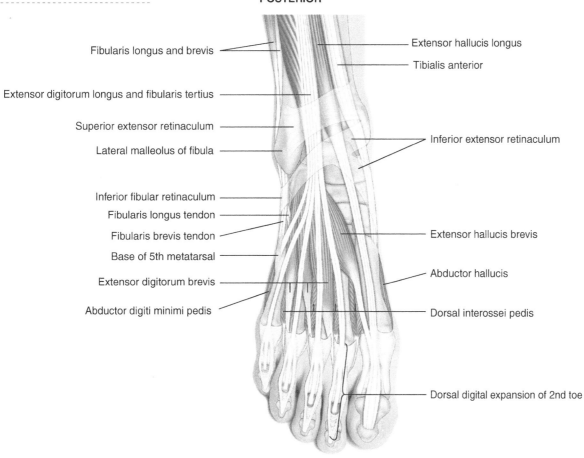

Fibularis longus and brevis

Extensor digitorum longus and fibularis tertius

Superior extensor retinaculum

Lateral malleolus of fibula

Inferior fibular retinaculum
Fibularis longus tendon
Fibularis brevis tendon
Base of 5th metatarsal
Extensor digitorum brevis
Abductor digiti minimi pedis

Extensor hallucis longus

Tibialis anterior

Inferior extensor retinaculum

Extensor hallucis brevis

Abductor hallucis

Dorsal interossei pedis

Dorsal digital expansion of 2nd toe

FIGURE 11-5 Dorsal view of the right foot.

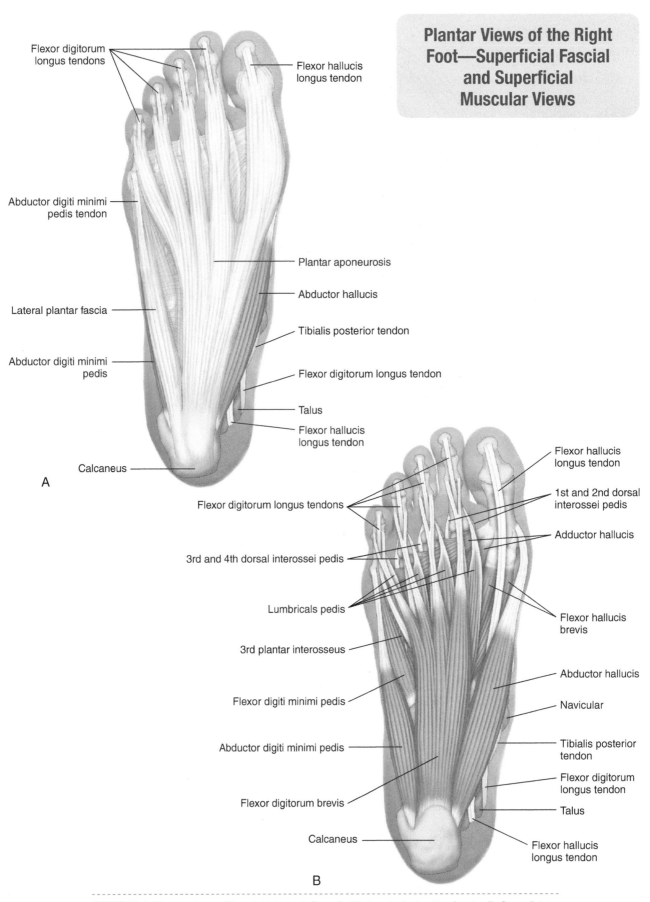

Flexor digitorum longus tendons

Flexor hallucis longus tendon

Abductor digiti minimi pedis tendon

Plantar aponeurosis

Abductor hallucis

Tibialis posterior tendon

Lateral plantar fascia

Flexor digitorum longus tendon

Abductor digiti minimi pedis

Talus

Flexor hallucis longus tendon

Calcaneus

A

Flexor hallucis longus tendon

1st and 2nd dorsal interossei pedis

Flexor digitorum longus tendons

Adductor hallucis

3rd and 4th dorsal interossei pedis

Lumbricals pedis

Flexor hallucis brevis

3rd plantar interosseus

Abductor hallucis

Navicular

Flexor digiti minimi pedis

Tibialis posterior tendon

Abductor digiti minimi pedis

Flexor digitorum longus tendon

Talus

Flexor digitorum brevis

Flexor hallucis longus tendon

Calcaneus

B

FIGURE 11-6 Plantar views of the right foot. **A,** Superficial view, including the fascia. **B,** Superficial muscular view.

1st and 2nd dorsal interossei pedis

3rd and 4th dorsal interossei pedis

3rd plantar interosseus

Flexor digiti minimi pedis

Base of 5th metatarsal

Fibularis longus tendon

Cuboid

Quadratus plantae

Calcaneus

Adductor hallucis

Flexor hallucis brevis

Lumbricals pedis

1st metatarsal

Tibialis anterior tendon

Flexor digitorum longus tendon

Navicular

Tibialis posterior tendon

Flexor hallucis longus tendon

Talus

C

2nd, 3rd, and 4th dorsal interossei pedis

1st and 2nd plantar interossei

3rd plantar interosseus

Flexor digiti minimi pedis

Base of 5th metatarsal

Fibularis longus tendon

Cuboid

1st dorsal interosseus pedis

Adductor hallucis

Flexor hallucis brevis

1st metatarsal

Tibialis anterior tendon

Navicular

Tibialis posterior tendon

Flexor digitorum longus tendon (cut)

Flexor hallucis longus tendon (cut)

D

FIGURE 11-6, cont'd Plantar views of the right foot. **C,** Intermediate view. **D,** Deep view.

MUSCLES OF THE LEG AND FOOT
Tibialis Anterior

Pronunciation **tib-ee-A-lis an-TEE-ri-or**

The tibialis anterior is a superficial muscle in the anterior compartment of the leg. It lies immediately lateral to the shaft of the tibia (Figure 11-7).

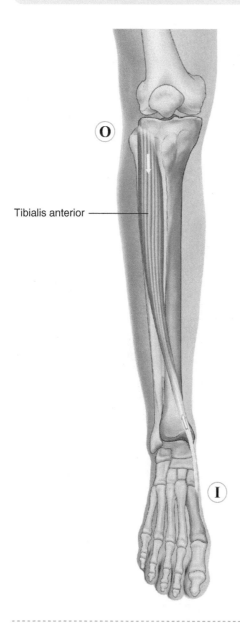

Tibialis anterior

FIGURE 11-7 Anterior view of the right tibialis anterior. *O*, Origin; *I*, insertion.

WHAT'S IN A NAME?

The name, *tibialis anterior*, tells us that this muscle attaches to the tibia and is located anteriorly.

✳ **Derivation:**
tibialis: L. refers to the tibia
anterior: L. before, in front of

ATTACHMENTS

Origin (Proximal Attachment)
- Anterior tibia

Insertion (Distal Attachment)
- Medial foot

ACTIONS

- Dorsiflexes the foot at the ankle joint.
- Inverts the foot at the subtalar joint.

STABILIZATION

Stabilizes the ankle and subtalar joints.

INNERVATION

- Deep fibular nerve

PALPATION

1. The client is supine. Place your resistance hand on the medial side of the distal foot.
2. Resist the client from dorsiflexing and inverting the foot. Look for the distal tendon of the tibialis anterior on the medial side of the ankle joint and foot; it is usually visible (Figure 11-8, *A*).
3. Palpate the distal tendon by strumming perpendicular across it. Continue palpating the tibialis anterior proximally to the lateral tibial condyle by strumming perpendicular to the fibers (Figure 11-8, *B*).
4. Once the tibialis anterior has been located, have the client relax it and palpate to assess its baseline tone.

11

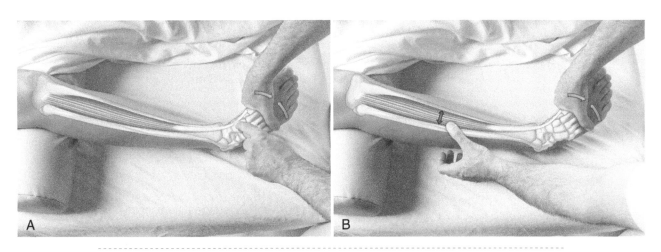

FIGURE 11-8 *A,* With resisted dorsiflexion and inversion of the foot, the distal tendon of the tibialis anterior is usually easily visible. *B,* The belly of the right tibialis anterior is palpated.

TREATMENT CONSIDERATIONS

- The tibialis anterior has a very prominent distal tendon.

- The tibialis anterior and the fibularis longus are known as the *stirrup muscles*. These two muscles both attach at the same location on the medial foot and may be viewed as a stirrup to support the arch structure of the foot.

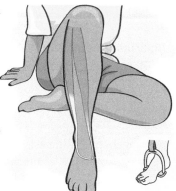

- When the tibialis anterior is tight and painful, especially along its tibial attachment, this condition is usually called *shin splints* or *anterior shin splints*.

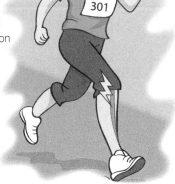

MUSCLES OF THE LEG AND FOOT
Extensor Hallucis Longus

Pronunciation **eks-TEN-sor hal-OO-sis LONG-us**

The extensor hallucis longus is a long extensor of the big toe that is located in the anterior compartment of the leg. Most of its belly is deep to the tibialis anterior and extensor digitorum longus, but its distal tendon is superficial as it crosses the ankle joint and on the dorsal surface of the foot (Figure 11-9).

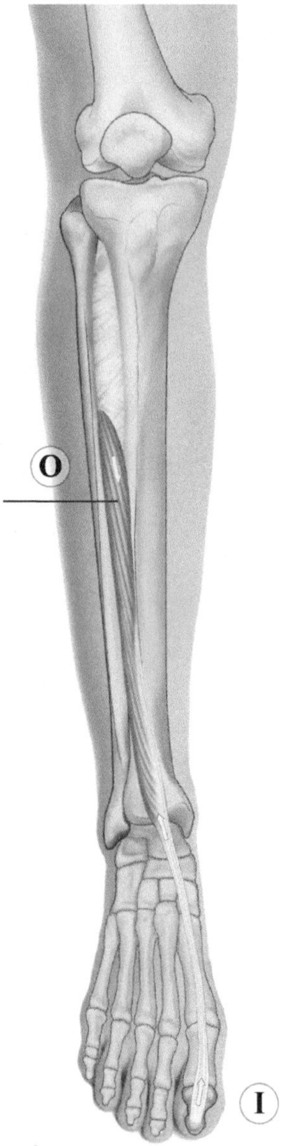

WHAT'S IN A NAME?

The name, *extensor hallucis longus,* tells us that this muscle extends the big toe and is longer than the extensor hallucis brevis.

✳ **Derivation:**
extensor: L. muscle that extends a body part
hallucis: L. refers to the big toe
longus: L. longer

ATTACHMENTS

Origin (Proximal Attachment)
■ Middle anterior fibula

Insertion (Distal Attachment)
■ Dorsal surface of the big toe (toe one)

ACTIONS

The extensor hallucis longus moves the foot at the ankle and subtalar joints and the big toe at the metatarsophalangeal (MTP) and interphalangeal (IP) joints.

■ Extends the big toe.
■ Dorsiflexes the foot (ankle joint).
■ Everts the foot (subtalar joint).

STABILIZATION

Stabilizes the ankle and subtalar joints and the MTP and IP joints of the big toe.

INNERVATION

■ Deep fibular nerve

PALPATION

1. The client is supine. Place the fingers of the resistance hand on the dorsal surface of the distal phalanx of the big toe.

2. Resist the client from extending the big toe at the MTP and IP joints. Look for the tendon of the extensor hallucis longus to become visible.

Extensor hallucis longus

O

I

FIGURE 11-9 Anterior view of the right extensor hallucis longus. *O,* Origin; *I,* insertion.

11

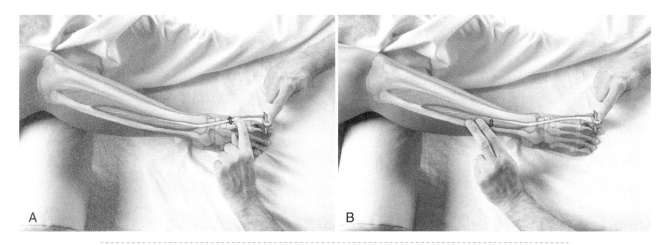

FIGURE 11-10 Palpation of the right extensor hallucis longus as the client extends the big toe against resistance. **A,** Palpation of the distal tendon on the dorsum of the foot. **B,** Palpation of the belly in the anterolateral leg.

3. Palpate the distal tendon by strumming perpendicular across it (Figure 11-10, *A*).

4. Continue palpating the extensor hallucis longus proximally. Once it goes deep to the adjacent musculature, do not strum perpendicular to it. Instead, gently place your finger pads over it, and feel for its contraction when the big toe extends (Figure 11-10, *B*).

▌ TREATMENT CONSIDERATION

- When we swing forward during the gait cycle, we usually extend our toes so they do not drag on the ground.

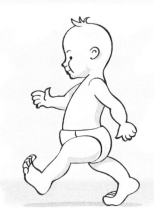

11

MUSCLES OF THE LEG AND FOOT
Extensor Digitorum Longus

Pronunciation   **eks-TEN-sor dij-i-TOE-rum LONG-us**

The extensor digitorum longus is a long extensor of toes two through five that is located in the anterior compartment of the leg. Most of it is superficial except for a small aspect of its proximal belly, which is deep to the tibialis anterior and fibularis longus (Figure 11-11).

WHAT'S IN A NAME?

The name, *extensor digitorum longus,* tells us that this muscle extends the digits (i.e., toes two through five) and is longer than the extensor digitorum brevis.

* **Derivation:**
  extensor: L. muscle that extends a body part
  digitorum: L. refers to a digit (toe)
  longus: L. longer

ATTACHMENTS

Origin (Proximal Attachment)
- Proximal anterior fibula

Insertion (Distal Attachment)
- Dorsal surface of toes two through five

ACTIONS

The extensor digitorum longus moves the foot at the ankle and subtalar joints and toes two through five at the metatarsophalangeal (MTP) and interphalangeal (IP–proximal interphalangeal [PIP] and distal interphalangeal [DIP] joints).

- Extends toes two through five at the MTP and IP joints.
- Dorsiflexes the foot at the ankle joint.
- Everts the foot at the subtalar joint.

STABILIZATION

Stabilizes the ankle and subtalar joints, and the MTP and IP joints of toes two through five.

INNERVATION

- Deep fibular nerve

PALPATION

1. The client is supine. Place your finger pads of the resistance hand on the dorsal surfaces of toes two to five.

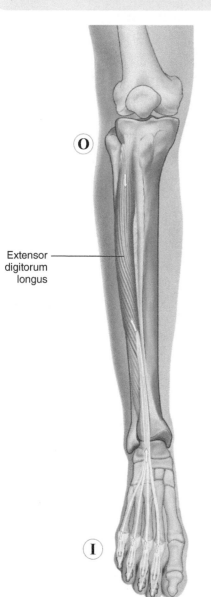

Extensor digitorum longus

O

I

FIGURE 11-11 Anterior view of the right extensor digitorum longus. The fibularis tertius has been ghosted in. *O,* Origin; *I,* insertion.

11

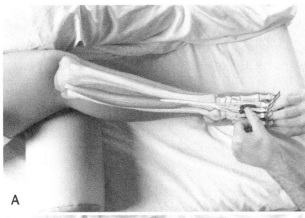

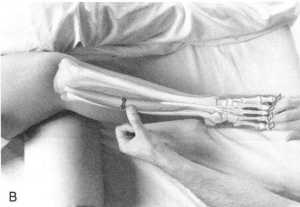

A

B

FIGURE 11-12 The right extensor digitorum longus is palpated as the client extends toes two to five against resistance. *A,* Palpation of the distal tendons on the dorsum of the foot. *B,* Palpation of the belly in the anterolateral leg.

2. Resist the client from extending toes two to five at the MTP and IP joints. Look for the tendons of the extensor digitorum longus to become visible on the dorsum of the foot.

3. Palpate the distal tendons by strumming perpendicularly across them (Figure 11-12, *A*).

4. Continue palpating the extensor digitorum longus proximally by strumming perpendicular to the fibers (Figure 11-12, *B*).

TREATMENT CONSIDERATIONS

■ The distal attachment of the extensor digitorum longus spreads out to become a fibrous aponeurotic expansion that covers much of the dorsal, medial, and lateral sides of the toes. This structure is called the *dorsal digital expansion* (see page 391) and is an attachment site for many intrinsic foot muscles.

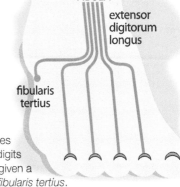

■ The most distal and lateral parts of the extensor digitorum longus (which arises from the distal one-third of the fibula) does not attach onto the digits (toes); therefore it is given a separate name, the *fibularis tertius*.

11

MUSCLES OF THE LEG AND FOOT: Fibularis Group
Fibularis Longus; Fibularis Brevis; Fibularis Tertius

Pronunciation   **fib-you-LA-ris LONG-us • fib-you-LA-ris BRE-vis • fib-you-LA-ris TER-she-us**

The fibularis group is located laterally on the leg, attached to the fibula. It is composed of the fibularis longus, brevis, and tertius (Figure 11-13). All three fibularis muscles evert the foot at the subtalar joint. The fibularis longus and brevis are located in the lateral compartment; the longus is superficial to the brevis; the fibularis tertius is superficial and located in the anterior compartment. The fibularis muscles used to be called the *peroneus muscles*.

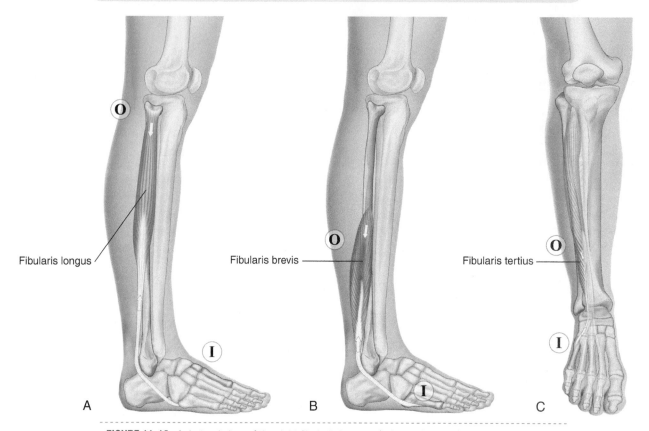

Fibularis longus

Fibularis brevis

Fibularis tertius

A   B   C

FIGURE 11-13 A, Lateral view of the right fibularis longus. **B,** Lateral view of the right fibularis brevis. **C,** Anterior view of the right fibularis tertius. The extensor digitorum longus has been ghosted in. *O,* Origin; *I,* insertion.

WHAT'S IN A NAME?

The name, *fibularis longus,* tells us that this muscle attaches to the fibula and is longer than the fibularis brevis.

The name, *fibularis brevis,* tells us that this muscle attaches onto the fibula and is shorter than the fibularis longus.

The name, *fibularis tertius,* tells us that this muscle attaches to the fibula and is the third fibularis muscle.

✳ **Derivation:**
fibularis: L. refers to the fibula
longus: L. longer
brevis: L. shorter
tertius: L. third

ATTACHMENTS

Fibularis Longus

Origin (Proximal Attachment)
- Proximal lateral fibula

Insertion (Distal Attachment)
- Medial foot

Fibularis Brevis

Origin (Proximal Attachment)
- Distal lateral fibula

Insertion (Distal Attachment)
- Fifth metatarsal

Fibularis Tertius

Origin (Proximal Attachment)
- Distal anterior fibula

Insertion (Distal Attachment)
- Fifth metatarsal

ACTIONS

Fibularis Longus and Fibularis Brevis
- Evert the foot at the subtalar joint.
- Plantarflex the foot at the ankle joint.

Fibularis Tertius
- Everts the foot at the subtalar joint.
- Dorsiflexes the foot at the ankle joint.

STABILIZATION

Stabilize the ankle and subtalar joints.

INNERVATION

- Superficial fibular nerve (longus and brevis)
- Deep fibular nerve (tertius)

PALPATION

Fibularis Longus and Fibularis Brevis

1. The client is side lying. Place your palpating finger pads on the lateral side of the fibula, just distal to the head of the fibula. Place the resistance hand on the lateral side of the foot.
2. Resist the client from everting the foot at the subtalar joint. Feel for the contraction of the fibularis longus (Figure 11-14, *A*).
3. Continue palpating the fibularis longus distally by strumming perpendicular to the fibers. The fibularis longus becomes tendon approximately halfway down the leg. The distal tendon can usually be seen immediately posterior to the lateral malleolus of the fibula (Figure 11-14, *B*).
4. To palpate the fibularis brevis, palpate on either side of the fibularis longus in the distal half of the leg (Figure 11-15, *A*).
5. The distal tendon of the fibularis brevis is often visible and palpable in the proximal foot distal to the lateral malleolus of the fibula (Figure 11-15, *B*).

11

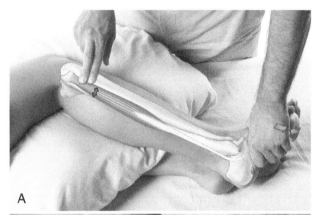

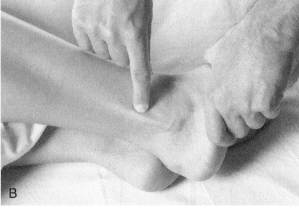

FIGURE 11-14 *A,* The belly of the fibularis longus is palpated as the client everts the foot against resistance. ***B,*** When resistance is applied to eversion of the foot, the distal tendon of the fibularis longus is often visible just proximal to the lateral malleolus of the fibula.

Turn page to ◉ more.

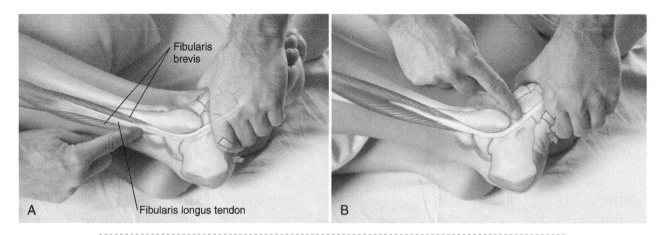

FIGURE 11-15 The right fibularis brevis is palpated as the client everts the foot against resistance. **A,** The fibularis brevis belly is palpated immediately posterior to the fibularis longus tendon. **B,** Its distal tendon is palpated distal to the lateral malleolus.

11

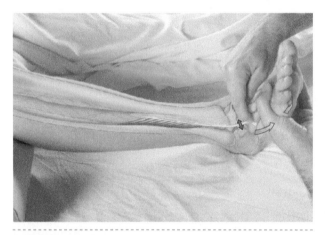

FIGURE 11-16 Anterolateral view of the right fibularis tertius demonstrates palpation of the distal tendon of the fibularis tertius as the client everts and dorsiflexes the foot against resistance. The extensor digitorum longus has been ghosted in.

Fibularis Tertius

1. To palpate the fibularis tertius, find the distal tendon of the extensor digitorum longus on the dorsum of the foot that goes to the little toe; then palpate directly lateral to it, feeling for a tendon that goes to the fifth metatarsal. It may not be visible; therefore you may need to strum perpendicular to its fiber direction to feel for it; it may even be necessary to gently use a fingernail to feel it.

2. If the fibularis tertius is not readily palpable, then resist the client from everting and dorsiflexing the foot and palpate again for its tendon (Figure 11-16).

TREATMENT CONSIDERATIONS

- The distal tendon of the fibularis longus follows an unusual path; it crosses posterior to the lateral malleolus to enter the lateral side of the foot, where it crosses posterior to the cuboid and then dives deep into the plantar side of the foot. It finally attaches onto the medial side of the foot at the same location as the attachment of the tibialis anterior (first cuneiform and first metatarsal).

- The fibularis longus and the tibialis anterior are known as the *stirrup muscles.* These two muscles both attach at the same location on the medial foot and may be viewed to act as a stirrup to support the arch structure of the foot.

- The fibularis longus and the fibularis brevis should be strengthened in people who have had inversion sprains of the ankle joint.

- The fibularis tertius is actually the most distal and lateral part of the extensor digitorum longus. Its fibers do not attach onto a digit (a phalanx); for this reason the fibularis tertius is given a separate name and considered to be a separate muscle from the extensor digitorum longus.

- The fibularis tertius is sometimes missing.

Notes

MUSCLES OF THE LEG AND FOOT: Triceps Surae Group
Gastrocnemius; Soleus

Pronunciation GAS-trok-NEE-me-us • SO-lee-us

11

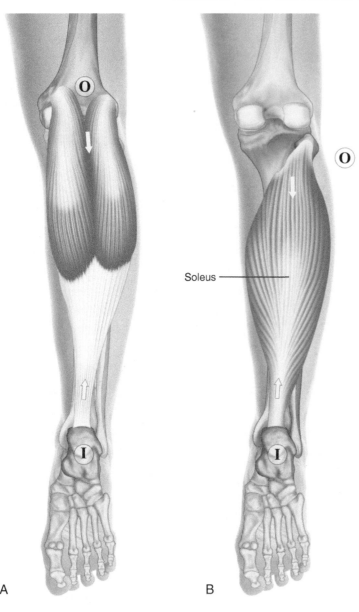

Soleus

A

B

The triceps surae group of the superficial posterior compartment of the leg is composed of the soleus and the two heads (medial and lateral) of the gastrocnemius (Figure 11-17). The gastrocnemius and soleus are grouped together as the triceps surae because they attach together onto the calcaneus via the calcaneal (Achilles) tendon. From the posterior perspective, the gastrocnemius is superficial to the soleus. However, the soleus is superficial in the lateral and medial leg.

FIGURE 11-17 *A,* Posterior view of the right gastrocnemius, *B,* Posterior view of the right soleus. *O,* Origin; *I,* insertion.

WHAT'S IN A NAME?

The name, *gastrocnemius,* tells us that this muscle gives the posterior leg its belly shape. (The contour of the posterior leg is the result of the two bellies of the gastrocnemius.)

The name, *soleus,* tells us that this muscle attaches onto the sole (calcaneus) of the foot.

✳ **Derivation:**
gastro: Gr. stomach
nemius: Gr. leg
soleus: L. sole of the foot

ATTACHMENTS

Gastrocnemius

Origin (Proximal Attachment)

■ Medial and lateral femoral condyles

Insertion (Distal Attachment)

■ Calcaneus via the calcaneal (Achilles) tendon

Soleus

Origin (Proximal Attachment)

■ Posterior tibia and fibula

Insertion (Distal Attachment)

■ Calcaneus via the calcaneal (Achilles) tendon

ACTIONS

■ Plantarflex the foot at the ankle joint (gastrocnemius and the soleus)

■ Flexes the leg at the knee joint (gastrocnemius only)

STABILIZATION

Both the gastrocnemius and the soleus stabilize the ankle and subtalar joints. The gastrocnemius also stabilizes the knee joint.

INNERVATION

■ Tibial nerve

PALPATION

Gastrocnemius

1. The client is prone with the knee joint fully or nearly fully extended. Place your palpating finger pads on the proximal posterior leg. Place the resistance hand on the plantar surface of the foot.

2. Ask the client to plantarflex the foot against your resistance. Feel for the contraction of the gastrocnemius (Figure 11-18, *A*). Palpate the medial and lateral bellies of the gastrocnemius in the proximal posterior leg.

3. Approximately halfway down the leg, the gastrocnemius becomes tendon. Palpate the tendon all the way to its attachment on the posterior surface of the calcaneus via the Achilles tendon (Figure 11-18, *B*).

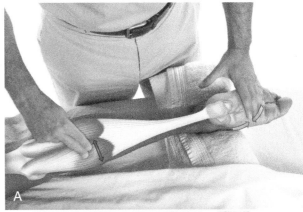

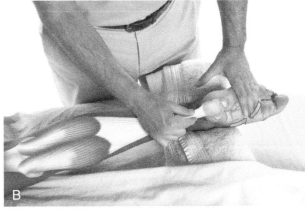

FIGURE 11-18 Palpation of the right gastrocnemius as the client plantarflexes the foot against resistance. *A,* Palpation of the medial belly. *B,* Palpation of the calcaneal (Achilles) tendon with two fingers on either side of the tendon just proximal to the calcaneus.

Soleus

1. The client is prone with the knee joint flexed to approximately 90 degrees. Place your palpating finger pads on the proximal posterior leg. Place the resistance hand on the plantar surface of the foot.

2. Ask the client to plantarflex the foot against gentle resistance. Feel for the contraction of the soleus deep to (through) the gastrocnemius (Figure 11-19, *A*).

3. Palpate the soleus to its proximal attachment, and palpate it distally to its distal attachment on the posterior calcaneus via the Achilles tendon.

4. The soleus is superficial and can be palpated in the lateral leg (Figure 11-19, *B*).

   Note: A portion of the soleus is also superficial and can also be palpated on the medial side of the proximal leg.

Turn page to more.

11

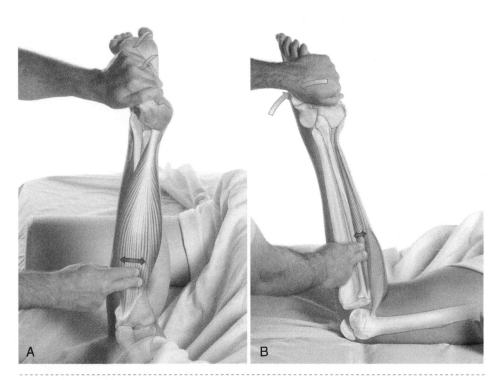

FIGURE 11-19 Palpation of the right soleus as the client plantarflexes the foot against gentle resistance with the knee joint flexed. *A,* Palpation of the posterior aspect through the gastrocnemius. *B,* Palpation of the lateral aspect where the soleus is superficial.

TREATMENT CONSIDERATIONS

- The Achilles tendon derives its name from the Greek myth in which Achilles went into battle to rescue Helen of Troy. When he was young, to make him invulnerable to poison arrows, his mother dipped him into the River Styx. However, she held him by his posterior ankle (i.e., heel). Therefore he was vulnerable in that one spot; hence, the expression *Achilles' heel* denotes a person's weakness. Unfortunately, Paris hit him with a poison arrow in his heel and he died. The relevance to anatomy is that if the Achilles tendon ruptures, an individual loses the ability to walk and/or run, which makes him or her vulnerable and weak.

- Excessive use of high-heeled shoes can result in chronically shortened triceps surae muscles.

- The gastrocnemius and soleus muscles are both stretched by dorsiflexing the ankle joint. Keeping the knee joint extended preferentially stretches the gastrocnemius; flexing the knee joint preferentially stretches the soleus.

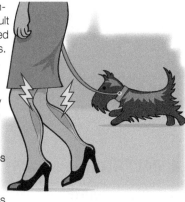

- The soleus is a thick muscle, largely accounting for the contours of the gastrocnemius being so visible. ("Behind every great gastrocnemius is a great soleus." ☺)

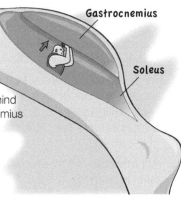

Notes

MUSCLES OF THE LEG AND FOOT
Plantaris

Pronunciation **plan-TA-ris**

The plantaris is a small muscle in the superficial posterior compartment of the leg. It has a very small belly with an extremely long tendon (Figure 11-20). Most of the plantaris is deep to the soleus.

WHAT'S IN A NAME?

The name, *plantaris,* tells us that this muscle attaches onto the calcaneus, a bone of the plantar surface of the foot.

✳ **Derivation:**
plantaris: L. refers to the plantar side of the foot

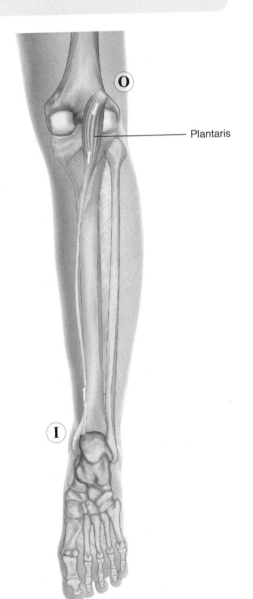

Plantaris

ATTACHMENTS

Origin (Proximal Attachment)
■ Distal posterolateral femur

Insertion (Distal Attachment)
■ Calcaneus

ACTIONS
■ Plantarflexes the foot at the ankle joint.
■ Flexes the leg at the knee joint.

STABILIZATION
Stabilizes the ankle, subtalar, and knee joints.

INNERVATION
■ Tibial nerve

PALPATION

1. To palpate the plantaris, begin with gentle palpation in the center of the popliteal fossa and gradually move laterally until you feel the presence of the muscle tissue that contracts with plantarflexion of the foot at the ankle joint (Figure 11-21). You are now on the plantaris. Discerning the plantaris from the lateral head of the gastrocnemius is difficult because these two muscles have identical actions.

FIGURE 11-20 Posterior view of the right plantaris. The popliteus has been ghosted in. *O,* Origin; *I,* insertion.

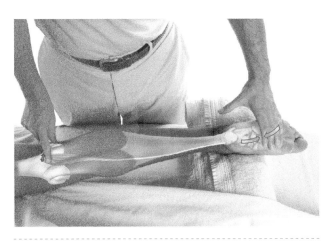

FIGURE 11-21 Palpation of the plantaris as the client plantarflexes the foot against resistance.

TREATMENT CONSIDERATIONS

■ The name plantaris is misleading, because this muscle does not attach onto the plantar surface of the foot in humans (although it does attach onto the posterior calcaneus, which is near the plantar surface). In other primates, the plantaris curves around the calcaneus to attach into the plantar fascia, thereby actually attaching onto the plantar surface of the foot.

■ The distal tendon of the plantaris muscle also attaches into the calcaneus, next to the Achilles tendon. Some sources group the two heads of the gastrocnemius, the soleus, and the plantaris as the quadriceps surae group.

11

MUSCLES OF THE LEG AND FOOT:
Tom, Dick, and Harry Group
Tibialis Posterior; Flexor Digitorum Longus; Flexor Hallucis Longus

Pronunciation   **tib-ee-A-lis pos-TEE-ri-or • FLEKS-or dij-i-TOE-rum LONG-us •
FLEKS-or hal-OO-sis LONG-us**

The Tom, Dick, and Harry group is located in the deep posterior compartment of the leg and is composed of the tibialis posterior, flexor digitorum longus, and flexor hallucis longus (Figure 11-22). Posteriorly, they are deep to the soleus, but they do have some superficial exposure in the distal medial leg. They are grouped together because all of their distal tendons cross posterior and distal to the medial malleolus of the tibia; therefore they all perform inversion and plantarflexion of the foot.

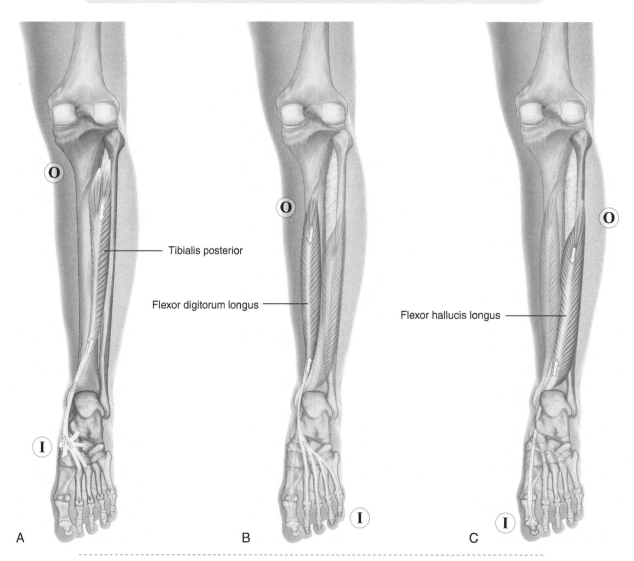

Tibialis posterior

Flexor digitorum longus

Flexor hallucis longus

A

B

C

FIGURE 11-22 *A,* Posterior view of the right tibialis posterior. *B,* Posterior view of the right flexor digitorum longus. The flexor hallucis longus has been ghosted in. *C,* Posterior view of the right flexor hallucis longus. The flexor digitorum longus has been ghosted in. *O,* Origin; *I,* insertion.

11

The name, *tibialis posterior,* tells us that this muscle attaches to the tibia and is located in the posterior leg.

The name, *flexor digitorum longus,* tells us that this muscle flexes the digits (toes) and is longer than the flexor digitorum brevis.

The name, *flexor hallucis longus,* tells us that this muscle flexes the big toe and is longer than the flexor hallucis brevis.

✳ Derivation:
tibialis: L. refers to the tibia
posterior: L. behind, toward the back
flexor: L. muscle that flexes a body part
digitorum: L. refers to a digit (toe)
hallucis: L. big toe
longus: L. longer

ATTACHMENTS

Tibialis Posterior

Origin (Proximal Attachment)
- Posterior tibia and fibula

Insertion (Distal Attachment)
- Navicular tuberosity

Flexor Digitorum Longus

Origin (Proximal Attachment)
- Middle posterior tibia

Insertion (Distal Attachment)
- Plantar surface of toes two through five

Flexor Hallucis Longus

Origin (Proximal Attachment)
- Distal posterior fibula

Insertion (Distal Attachment)
- Plantar surface of the big toe (toe one)

ACTIONS

All three muscles of this group plantarflex the foot at the ankle joint and invert the foot at the subtalar joint. The flexor digitorum longus also moves toes two through five at the metatarsophalangeal (MTP) and interphalangeal (IP–proximal interphalangeal [PIP] and distal interphalangeal [DIP] joints). The flexor hallucis longus also moves the big toe (toe one) at the IP joint.

Tibialis Posterior
- Plantarflexes the foot.
- Inverts the foot.

Flexor Digitorum Longus
- Flexes toes two through five at the MTP and IP joints.
- Plantarflexes the foot.
- Inverts the foot.

Flexor Hallucis Longus
- Flexes the big toe at the MTP and IP joints.
- Plantarflexes the foot.
- Inverts the foot.

STABILIZATION
- All three stabilize the ankle and subtalar joints.
- The flexor digitorum longus and flexor hallucis longus also stabilize the MTP and IP joints of the toes.

INNERVATION
- Tibial nerve

PALPATION

Tibialis Posterior
1. The client is prone with a roll under the ankles. If resistance is needed, place your resistance hand on the foot.
2. Ask the client to plantarflex the foot at the ankle joint and invert the foot at the subtalar joint. Look for the distal tendon of the tibialis posterior immediately posterior and distal to the medial malleolus of the tibia. If needed, resistance can be added (Figure 11-23, *A*).
3. Once located, strum perpendicularly across the tendon as the client alternately contracts and relaxes the muscle. Palpate the tendon distally as far as possible.
4. The belly of the tibialis posterior is located very deep in the posterior compartment of the leg. Gently press over the belly in the midline of the posterior leg, and ask the client to invert the foot. Feel for its contraction (Figure 11-23, *B*).

Turn page to 👁 more.

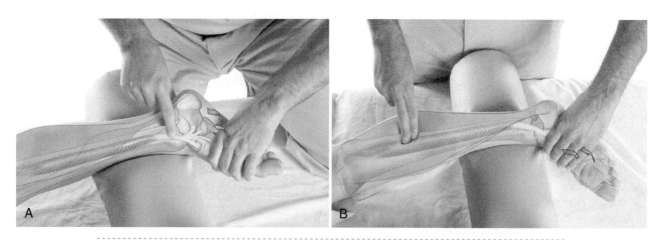

FIGURE 11-23 Palpation of the tibialis posterior as the client plantarflexes and inverts the foot against resistance. **A,** Visualization of the distal tendon near the medial malleolus. **B,** Palpation proximally of the belly deep to the gastrocnemius and soleus. Note: The gastrocnemius and soleus have been ghosted in both *A* and *B*.

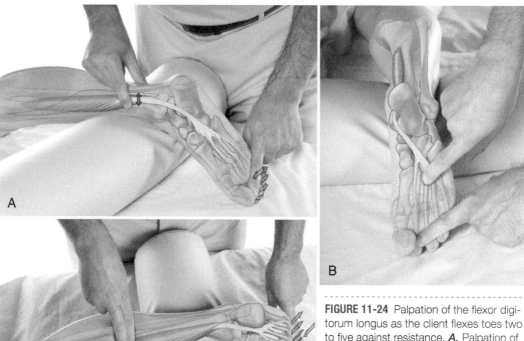

FIGURE 11-24 Palpation of the flexor digitorum longus as the client flexes toes two to five against resistance. **A,** Palpation of the belly in the distal medial leg. **B,** Palpation of the distal tendons in the plantar foot. **C,** Palpation proximally of the belly deep in the posterior leg. Note: The gastrocnemius and soleus have been ghosted in parts A and C.

Flexor Digitorum Longus

1. The client is prone with a roll under the ankles. If resistance is needed, place your resistance fingers on toes two through five.

2. Part of the belly of the flexor digitorum longus is superficial in the distal medial leg between the soleus and the shaft of the tibia (see Figure 11-3, *B*). Ask the client to flex toes two to five; feel for its contraction (Figure 11-24, *A*). If needed, resistance can be added.

3. Within the plantar foot, the distal tendons of the flexor digitorum longus are fairly superficial and can usually be palpated if the client alternately contracts and relaxes the muscle (Figure 11-24, *B*).

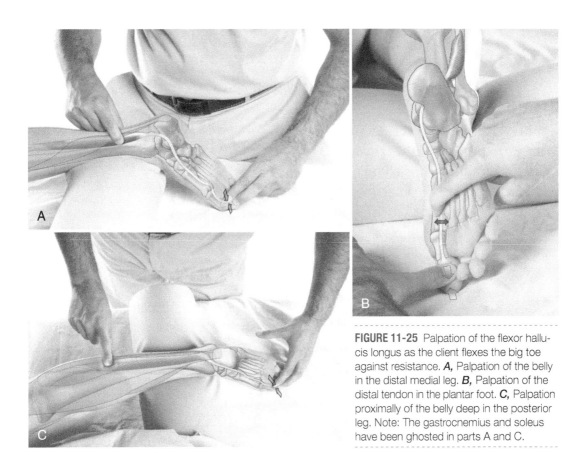

FIGURE 11-25 Palpation of the flexor hallucis longus as the client flexes the big toe against resistance. **A,** Palpation of the belly in the distal medial leg. **B,** Palpation of the distal tendon in the plantar foot. **C,** Palpation proximally of the belly deep in the posterior leg. Note: The gastrocnemius and soleus have been ghosted in parts A and C.

4. The belly of the flexor digitorum longus is located deep in the posterior compartment of the leg. To palpate its belly, press gently over it in the posterior medial leg, ask the client to flex toes two to five. Feel for its contraction (Figure 11-24, *C*).

Flexor Hallucis Longus

1. A small part of the distal belly of the flexor hallucis longus is superficial in the distal medial leg between the flexor digitorum longus and the calcaneal tendon (see Figure 11-3, *B*). Ask the client to flex the big toe. Feel for its contraction (Figure 11-25, *A*). If needed, resistance can be added.

2. Once the flexor hallucis longus has been found, strum perpendicular to its fibers and try to follow it as far distally as possible. At the level of the medial malleolus, its distal tendon runs quite deep and is difficult to palpate.

3. Within the plantar foot, the distal tendon of the flexor hallucis longus is fairly superficial and can usually be palpated if the client alternately contracts and relaxes the muscle by flexing the big toe (Figure 11-25, *B*).

4. The belly of the flexor hallucis longus is located deep in the posterior compartment of the leg. Gently press over it in the posterior lateral leg, and ask the client to flex the big toe. Feel for its contraction (Figure 11-25, *C*).

TREATMENT CONSIDERATIONS

■ It is worth noting that the location of the muscle bellies of the Tom, Dick, and Harry muscles in the posterior leg is, from medial to lateral, Dick, Tom, and Harry (i.e., flexor digitorum longus, tibialis posterior, and flexor hallucis longus).

■ The tibialis posterior plays an important role in supporting and stabilizing the arch structure of the foot. Because the tibialis posterior helps support the arch (medial longitudinal arch) of the foot, some sources consider it to be the medial stirrup muscle, instead of the tibialis anterior.

■ When the tibialis posterior is tight and painful, this condition is often called *shin splints* or *posterior shin splints.*

■ For the tendons of the flexor digitorum longus to reach their insertion (distal attachment) on the toes, the tendons of the flexor digitorum brevis split, and the tendons of the flexor digitorum longus then pass through these splits to continue on to the distal phalanges.)

■ Because the four individual distal tendons of the flexor digitorum longus split from one common distal tendon, the flexor digitorum longus does not allow for individual control of toes two through five.

MUSCLES OF THE LEG AND FOOT
Popliteus

Pronunciation   **pop-LIT-ee-us**

The popliteus is located in the deep posterior compartment of the leg, deep to the gastrocnemius and proximal to the soleus. It crosses the knee joint from lateral on the femur to medial on the tibia (Figure 11-26).

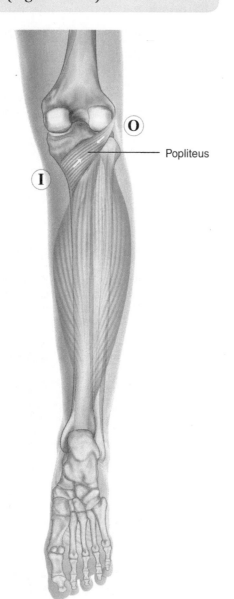

Popliteus

FIGURE 11-26 Posterior view of the right popliteus. The soleus has been ghosted in. *O,* Origin; *I,* insertion.

WHAT'S IN A NAME?

The name, *popliteus,* tells us that this muscle is located in the posterior knee.

✳ **Derivation:**
  popliteus: L. ham of the knee (refers to the posterior knee)

ATTACHMENTS

Origin (Proximal Attachment)
■ Distal posterolateral femur

Insertion (Distal Attachment)
■ Proximal posteromedial tibia

ACTIONS

The popliteus moves the leg or the thigh at the knee joint.
■ Medially rotates the leg.
■ Flexes the leg.
■ Laterally rotates the thigh (at the knee joint).

STABILIZATION

Stabilizes the knee joint.

INNERVATION

■ Tibial nerve

PALPATION

1. The client is prone with the leg flexed 90 degrees at the knee joint. Curl your palpating finger pads around the posterior side of the medial border of the proximal tibia. If resistance is given, place the resistance hand on the distal leg (just proximal to the ankle joint).

2. Ask the client to medially rotate the leg at the knee joint. Feel for the contraction of the popliteus. Resistance can be given if desired (Figure 11-27).

3. Once the tibial attachment of the popliteus has been felt, try to continue palpating the popliteus through the gastrocnemius toward its proximal attachment while the client is alternately contracting and relaxing it by medially rotating the leg at the knee joint.

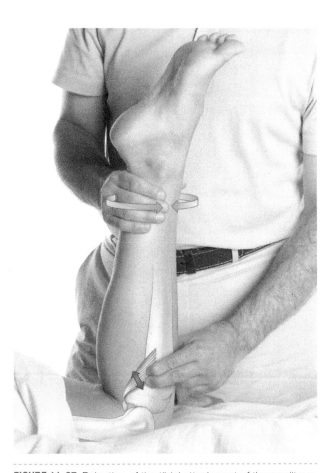

FIGURE 11-27 Palpation of the tibial attachment of the popliteus as the client medially rotates the leg against resistance.

TREATMENT CONSIDERATIONS

- The popliteus also attaches into the lateral meniscus of the knee joint. This attachment helps prevent impingement of the lateral meniscus between the femur and tibia during flexion of the knee joint.

11

MUSCLES OF THE LEG AND FOOT:
Intrinsic Foot—Dorsal Surface
Extensor Digitorum Brevis; Extensor Hallucis Brevis

Pronunciation **eks-TEN-sor dij-i-TOE-rum BRE-vis • eks-TEN-sor hal-OO-sis BRE-vis**

The extensor digitorum brevis and extensor hallucis brevis are two intrinsic foot muscles of the dorsal surface of the foot (Figure 11-28). Except for the distal tendons of the extensor digitorum longus and fibularis tertius, they are superficial.

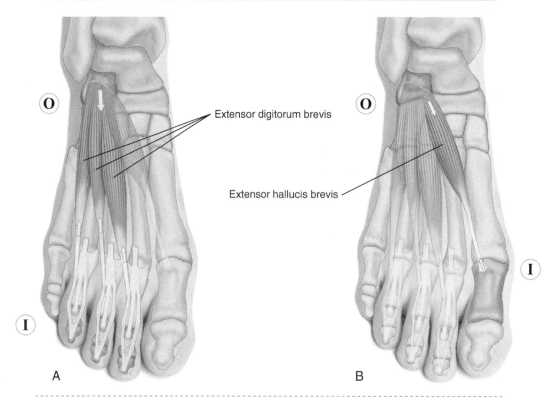

A B

FIGURE 11-28 *A*, Dorsal view of the right extensor digitorum brevis. The extensor hallucis brevis has been ghosted in. ***B*,** Dorsal view of the right extensor hallucis brevis. The extensor digitorum brevis has been ghosted in. *O*, Origin; *I*, insertion.

WHAT'S IN A NAME?

The name, *extensor digitorum brevis,* tells us that this muscle extends the digits (i.e., toes) and is shorter than the extensor digitorum longus.

The name, *extensor hallucis brevis,* tells us that this muscle extends the big toe and is shorter than the extensor hallucis longus.

✳ **Derivation:**
extensor: L. muscle that extends a body part
digitorum: L. refers to a digit (toe)
hallucis: L. refers to the big toe
brevis: L. shorter

ATTACHMENTS

Extensor Digitorum Brevis

Origin (Proximal Attachment)
■ Dorsal surface of the calcaneus

Insertion (Distal Attachment)
■ Toes two through four

Extensor Hallucis Brevis

Origin (Proximal Attachment)

■ Dorsal surface of the calcaneus

Insertion (Distal Attachment)

■ Dorsal surface of the big toe (toe one)

ACTIONS

The extensors digitorum and hallucis brevis move the toes at the metatarsophalangeal (MTP) and/or the proximal interphalangeal (PIP) and distal interphalangeal (DIP) joints.

Extensor Digitorum Brevis

■ Extends toes two through four at the MTP, PIP, and DIP joints.

Extensor Hallucis Brevis

■ Extends the big toe at the MTP joint.

STABILIZATION

Stabilizes the MTP, PIP, and DIP joints of the toes.

INNERVATION

■ Deep fibular nerve

PALPATION

1. The client is supine. First visualize the common belly in the proximal dorsolateral surface of the foot (approximately 1 inch distal to the lateral malleolus of the fibula).

2. Extensor digitorum brevis: Once visualized, place your palpating finger pads on the belly and place the fingers of the resistance hand on the proximal phalanges of toes two to four.

3. Resist the client from extending toes two to four; look for and then palpate the contraction of the belly of the extensor digitorum brevis (Figure 11-29, A).

4. Extensor hallucis brevis: Now move the finger pads of the resistance hand onto the proximal phalanx of the big toe. Resist the client from extending the big toe; look for and then palpate the contraction of the belly of the extensor hallucis brevis (Figure 11-29, B).

5. Ask the client to alternately contract and relax the extensors digitorum and hallucis brevis against resistance; try to follow each one distally toward its toe attachment by strumming perpendicularly to the tendon(s).

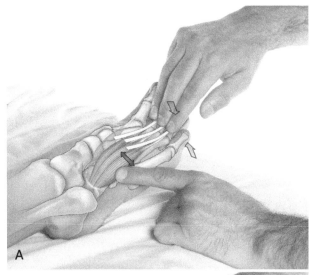

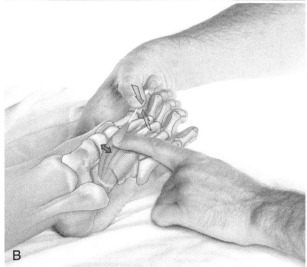

FIGURE 11-29 Palpation of the right extensor digitorum brevis (EDB) and extensor hallucis brevis (EHB). **A,** Palpation of the EDB as the client extends toes two to four against resistance. The EHB has been ghosted in. **B,** Palpation of the EHB as the client extends the big toe against resistance. The EDB has been ghosted in.

TREATMENT CONSIDERATIONS

■ The extensor digitorum brevis and extensor hallucis brevis are actually one muscle. However, they are separately named based on their distal attachments. Digitorum attaches to toes two through four; hallucis attaches to the big toe (toe one).

■ The common belly of the extensors digitorum and hallucis brevis is often visible on the proximal lateral surface of the dorsum of the foot.

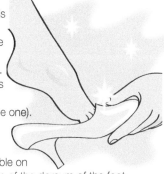

MUSCLES OF THE LEG AND FOOT:
Intrinsic Foot—Plantar Layer I
Abductor Hallucis; Abductor Digiti Minimi Pedis; Flexor Digitorum Brevis

Pronunciation   **ab-DUK-tor hal-OO-sis • ab-DUK-tor DIJ-i-tee MIN-i-mee PEED-us • FLEKS-or dij-i-TOE-rum BRE-vis**

Layer I of the plantar surface of the foot contains three muscles: the abductor hallucis on the big toe side, the abductor digiti minimi pedis on the little toe side, and the flexor digitorum brevis in between (Figure 11-30). They all originate on (attach proximally to) the tuberosity of the calcaneus and are superficial, except for being deep to the plantar fascia of the foot.

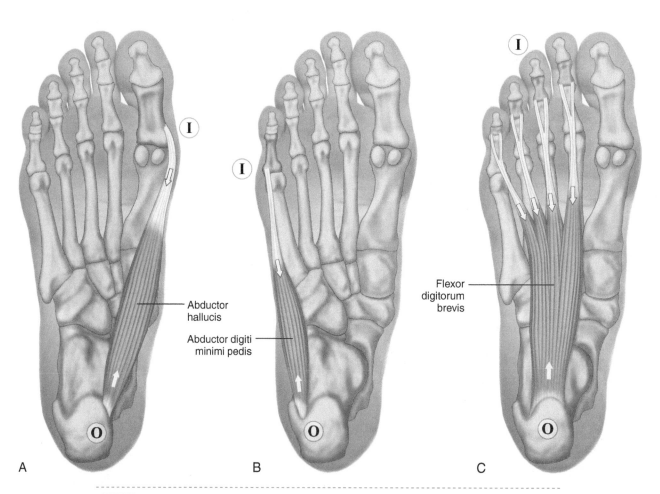

FIGURE 11-30 Plantar views of the intrinsic muscles of the right foot, Plantar Layer I. **A,** Abductor hallucis. **B,** Abductor digiti minimi pedis. **C,** Flexor digitorum brevis. *O,* Origin; *I,* insertion.

WHAT'S IN A NAME?

The name, *abductor hallucis,* tells us that this muscle abducts the big toe.

The name, *abductor digiti minimi pedis,* tells us that this muscle abducts the little toe.

The name, *flexor digitorum brevis,* tells us that this muscle flexes the digits (i.e., toes) and is shorter than the flexor digitorum longus.

❊ **Derivation:**
abductor: L. muscle that abducts a body part
hallucis: L. refers to the big toe
digitorum, digiti: L. refers to a digit (toe)
minimi: L. least
pedis: L. refers to the foot
flexor: L. muscle that flexes a body part
brevis: L. shorter

ATTACHMENTS

Abductor Hallucis

Origin (Proximal Attachment)
- Tuberosity of the calcaneus

Insertion (Distal Attachment)
- Big toe (toe one)

Abductor Digiti Minimi Pedis

Origin (Proximal Attachment)
- Tuberosity of the calcaneus

Insertion (Distal Attachment)
- Little toe (toe five)

Flexor Digitorum Brevis

Origin (Proximal Attachment)
- Tuberosity of the calcaneus

Insertion (Distal Attachment)
- Toes two through five

ACTIONS

All three muscles of plantar layer I move the toes at the metatarsophalangeal (MTP) and/or proximal interphalangeal (PIP) joints.

Abductor Hallucis
- Abducts the big toe at the MTP joint.

Abductor Digiti Minimi Pedis
- Abducts the little toe at the MTP joint.

Flexor Digitorum Brevis
- Flexes toes two through five at the MTP and PIP joints.

STABILIZATION
- The abductor hallucis and abductor digiti minimi pedis stabilize the MTP joints of the big and little toes, respectively.
- The flexor digitorum brevis stabilizes the MTP and PIP joints of toes two through five.

INNERVATION
- Medial plantar nerve (abductor hallucis and flexor digitorum brevis)
- Lateral plantar nerve (abductor digiti minimi pedis)

PALPATION

For all three palpations, have the client prone with a roll under the ankles.

Abductor Hallucis
1. Place your palpating finger pads on the medial side of the foot, close to the plantar surface.
2. Ask the client to abduct the big toe at the MTP joint. Feel for the contraction of the abductor hallucis. If desired, resistance can be given by placing a finger of the resistance hand on the medial side of the proximal phalanx of the big toe (Figure 11-31).
3. Once located, palpate the abductor hallucis proximally and distally toward its attachments by strumming perpendicular to its fibers.

Abductor Digiti Minimi Pedis
1. Move your palpating finger pads over to the lateral side of the distal foot, close to the plantar surface.
2. Ask the client to abduct the little toe at the MTP joint; feel for the contraction of the abductor digiti minimi pedis. If desired, resistance can be given by placing a finger of the resistance hand on the lateral side of the proximal phalanx of the little toe (Figure 11-32).

11

Turn page to 👁 more.

11

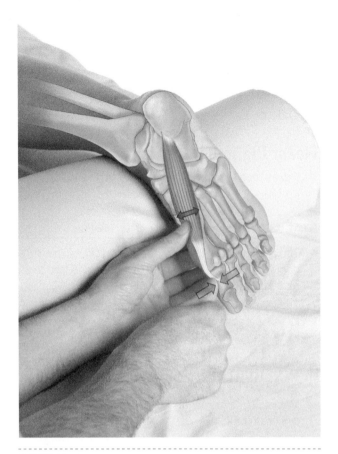

FIGURE 11-31 Palpation of the right abductor hallucis as the client abducts the big toe against resistance.

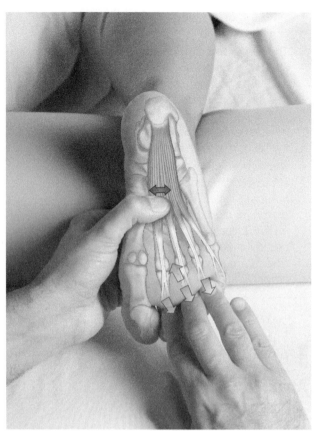

FIGURE 11-33 Palpation of the right flexor digitorum brevis as the client flexes toes two to five against resistance.

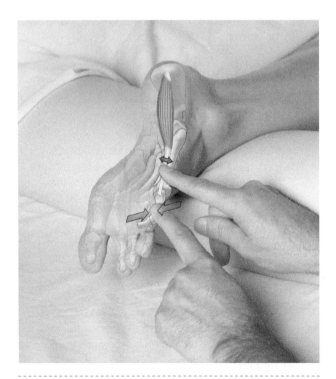

FIGURE 11-32 Palpation of the right abductor digiti minimi pedis as the client abducts the little toe against resistance.

3. Once located, palpate the flexor hallucis brevis proximally and distally toward its attachments by strumming perpendicular to its fibers.

Flexor Digitorum Brevis

1. Move your palpating finger pads to the midline of the plantar surface of the proximal foot.

2. Ask the client to flex toes two through five at the MTP joints; feel for the contraction of the flexor digitorum brevis. If desired, resistance can be given with the finger pads of the resistance hand on the plantar surface of the proximal or middle phalanges of toes two to five (Figure 11-33).

3. Once located, palpate the flexor digitorum brevis proximally to the calcaneus by strumming perpendicular to its fibers. Then palpate it distally as far as possible.

TREATMENT CONSIDERATIONS

■ In addition to their bony attachments, all three muscles in the first plantar layer of intrinsic muscles of the foot also attach into the plantar fascia of the foot. Therefore strengthening these muscles can help stabilize the plantar fascia and therefore the arch structure of the foot.

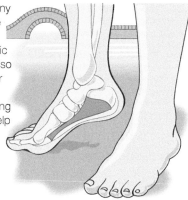

■ Each distal tendon of the flexor digitorum brevis splits to allow passage for the flexor digitorum longus' distal tendon to attach onto the distal phalanx of toes two through five.

MUSCLES OF THE LEG AND FOOT:
Intrinsic Foot—Plantar Layer II
Quadratus Plantae; Lumbricals Pedis

Pronunciation **kwod-RAY-tus PLAN-tee • LUM-bri-kuls PEED-us**

Layer II of the plantar surface of the foot contains one muscle, the quadratus plantae; and one muscle group, the lumbricals pedis group, which is composed of four lumbricals pedis muscles, named one, two, three, and four from medial to lateral (Figure 11-34). The quadratus plantae and lumbricals pedis muscles are located midline in the plantar foot and attach into the distal tendon of the flexor digitorum longus. The quadratus plantae is entirely deep to the flexor digitorum brevis; the lumbricals pedis muscles are partially deep to the flexor digitorum brevis.

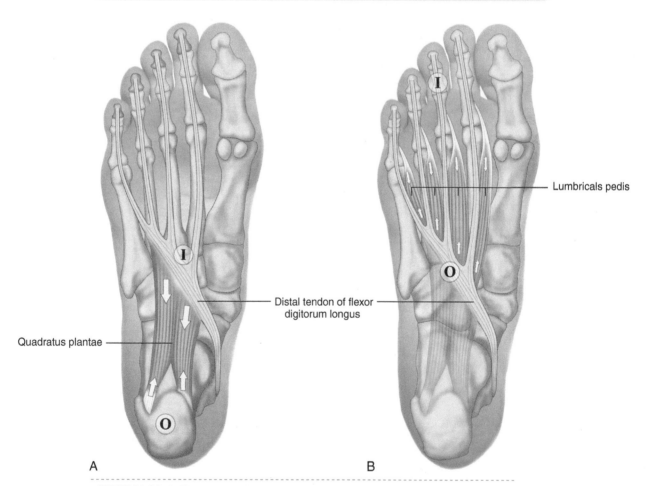

Lumbricals pedis

Distal tendon of flexor digitorum longus

Quadratus plantae

A   B

FIGURE 11-34 A, Plantar view of the right quadratus plantae. **B,** Plantar view of the right lumbricals pedis. The quadratus plantae has been ghosted in. *O,* Origin; *I,* insertion.

The name, *quadratus plantae,* tells us that this muscle has a square shape and is located on the plantar side of the foot.

The name, *lumbricals pedis,* tells us that these muscles are shaped like earthworms and are located in the foot. (The four lumbrical pedis muscles are named one, two, three, and four.)

✳ **Derivation:**
quadratus: L. squared
plantae: L. refers to the plantar surface of the foot
lumbricals: L. earthworms
pedis: L. refers to the foot

ATTACHMENTS

Quadratus Plantae

Origin (Proximal Attachment)
- Calcaneus

Insertion (Distal Attachment)
- Distal tendon of the flexor digitorum longus muscle

Lumbricals Pedis

Origin (Proximal Attachment)
- Distal tendons of the flexor digitorum longus muscle

Insertion (Distal Attachment)
- Dorsal digital expansion

ACTIONS

The quadratus plantae and lumbricals pedis move toes two through five at the metatarsophalangeal (MTP), proximal interphalangeal (PIP), and distal interphalangeal (DIP) joints.

Quadratus Plantae

- Flexes toes two through five at the MTP, PIP, and DIP joints.

Lumbricals Pedis

- Flex toes two through five at the MTP joints.
- Extend toes two through five at the PIP and DIP joints.

STABILIZATION

Plantar layer II muscles stabilize the MTP, PIP, and DIP joints of toes two through five.

INNERVATION

- Lateral plantar nerve (quadratus plantae)
- Medial and lateral plantar nerves (lumbricals pedis)

PALPATION

Quadratus Plantae

1. The client is supine. Place your palpating finger pads on the midline of the plantar surface of the proximal foot.
2. Ask the client to flex toes two to five; feel for the contraction of the quadratus plantae. Because the quadratus plantae lies immediately deep to the flexor digitorum brevis and both these muscles flex toes two to five, palpating and discerning the quadratus plantae from the flexor digitorum brevis can be very difficult.

Lumbricals pedis

1. Now place your palpating finger pads between the metatarsal bones on the plantar surface of the foot. Ask the client to flex toes two to five at the MTP joints and, if possible, keep the IP joints extended; feel for their contraction.

TREATMENT CONSIDERATIONS

- The quadratus plantae assists the flexor digitorum longus by both adding strength to the contraction and also by straightening out its line of pull. Because the flexor digitorum longus enters the foot from the medial side, it tends to pull the toes toward that side when it contracts. The quadratus plantae straightens out this line of pull to keep the toes straight when they flex.

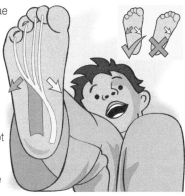

11

MUSCLES OF THE LEG AND FOOT:
Intrinsic Foot—Plantar Layer III
Flexor Hallucis Brevis; Flexor Digiti Minimi Pedis; Adductor Hallucis

Pronunciation   **FLEKS-or hal-OO-sis BRE-vis • FLEKS-or DIJ-i-tee MIN-i-mee PEED-us •**
ad-DUK-tor hal-OO-sis

Layer III of the plantar surface of the foot contains three muscles: the flexor hallucis brevis on the big toe side, the flexor digiti minimi pedis on the little toe side, and the adductor hallucis in between. The adductor hallucis has transverse and oblique heads (Figure 11-35). Although they are in the third plantar layer, much of the flexor hallucis brevis, flexor digiti minimi pedis, and transverse head of the adductor hallucis are deep only to the plantar fascia.

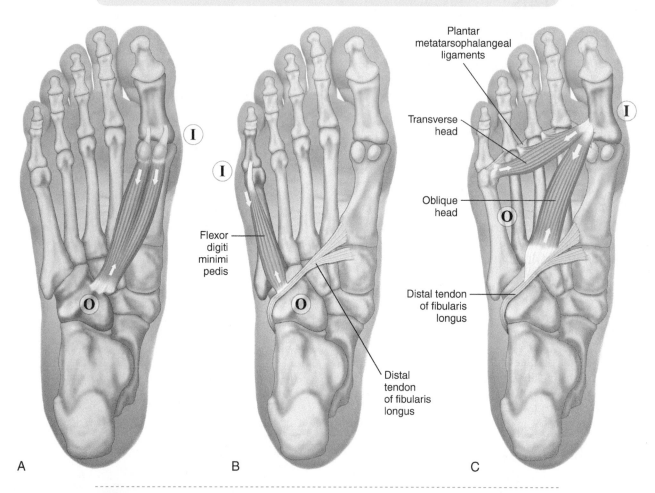

FIGURE 11-35 Plantar views of the intrinsic muscles of the right foot, Plantar Layer II. *A,* Flexor hallucis brevis. *B,* Flexor digiti minimi pedis. *C,* Adductor hallucis. O, Origin; I, insertion.

Turn page to 👁 more.

WHAT'S IN A NAME?

The name, *flexor hallucis brevis,* tells us that this muscle flexes the big toe and is shorter than the flexor hallucis longus.

The name, *flexor digiti minimi pedis,* tells us that this muscle flexes the little toe.

The name, *adductor hallucis,* tells us that this muscle adducts the big toe.

✳ Derivation:

flexor: L. muscle that flexes a body part
adductor: L. muscle that adducts a body part
hallucis: L. refers to the big toe
digiti: L. refers to a digit (toe)
brevis: L. shorter
minimi: L. least
pedis: L. refers to the foot

ATTACHMENTS

Flexor Hallucis Brevis

Origin (Proximal Attachment)
- Cuboid and the third cuneiform

Insertion (Distal Attachment)
- Big toe (toe one)

Flexor Digiti Minimi Pedis

Origin (Proximal Attachment)
- Fifth metatarsal

Insertion (Distal Attachment)
- Little toe (toe five)

Adductor Hallucis

Origin (Proximal Attachment)
- Metatarsals

Insertion (Distal Attachment)
- Big toe (toe one)

ACTIONS

The flexor hallucis brevis, flexor digiti minimi pedis, and adductor hallucis move the toes at the metatarsophalangeal (MTP) joints.

Flexor Hallucis Brevis
- Flexes the big toe at the MTP joint.

Flexor Digiti Minimi Pedis
- Flexes the little toe at the MTP joint.

Adductor Hallucis
- Adducts the big toe at the MTP joint.

STABILIZATION

Stabilizes the MTP joints of the big and little toes.

INNERVATION

- Medial plantar nerve (flexor hallucis brevis)
- Lateral plantar nerve (flexor digiti minimi pedis and adductor hallucis)

PALPATION

To palpate all three muscles of the third plantar layer, have the client prone with a roll under the ankles.

Flexor Hallucis Brevis

1. Place your palpating finger pads over the first metatarsal bone on the plantar side of the foot.
2. Now ask the client to flex the big toe at the MTP joint; feel for the contraction of the flexor hallucis brevis. If desired, resistance can be given with the fingers of the resistance hand on the plantar surface of the proximal phalanx of the big toe (Figure 11-36).
3. Once located, palpate it proximally and distally to its attachments by strumming perpendicular to its fibers.

Flexor Digiti Minimi Pedis

1. Move your palpating finger pads over the fifth metatarsal bone on the plantar side of the foot.
2. Ask the client to flex the little toe at the MTP joint; feel for the contraction of the flexor digiti minimi pedis. If desired, resistance can be given with a finger of the resistance hand on the plantar surface of the proximal phalanx of the little toe (Figure 11-37).
3. Once located, palpate it distally to the proximal phalanx of the little toe by strumming perpendicular to its fibers. Then palpate it proximally as far as possible.

11

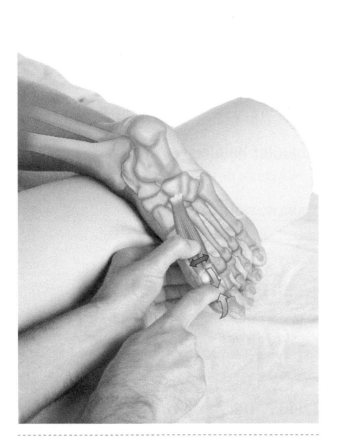

FIGURE 11-36 Palpation of the right flexor hallucis brevis as the client flexes the big toe against resistance.

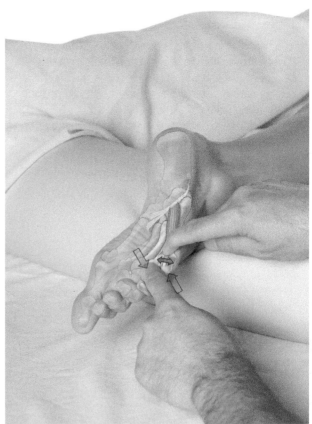

FIGURE 11-37 Palpation of the right flexor digiti minimi pedis as the client flexes the little toe against resistance.

Adductor Hallucis

1. Place your palpating finger pads over the heads of the metatarsals of the second, third, and fourth toes. Place the fingers of resistance hand on the lateral side of the proximal phalanx of the big toe.

2. Ask the client to adduct the big toe against resistance; feel for the contraction of the transverse head of the adductor hallucis. Try to palpate the oblique head in a similar manner.

   Note: This muscle can be challenging to palpate and discern.

TREATMENT CONSIDERATIONS

- A sesamoid bone is located distally in each of the medial and lateral tendons of the flexor hallucis brevis.

- The adductor hallucis occasionally has attachments onto the first metatarsal distally and can oppose the big toe toward the other toes. When this occurs, it is named the *opponens hallucis* of the foot. The flexor digiti minimi pedis occasionally has attachments onto the fifth metatarsal distally and can oppose the little toe. When this occurs, it is named the *opponens digiti minimi pedis.* These muscles are commonly found in apes, who have feet that are more handy than ours!

- The adductor hallucis stabilizes the arch structure of the foot.

Notes

MUSCLES OF THE LEG AND FOOT:
Intrinsic Foot—Plantar Layer IV
Plantar Interossei; Dorsal Interossei Pedis

Pronunciation **PLAN-tar in-ter-OSS-ee-eye • DOR-sul in-ter-OSS-ee-eye PEED-us**

Layer IV of the plantar surface of the foot contains two muscle groups: the plantar interossei and the dorsal interossei pedis. Three plantar interossei attach to toes three through five; they are named one, two, and three from the medial side. Four dorsal interossei pedis attach to toes two through four; they are named one, two, three, and four from the medial side (Figure 11-38). The plantar interossei are very deep in the plantar foot. Although the dorsal interossei pedis are considered plantar muscles, they are accessible to palpation on the dorsal side of the foot.

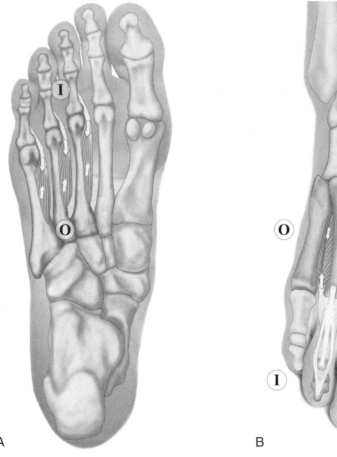

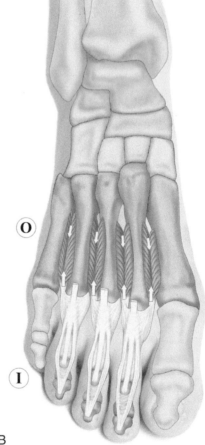

A

B

FIGURE 11-38 A, Plantar view of the right plantar interossei. **B,** Dorsal view of the right dorsal interossei pedis. *O,* Origin; *I,* insertion.

WHAT'S IN A NAME?

The name, *plantar interossei,* tells us that these muscles are located between bones (metatarsals) on the plantar side.

The name, *dorsal interossei pedis,* tells us that these muscles are located between bones (metatarsals) on the dorsal side and located in the foot.

✷ **Derivation:**
plantar: L. refers to the plantar side of the foot
dorsal: L. refers to the dorsal side
interossei: L. between bones
pedis: L. refers to the foot

ATTACHMENTS

Plantar Interossei

Origin (Proximal Attachment)
- Metatarsals

Insertion (Distal Attachment)
- Second-toe sides of the proximal phalanges of toes three through five

Dorsal Interossei Pedis

Origin (Proximal Attachment)
- Metatarsals

Insertion (Distal Attachment)
- Sides of the phalanges (the sides away from the center of the second toe) of toes two through four

ACTIONS

The dorsal interossei manus and plantar interossei move the toes at the metatarsophalangeal (MTP) joints.

Plantar Interossei

- Adduct toes three through five at the MTP joints.

Dorsal Interossei Pedis

- Abduct toes two through four at the MTP joints.

STABILIZATION

Stabilize toes two through five.

INNERVATION

- Lateral plantar nerve

PALPATION

Plantar Interossei

1. The client is prone with a roll under the ankles. Place your palpating finger pads between metatarsals (second through fifth) on the plantar side.
2. Resist the client from adducting toes three through five; feel for the contraction of the plantar interossei.
3. Given their depth and the difficulty that most people have isolating the action of this muscle group, the plantar interossei are usually difficult to palpate and discern from adjacent soft tissues.

Dorsal Interossei Pedis

1. The client is supine. Place your palpating finger pads on the dorsal side of the foot between the metatarsal bones.
2. The first dorsal interosseus is palpated between the first and second metatarsals (Figure 11-39, *A*).

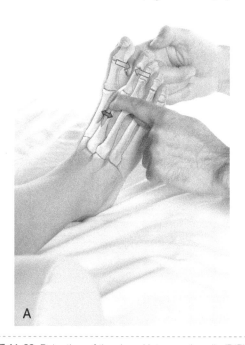

A

FIGURE 11-39 Palpation of the dorsal interossei pedis (DIP). *A,* Palpation of the first DIP as the client does tibial abduction of the second toe against resistance. *Continued*

11

Turn page to more.

11

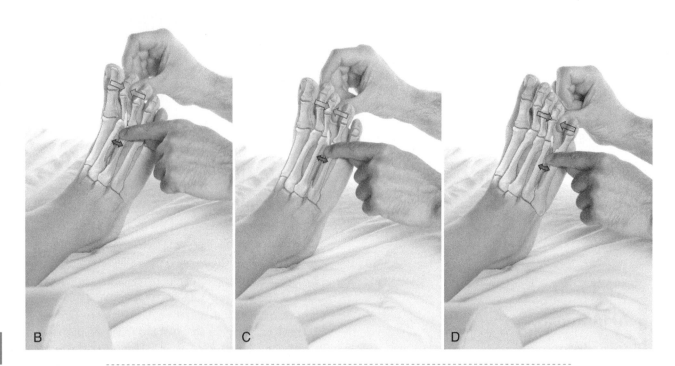

FIGURE 11-39, cont'd   Palpation of the dorsal interossei pedis (DIP). **B,** Palpation of the second DIP as the client does fibular abduction of the second toe against resistance. **C,** Palpation of the third DIP as the client abducts the third toe against resistance. **D,** Palpation of the fourth DIP as the client abducts the fourth toe against resistance.

3. The second dorsal interosseus is palpated between the second and third metatarsals (Figure 11-39, *B*).

4. The third dorsal interosseus is palpated between the third and fourth metatarsals (Figure 11-39, *C*).

5. The fourth dorsal interosseus is palpated between the fourth and fifth metatarsals (Figure 11-39, *D*).

TREATMENT CONSIDERATIONS

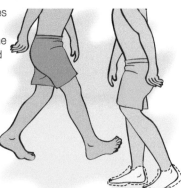

- Because we wear shoes so often, we rarely use our toes. As a result, the interossei muscles tend to be weak and poorly coordinated.

- The big toe gets its own adductor, and toe number two cannot adduct (its movement is described as being either tibial abduction or fibular abduction). That leaves toes three, four, and five that can adduct. The result is that three plantar interossei muscles attach to toes three, four, and five.

- The big toe and the little toe each get their own abductor muscle. That leaves toes two, three, and four to have dorsal interossei pedis muscles attached. However, toe number two can abduct in the tibial (medial) direction and in the fibular (lateral) direction; therefore it gets two dorsal interossei pedis muscles attached to it (one on each side). The result is that of the four dorsal interossei pedis muscles, one attaches to toe number four, one attaches to toe number three, and two attach to toe number two.

REVIEW QUESTIONS

Circle or fill in the correct answer for each of the following questions. More study resources, including audio pronunciations of muscle names, are provided on the Evolve website at http://evolve.elsevier.com/Muscolino/knowthebody.

1. **What are the three muscles of the Tom, Dick, and Harry group?**

   _____

   _____

   _____

2. **What are the three muscles in plantar layer 1 of the foot?**

   _____

   _____

   _____

3. **What are the muscles of the triceps surae group?**

   _____

   _____

4. **Which of the following muscles dorsiflexes and inverts the foot?**
   a. Tibialis anterior
   b. Tibialis posterior
   c. Extensor digitorum longus
   d. Gastrocnemius

5. **Which of the following muscles plantarflexes and everts the foot?**
   a. Tibialis anterior
   b. Tibialis posterior
   c. Fibularis longus
   d. Fibularis tertius

6. **Which of the following muscles crosses the knee joint?**
   a. Quadratus plantae
   b. Tibialis anterior
   c. Soleus
   d. Gastrocnemius

7. **Which of the following muscles adducts the big toe?**
   a. Popliteus
   b. Abductor hallucis
   c. Adductor hallucis
   d. Quadratus plantae

8. **Which of the following muscles are often referred to as stirrup muscles?**
   a. Tibialis anterior and extensor digitorum longus
   b. Fibularis brevis and fibularis longus
   c. Gastrocnemius and soleus
   d. Fibularis longus and tibialis anterior

9. **Which of the following muscles attach into the tuberosity of the calcaneus?**
   a. Flexor digitorum brevis and lumbricals pedis
   b. Plantaris and gastrocnemius
   c. Abductor hallucis and abductor digiti minimi pedis
   d. Flexor digitorum longus and fibularis tertius

10. **What muscles attach into the Achilles tendon?**
    a. Gastrocnemius and soleus
    b. Soleus and fibularis longus
    c. Fibularis longus and tibialis anterior
    d. Tibialis anterior and gastrocnemius

11

CASE STUDY 1

A 34-year-old female client has pain and muscle cramps in the back of her right leg (calf). Her pain intensity is 5 to 6 on a scale of 0 to 10. The client is a long-distance runner and has trained 70 to 80 miles per week for the past 10 years. She warms up before running and stretches afterward. Her gait has been professionally evaluated with no reported problems. The client has no history of traumatic injuries to the region.

Verbal history reveals no life style changes or major changes to her training regimen. She trains with a running club once a week. She finished a half marathon 1 month earlier. No difference was noted in her pain level or muscle tension after the marathon versus what she has experienced after previous races. Continued questioning revealed that the client recently took a 2-week vacation driving across the United States.

QUESTIONS

1. Considering the location of her pain, what musculature do you expect to find tight on this client?

_____

_____

_____

_____

_____

_____

2. How would her activities contribute to this musculature being tight?

_____

_____

_____

_____

_____

_____

_____

_____

_____

3. What would be the best treatment plan?

_____

_____

_____

_____

_____

_____

_____

11

CASE STUDY 2

A regular client recently made a life-style change by losing weight, exercising, and meditation. Her exercise includes running and weight lifting. The client is now experiencing constant pain on the anterior side of the right leg; the pain intensity varies from a 3 to 6 on a scale of 0 to 10. At first, the pain occurred only when running; now it occurs with walking. The client's medical physician ordered an x-ray examination; the results were negative for fracture or any other osseous pathologic condition. The physician suggested that the client reduce the amount of running and recommended the use an over-the-counter pain medication.

Physical examination of the client's leg revealed significant tenderness along the lateral border of the shaft of the tibia. Passive range of motion (ROM), active ROM, and manual resistance to motion of the foot were performed. The following results were positive with pain in the anterior leg: (1) Passive ROM into extension caused slight pain in the anterior leg. (2) Active ROM into dorsiflexion caused moderate pain in the anterior leg. (3) Manual resistance to dorsiflexion and inversion caused strong pain at a level of 6 in the anterior leg.

Physical examination shows that the client has a dropped arch on the right side when weight bearing. Her left arch is normal and healthy.

QUESTIONS

1. **What condition do you suspect the client has? What musculature do you palpate to confirm this?**

   _____

   _____

2. **What role did running play in this condition?**

   _____

   _____

   _____

   _____

   _____

   _____

   _____

   _____

   _____

3. **What role does her dropped arch on weight bearing have?**

   _____

   _____

   _____

   _____

   _____

   _____

   _____

11

Appendix: Stretching Atlas

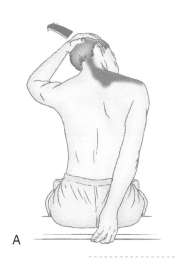

A

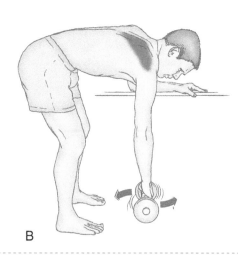

B

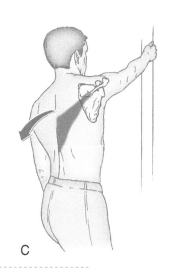

C

FIGURE 1 Trapezius.

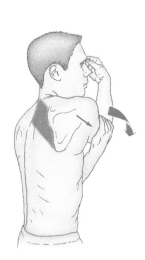

FIGURE 2 Rhomboids.

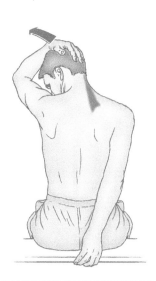

FIGURE 3 Levator scapulae.

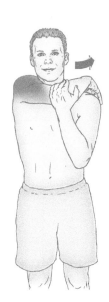

FIGURE 4 Posterior deltoid.

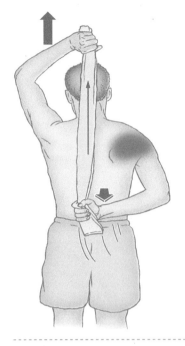

FIGURE 5 Infraspinatus and teres minor.

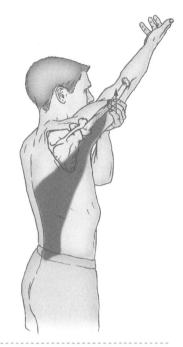

FIGURE 6 Teres major and latissimus dorsi.

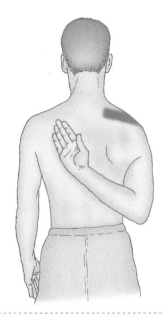

FIGURE 7 Supraspinatus.

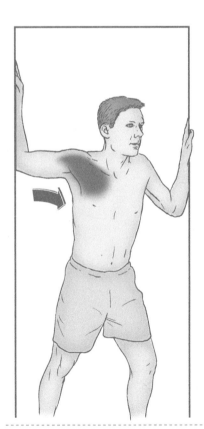

FIGURE 8 Anterior deltoid and pectoralis major.

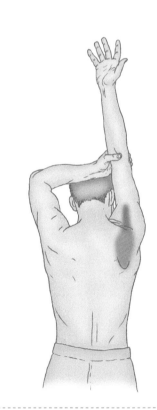

FIGURE 9 Subscapularis.

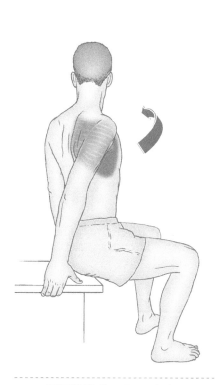

FIGURE 10 Serratus anterior.

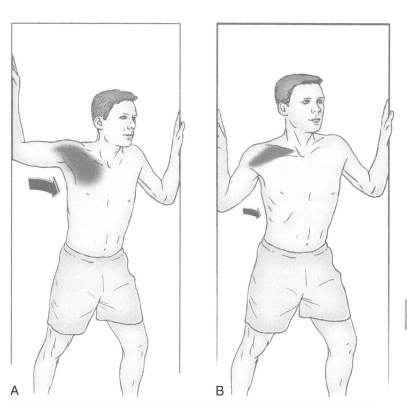

A   B

FIGURE 11 *A,* Pectoralis major, sternocostal head. *B,* Pectoralis major, clavicular head.

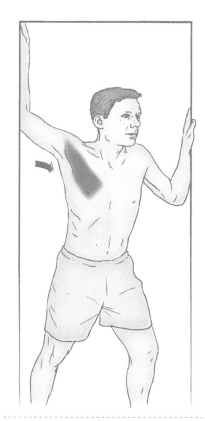

FIGURE 12 Pectoralis minor.

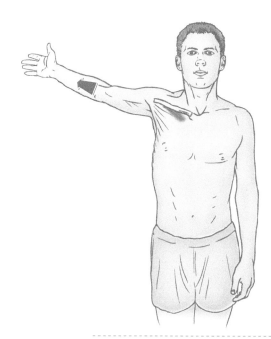

FIGURE 13 Subclavius.

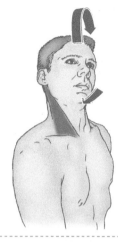

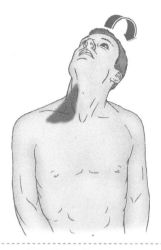

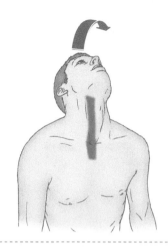

FIGURE 14 Sternocleidomastoid. The client left laterally flexes and right rotates the head and neck and extends the lower neck but tucks the chin (flexes the head).

FIGURE 15 Scalene group.

FIGURE 16 Longus colli. The client's head and neck are extended and laterally flexed to the opposite side.

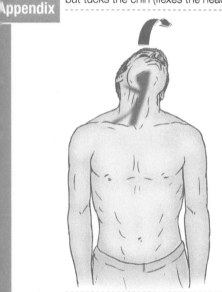

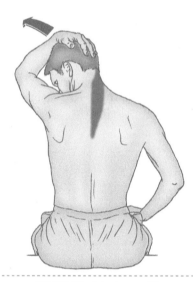

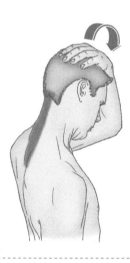

FIGURE 17 Hyoid group. The client's neck is extended and left laterally flexed.

FIGURE 18 Splenius capitis.

FIGURE 19 Semispinalis capitis. **Note:** Flexion is the most important component of this stretch.

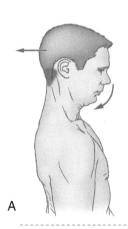

A

B

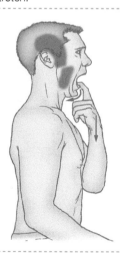

FIGURE 20 Suboccipitals.

FIGURE 21 Temporalis.

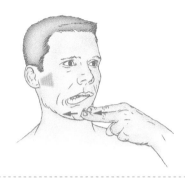

FIGURE 22 Lateral pterygoid.

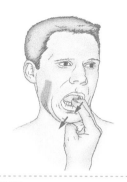

FIGURE 23 Medial pterygoid.

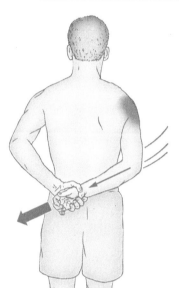

FIGURE 24 Deltoid.

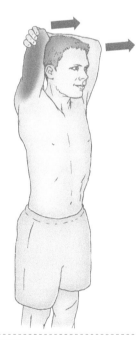

FIGURE 25 Biceps brachii.

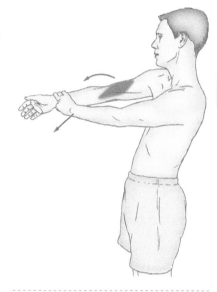

FIGURE 26 Brachialis. The client's elbow joint is fully extended with the forearm in position half way between full supination and full pronation.

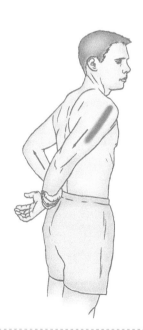

FIGURE 27 Coracobrachialis.

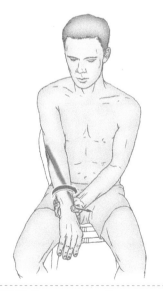

FIGURE 28 Triceps brachii.

FIGURE 29 Brachioradialis. The client's forearm is fully extended.

Appendix

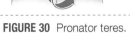

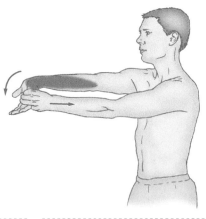

FIGURE 30 Pronator teres.

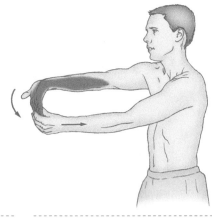

FIGURE 31 Wrist flexor group. If ulnar deviation is added to the extension, the stretch of the flexor carpi radialis will be enhanced. If radial deviation is added to the extension, the stretch of the flexor carpi ulnaris will be enhanced.

FIGURE 32 Flexors digitorum superficialis and profundus.

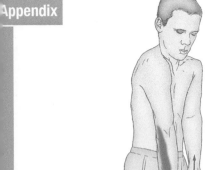

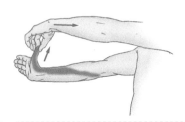

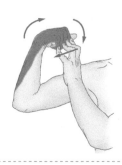

FIGURE 33 Radial group.

FIGURE 34 Flexor pollicis longus.

FIGURE 35 Extensor digitorum, extensor digiti minimi, and extensor indicis.

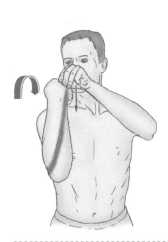

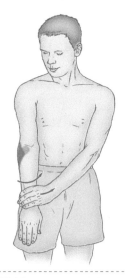

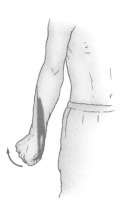

FIGURE 36 Extensor carpi ulnaris.

FIGURE 37 Supinator. **Note:** It is easy to confuse pronation of the forearm at the radioulnar joints with medial rotation of the arm at the glenohumeral joint. Be sure that forearm pronation is being done.

FIGURE 38 Deep distal four group.

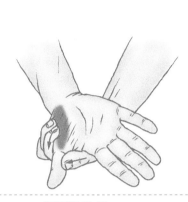

FIGURE 39 Thenar group.

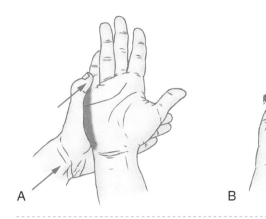

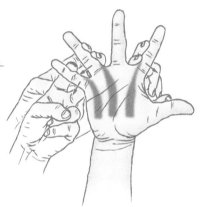

FIGURE 40 Hypothenar group. ***A,*** Abductor digiti minimi manus. ***B,*** Flexor digiti minimi manus and opponens digiti minimi.

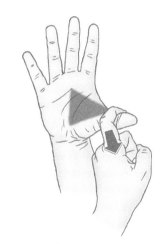

FIGURE 41 Adductor pollicis.

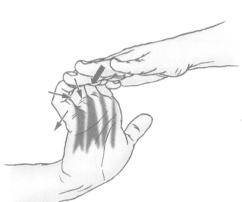

FIGURE 42 Lumbricals manus.

FIGURE 43 Palmer interossei.

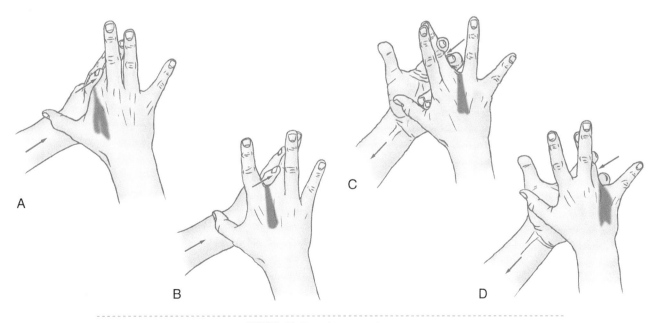

FIGURE 44 Dorsal interossei manus.

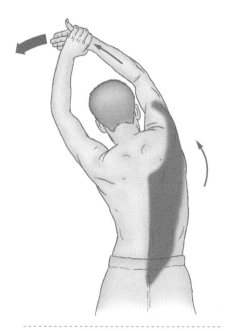

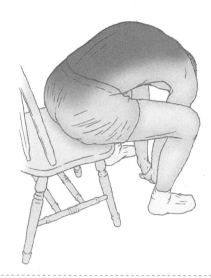

FIGURE 45 Latissimus dorsi.

FIGURE 46 Erector spinae group. **Note:** When returning to the seated position, it is best for the client to place the forearms on the thighs, using them to push him or herself back up.

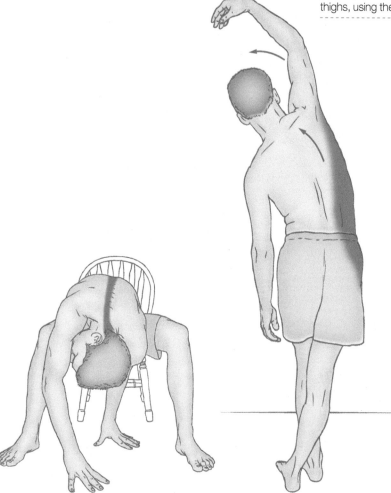

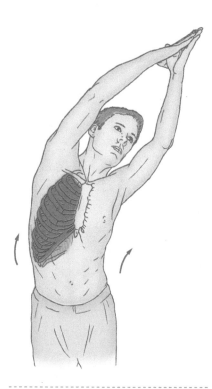

FIGURE 47 Transversospinalis group.

FIGURE 48 Quadratus lumborum.

FIGURE 49 Intercostals. Isolating the bending to the thoracic region as much as possible is important.

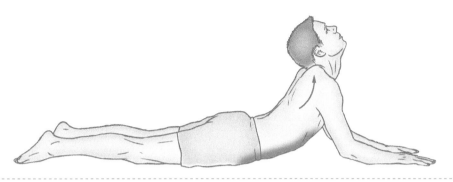

FIGURE 50 Rectus abdominis. The stretch of one side muscle can be enhanced by adding some lateral flexion to the opposite side.

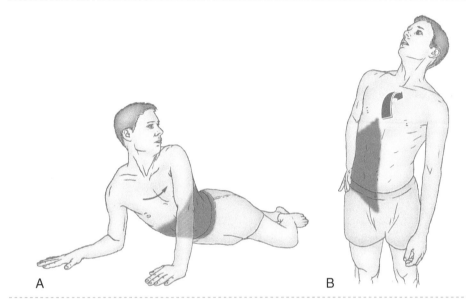

A   B

FIGURE 51 Abdominal obliques.

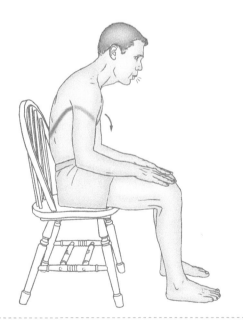

FIGURE 52 Diaphragm.

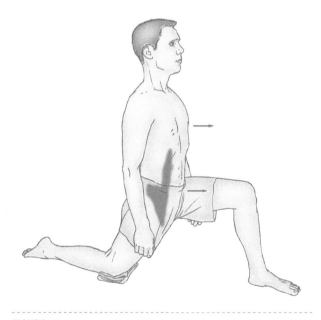

FIGURE 53 Iliopsoas. **Note:** Keeping the trunk straight or slightly extended is important.

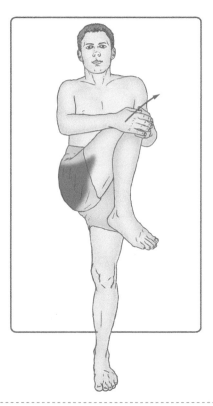

FIGURE 54 Gluteus maximus. **Note:** If the client experiences a pinching sensation in the groin with this stretch, it is helpful to either first stretch the hip flexors (especially the sartorius and iliopsoas) before doing this stretch or to first laterally rotate and abduct the thigh at the hip joint to untwist and slacken the hip joint capsule before performing the stretch.

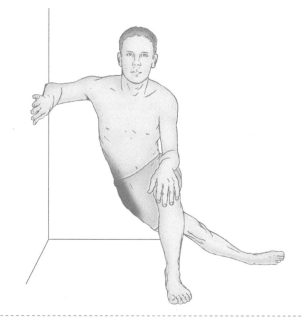

FIGURE 55 Gluteus medius and tensor fasciae latae. **Note:** It is important to avoid placing too much weight on the ankle joint of the foot in back.

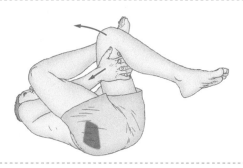

FIGURE 56 Piriformis.

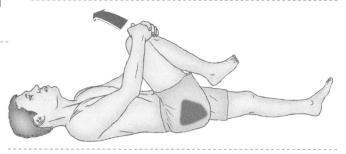

FIGURE 57 Quadratus femoris. **Note:** If the client experiences a pinching sensation in the groin with this stretch, it is helpful to first stretch the hip flexors (especially the sartorius and illiopsoas) before stretching or to first laterally rotate and abduct the thigh at the hip joint to untwist and slacken the hip joint capsule before doing this stretch.

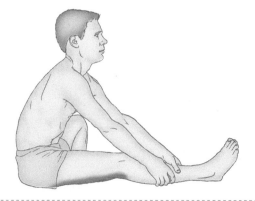

FIGURE 58 Hamstring group. **Note:** The spine does not need to bend in this stretch.

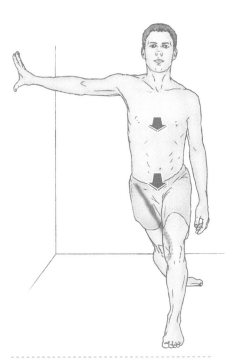

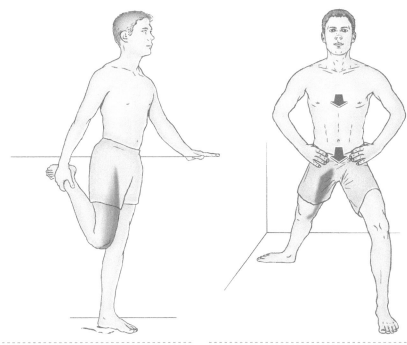

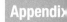

FIGURE 59 Sartorius. **Note:** Not allowing the pelvis to fall into an anterior tilt and ensuring that excessive weight is not placed on the ankle joint of the foot in back are important.

FIGURE 60 Quadriceps femoris. **Note:** When performing this stretch, ensuring that the knee joint is not rotated is important.

FIGURE 61 Pectineus and gracilis. **Note:** Not allowing the pelvis to fall into anterior tilt and ensuring that excessive weight is not placed on the ankle joint of the foot in back are important.

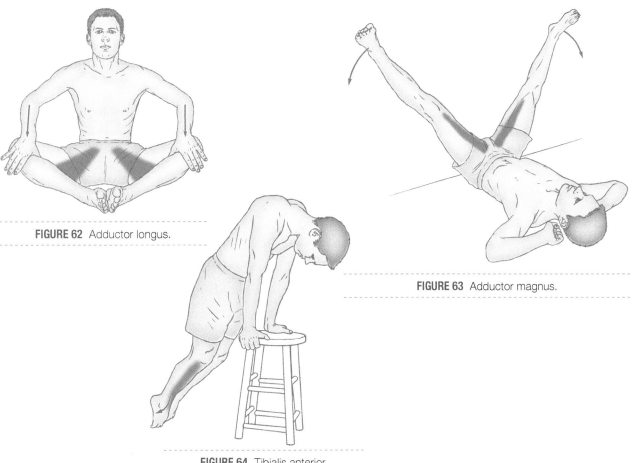

FIGURE 62 Adductor longus.

FIGURE 63 Adductor magnus.

FIGURE 64 Tibialis anterior.

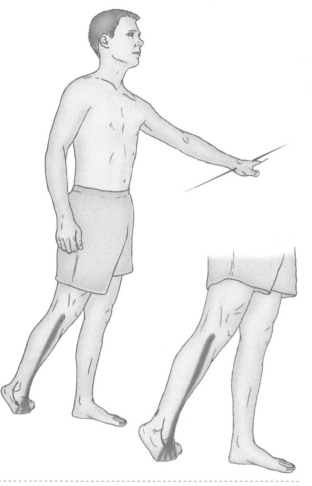

FIGURE 65 Extensor digitorum longus.

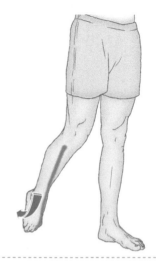

FIGURE 66 Extensor hallucis longus.

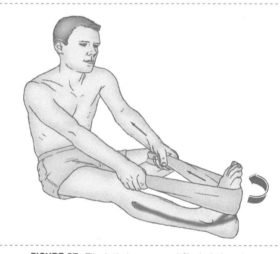

FIGURE 67 Fibularis longus and fibularis brevis.

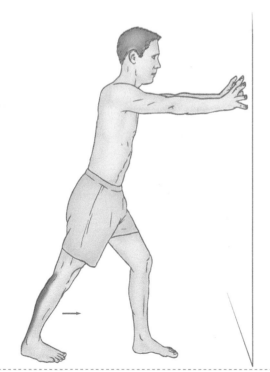

FIGURE 68 Gastrocnemius.

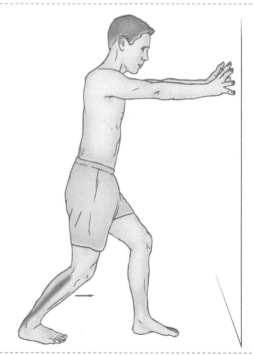

FIGURE 69 Soleus.

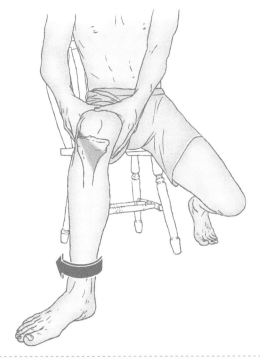

FIGURE 70 Popliteus.

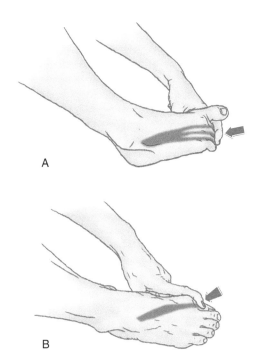

FIGURE 71 *A,* Extensor digitorum brevis. *B,* Extensor hallucis brevis.

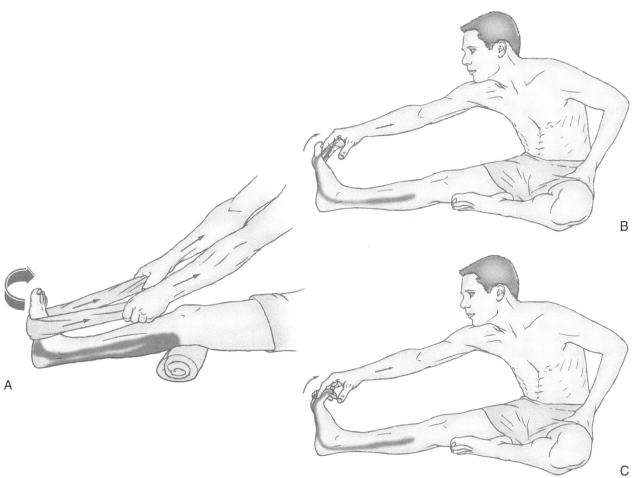

FIGURE 72 *A,* Tibialis posterior. *B,* Flexor digitorum longus. *C,* Flexor hallucis longus.

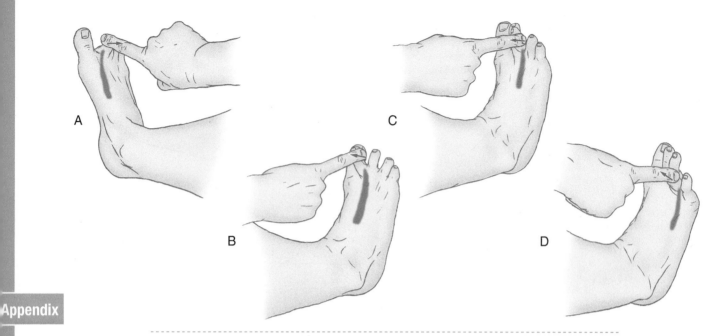

FIGURE 73 Dorsal interossei pedis (DIP). **A,** First DIP. **B,** Second DIP. **C,** Third DIP. **D,** Fourth DIP.

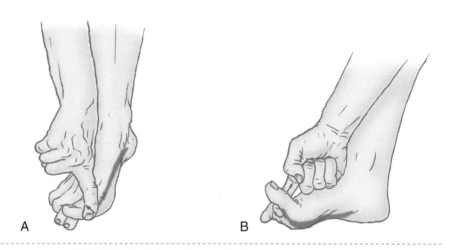

FIGURE 74 A, Abductor hallucis. **B,** Flexor hallucis brevis.

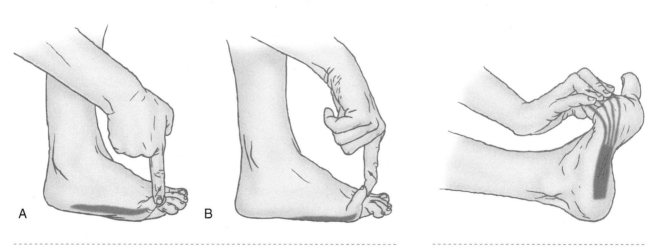

FIGURE 75 A, Abductor digiti minimi pedis. **B,** Flexor digiti minimi pedis.

FIGURE 76 Flexor digitorum brevis.

Bibliography

Aaberg E: *Muscle mechanics,* ed 2, Champaign, IL, 2006, Human Kinetics.

Abrahams PH, Marks Jr SC, Hutchings RT: *McMinn's color atlas of human anatomy,* ed 5, Edinburgh, 2003, Mosby–Elsevier.

Anderson JE: *Grant's atlas of anatomy,* ed 7, Baltimore, 1980, Williams & Wilkins.

Atlas of anatomy, Germany, 2005, Thieme.

Bandy WD, Reese NB: *Joint range of motion and muscle length testing,* Philadelphia, 2002, Saunders–Elsevier.

Basmajian JV, De Luca CJ: *Muscles alive: their functions revealed by electromyography,* ed 5, Baltimore, 1985, Williams & Wilkins.

Biel A: *Trail guide to the body,* ed 4, Boulder, CO, 2010, Books of Discovery.

Biel A: *Student handbook: trail guide to the body,* Boulder, CO, 2005, Books of Discovery.

Bisschop P, Ombregt L: *Atlas of orthopedic examination of the peripheral joints,* Edinburgh, 1999, Saunders.

Burkel WE, Woodburne RT: *Essentials of human anatomy,* ed 9, New York, 1994, Oxford University Press.

Cailliet R: *Neck and arm pain,* ed 2, Philadelphia, 2001, F.A. Davis.

Calais-Germain B: *Anatomy of movement,* Seattle, 1993, Eastland Press.

Chaitow L: *Palpation and assessment skills,* ed 2, Edinburgh, 2003, Churchill Livingstone.

Cipriano JJ: *Photographic manual of regional orthopaedic and neurological tests,* ed 4, Philadelphia, 2003, Lippincott Williams & Wilkins.

Clay JH, Pounds DM: *Basic clinical massage therapy,* ed 2, Philadelphia, 2008, Lippincott Williams & Wilkins.

Clemente CD: *Clemente anatomy,* ed 4, Philadelphia, 1997, Lippincott Williams & Wilkins.

Cohen BJ: *Structure and function of the human body,* ed 8, Philadelphia, 2005, Lippincott Williams & Wilkins.

Cramer GD, Darby SA: *Basic and clinical anatomy of the spine, spinal cord, and ANS,* St Louis, 1995, Mosby.

Deutsch H, Hamilton N, Luttgens K: *Kinesiology: scientific basis of human motion,* ed 8, Madison, WI, 1992, WCB Brown U Benchmark.

Dixon M: *Joint play the right way: axial skeleton,* Port Moody, BC, 2006, Arthrokinetic Publishing.

Dixon M: *Joint play the right way: for the peripheral skeleton,* Port Moody, BC, 2003, Arthrokinetic Publishing.

Earls J, Myers T: *Fascial release for structural balance,* Chichester, England, 2010, Lotus Publishing.

Enoka RM: *Neuromechanics of human movement,* ed 3, Champaign, IL, 2002, Human Kinetics.

Field D, Palastanga N, Soames R: *Anatomy and human movement,* ed 4, Oxford, 2002, Butterworth Heinemann.

Findley TW, Schleip R: *Fascia research: basic science and implications for conventional and complementary health care,* Munich, Germany, 2007, Elsevier.

Frankel VH, Nordin M: *Basic biomechanics of the musculoskeletal system,* ed 3, Philadelphia, 2001, Lippincott Williams & Wilkins.

Gardiner PF, MacIntosh BR, McComas AJ: *Skeletal muscle: form and function,* ed 2, Champaign, IL, 2006, Human Kinetics.

Gosling JA, Harris PF, Whitmore I, Willan PLT: *Human anatomy: color atlas and text,* ed 4, Edinburgh, 2002, Mosby–Elsevier.

Greene DP, Roberts SL: *Kinesiology: movement in the context of activity,* ed 2, St Louis, 2005, Mosby–Elsevier.

Gray's anatomy for students, New York, 2005, Churchill Livingstone.

Gray's anatomy, ed 40, New York, 2008, Churchill Livingstone.

Greene DP, Roberts SL: *Kinesiology: movement in the context of activity,* ed 2, St Louis, 2005, Elsevier.

Gunn C: *Bones & joints: a guide for students,* ed 4, Edinburgh, 2002, Churchill Livingstone.

Hamill J, Knutzen JM: *Biomechanical basis of human movement,* ed 2, Philadelphia, 2003, Lippincott Williams & Wilkins.

Hoppenfeld S: *Physical examination of the spine and extremities,* New York, 1976, Appleton-Century-Crofts.

Jenkins DB: *Hollinshead's functional anatomy of the limbs and back,* ed 8, Philadelphia, 2002, Saunders–Elsevier.

Juhan D: *Job's body: a handbook for bodywork,* New York, 1987, Station Hill Press.

Kapandji IA: *The physiology of the joints,* vol 1, ed 5, Edinburgh, 2002, Churchill Livingstone.

Kapandji IA: *The physiology of the joints,* vol 3, ed 2, Edinburgh, 1980, Churchill Livingstone.

Kendall FP, McCreary EK, Provance PG: *Muscles: testing and function,* ed 4, Baltimore, 1993, Williams & Wilkins.

Lehmkuhl LD, Smith LK, Weiss EL: *Brunnstrom's clinical kinesiology,* ed 5, Philadelphia, 1996, F.A. Davis.

Leonard CT: *The neuroscience of human movement,* St Louis, 1998, Mosby.

Levangie PK, Norkin CC: *Joint structure and function: a comprehensive analysis,* ed 3, Philadelphia, 2001, F.A. Davis.

Liebenson C: *Rehabilitation of the spine: a practitioner's manual,* Philadelphia, 1996, Lippincott Williams & Wilkins.

Lieber RL: *Skeletal muscle, structure, function & plasticity,* ed 2, Baltimore, 2002, Lippincott Williams & Wilkins.

Lowe W: *Orthopedic assessment in massage therapy,* Sisters, OR, 2006, Daviau Scott Publishers.

Ludwig L, Rattray F: *Clinical massage therapy: understanding, assessing and treating over 70 conditions,* Toronto, 2000, Talus.

Lutjen-Drecoll E, Rohen JW, Yokochi C: *Color atlas of anatomy: a photographic study of the human body,* ed 5, Philadelphia, 2002, Lippincott Williams & Wilkins.

Magee DJ: *Orthopedic physical assessment,* ed 4, Philadelphia, 2002, Saunders–Elsevier.

Magill RA: *Motor learning and control: concepts and applications,* ed 9, New York, 2011, McGraw Hill.

Mense S, Simons DG: *Muscle pain: understanding its nature, diagnosis, and treatment,* Baltimore, 2001, Lippincott Williams & Wilkins.

Muscolino JE: *Kinesiology: the skeletal system and muscle function,* ed 2, St Louis, 2011, Mosby–Elsevier.

Muscolino JE: *The muscle and bone palpation manual,* St Louis, 2009, Mosby–Elsevier.

Muscolino JE: *The Muscular system manual: the skeletal muscles of the human body,* ed 3, St Louis, 2010, Mosby–Elsevier.

Myers TM: *Anatomy trains,* ed 2, New York, 2009, Churchill Livingstone.

Netter FH: *Atlas of human anatomy,* ed 3, Teterboro, NJ, 2003, ICON Learning Systems.

Neumann DA: *Kinesiology of the musculoskeletal system: foundations for physical rehabilitation*, ed 2, St Louis, 2010, Mosby–Elsevier.

Norkin CC, White DJ: *Measurement of join motion: a guide to goniometry*, ed 3, Philadelphia, 2003, F.A. Davis.

Oatis CA: *Kinesiology: the mechanics & pathomechanics of human movement*, Philadelphia, 2004, Lippincott Williams & Wilkins.

Olson TR: *A.D.A.M. student atlas of anatomy*, Baltimore, 1996, Williams & Wilkins.

Patton KT, Thibodeau GA: *Anatomy & physiology*, ed 7, St Louis, 2010, Mosby–Elsevier.

Simons DG, Travell JG: *Myofascial pain and dysfunction: the trigger point manual—the lower extremities*, vol 2, Baltimore, 1999, Williams & Wilkins.

Simons DG, Travell JG: *Myofascial pain and dysfunction: the trigger point manual—the upper half of the body*, vol 1, ed 2, Baltimore, 1999, Williams & Wilkins.

Stone JA, Stone RJ: *Atlas of skeletal muscles*, ed 4, Boston, 2003, McGraw-Hill.

Tixa S: *Atlas of palpatory anatomy of limbs and trunk*, Teterboro, NJ, 2003, ICON Learning Systems.

Warfel JH: *The extremities*, ed 4, Philadelphia, 1981, Lea & Febiger.

Warfel JH: *The head, neck and trunk*, ed 4, Philadelphia, 1978, Lea & Febiger.

Watkins J: *Structure and function of the musculoskeletal system*, Champaign, IL, 1999, Human Kinetics.

White TD: *Human osteology*, ed 2, San Diego, 2000, Academic Press.

Index